NEUROLOGY OF
CRITICAL ILLNESS

CONTEMPORARY NEUROLOGY SERIES AVAILABLE:

NEUROLOGY OF CRITICAL ILLNESS

EELCO F. M. WIJDICKS, M.D., Ph.D., F.A.C.P.

Associate Professor of Neurology
Mayo Medical School
Co-Director, Neurology-Neurosurgery Intensive Care Unit

Senior Associate Consultant
Department of Neurology
Mayo Clinic and Mayo Foundation
Rochester, Minnesota

 F. A. DAVIS COMPANY • Philadelphia

F. A. Davis Company
1915 Arch Street
Philadelphia, PA 19103

Printed in the United States of America

Last digit indicates print number: 10 9 8 7 6 5 4 3 2 1

Medical Editor: Robert W. Reinhardt
Medical Developmental Editor: Bernice M. Wissler
Production Editor: Marianne Fithian
Cover Design by: Donald B. Freggens, Jr.

As new scientific information becomes available through basic and clinical research, recommended treatments and drug therapies undergo changes. The au-
thor(s) and publisher have done everything possible to make this book accurate, up
to date, and in accord with accepted standards at the time of publication. The au-
thors, editors, and publisher are not responsible for errors or omissions or for consequences from application of the book, and make no warranty, expressed or implied,
in regard to the contents of the book. Any practice described in this book should be
applied by the reader in accordance with professional standards of care used in regard to the unique circumstances that may apply in each situation. The reader is
advised always to check product information (package inserts) for changes and new
information regarding dose and contraindications before administering any drug.
Caution is especially urged when using new or infrequently ordered drugs.

Library of Congress Cataloging-in-Publication Data

Wijdicks, Eelco F. M., 1954–
    Neurology of critical illness / Eelco F.M. Wijdicks.
      p.   cm. — (Contemporary neurology series ; 43)
    Includes bibliographical references and index.
    ISBN 0-8036-9316-8 (hard cover : alk. paper)
    1. Neurological intensive care.   2. Neurological manifestations of general
diseases.   I. Title.   II. Series.
    [DNLM: 1. Nervous System Diseases.   2. Critical Illness.   3. Intensive
Care Units.   W1 W0769N v. 43 1994 / WL W662n 1994]
RC350.N49W55   1995
616.8′0428 — dc20
DNLM/DLC
for Library of Congress   94-12407
                                                                         CIP

To my wife, Barbara-Jane, my children, Coen and Marilou
—my everything.

FOREWORD

Neurologic intensive care has indeed come far as a distinctive specialty in its 15 or so years of existence. When critical care was in its adolescence, few internists felt the need to have neurologic assistance for their patients with hepatic or renal encephalopathies or seizures. Even the practice of asking neurologists to see comatose patients after cardiac arrest is relatively new and arises from the perception that these clinical states are too complex to understand confidently and that alternative and secondary neurologic problems potentially complicate the management picture. The current situation is quite different. As the neurologic aspects of medicine have been omitted from many medical training programs and the tools of neurology, particularly imaging and electrophysiology, have been refined, the neurologic state has become even more mysterious to the non-neurologist. Moreover, a panoply of new neurologic problems has been produced by organ transplantation. The system has stayed balanced, however, as neurologists have assumed the task of educating themselves about aspects of acute medical illness that affect neurologic care and, recently, about neurologic features of acute but primarily systemic diseases. Neurologists like Dr. Wijdicks are to be found heading large neurologically and neurosurgically oriented intensive care units and playing a large role in the clinical advice and procedures in other critical care units throughout the hospital. They have become the arbiters of such diverse problems as brain death, postoperative neurologic complications, and respiratory and medical decisions in patients with Guillain-Barré syndrome and myasthenia gravis.

By building on the impressive advances of the original field of neurointensive care, involving intracranial pressure and acute stroke management, from what was essentially a subsidiary part of neurosurgical practice, Dr. Wijdicks has greatly expanded the purview of the neurologist with this book and provided for the first time a comprehensive guide to neurologic problems in general intensive care. A recent survey by Dr. Thomas Bleck and colleagues (Crit Care Med 21:98–103, 1993) emphasizes the importance of this subject by pointing out that 12% of 1758 consecutive patients in a general intensive care unit had major neurologic complications of their illness, many unrecognized.

The chapters herein are comprehensive and very practical and provide the reader with ample citations to pursue finer points of management. The style of giving sensible advice when any of several courses of action is possible is commendable, particularly because so much of the material is original work that addresses crucial problems in the field. This book will be devoured not only by clinically oriented neurologists but also, it is hoped, by intensive care specialists of every sort, so that the field will be viewed as more unified than before the book was written and a new basis for neurologic practice in medical and surgical intensive care will be established.

Allan H. Ropper, M.D.
Chief of Neurology
St. Elizabeth's Hospital
Boston, MA

PREFACE

Neurologic critical care has emerged from the practical management issues of acute stroke care, increased intracranial pressure, and neuromuscular weakness. At Saint Marys Hospital, one of the hospitals affiliated with the Mayo Clinic, the neurology critical care service provides primary care for all neurology patients in the neurology-neurosurgery intensive care unit. Operating under the aegis of the Department of Neurology and the Division of Pulmonary and Critical Care Medicine, the service also manages neurologic complications in critically ill patients in medical and surgical intensive care units. Many anesthesiologists and pulmonologists in critical care play a major part in the daily care of these very sick patients. It is unfortunate that even today, many excellent textbooks and monographs on critical care tend to be superficial (and certainly not focused) in their discussion of neurologic complications.

This monograph introduces the neurology of critical illness within the field of neurologic critical care and reflects the continuing shift in the orientation of the field. The orientation of this book is clinical, and the management protocols in each clinical chapter should emphasize this orientation. The book is divided into four parts. The first part focuses on general clinical neurologic problems in patients in intensive care units. It deals with the most frequent consultations in critically ill patients. Parts II and III, the core of the book, provide full accounts of major clinical syndromes organized by specialized intensive care units. Every experienced neurologist knows that a neurologic complication in a critically ill patient occurs in a complex clinical situation that requires a broad basic knowledge of many of the subspecialities. Every chapter provides a representative selection of the state of the art in the intensive care unit, necessary for an understanding of critical care medicine. The chapters attempt to be comprehensive but concentrate on the most important issues in critical care medicine. The diagnostic approach is the theme of each chapter, but emergency management and salvation of the patient with a neurologic catastrophe are also considered.

A common misunderstanding is that a serious neurologic complication will put an end to the aggressive care of the very sick patient. In many instances, neurologists do not share this pessimism. It is true that at times no recovery can be anticipated, but the outcome need not always be grim.

Thus, part IV of the book covers the prognostication of neurologic complications and provides guidelines in common clinical neurologic problems facing the intensive care specialist and consulting neurologist in everyday decisions.

A good deal of what follows is new. I hope this book is useful to neurologists, medical and surgical intensive care specialists, critical care nurses, and many other specialized physicians who manage the pressing problems in intensive care units.

E.F.M. Wijdicks, M.D., Ph.D., F.A.C.P.

ACKNOWLEDGMENTS

Many people have contributed to the composition, assembly, and editing of this book. It is no exaggeration to say that I could not have achieved this book without the hard work of the Mayo Clinic Section of Publications (Roberta Schwartz, John Prickman, Sharon Wadleigh, Renée Van Vleet, and Jen Schlotthauer), Computer Graphics, and Medical Illustration (Alice McKinney and her invaluable assistants). My particular appreciation is due to my colleagues in the Division of Pulmonary and Critical Care Medicine and colleagues in liver transplantation, who continue to call me when neurologic problems emerge. My good friend Dr. Allan Ropper, a pioneer in neurologic critical care, was asked to muse about the portrayal of this field, and he always provided inspiration and support. I specifically thank the staff of F. A. Davis for reviewing and editing the entire text with much enthusiasm.

CONTENTS

Part I

GENERAL CLINICAL NEUROLOGIC PROBLEMS IN THE INTENSIVE CARE UNIT

Chapter 1

NEUROLOGIC MANIFESTATIONS OF PHARMACOLOGIC AGENTS COMMONLY USED IN THE INTENSIVE CARE UNIT

EFFECT OF DRUGS ON NEUROMUSCULAR FUNCTION
EFFECT OF DRUGS ON PUPILS
EFFECT OF DRUGS ON LEVEL OF CONSCIOUSNESS
COMMONLY USED DRUGS WITH DIRECT NEUROTOXIC EFFECTS

The interpretation of neurologic findings may be inaccurate in critically ill patients receiving multiple drug regimens. Many of these patients are sedated to facilitate mechanical ventilation, to overcome anxiety, and to support sleep. To some extent, these circumstances reflect the occasional reluctance of neurologists to consult in the intensive care unit (ICU). Neurologic assessment in heavily sedated patients is less accurate, but with knowledge of the pharmacokinetics of each agent, a reasonable estimate is possible. Certainly in the ideal situation, sedation is simply discontinued or reversed, but the severity of illness often dictates prolonged use. This chapter describes drugs commonly used in the ICU that can influence level of alertness, affect pupil size and eye movement, and impair motor responses. Another section

of this chapter deals with the direct neurotoxic effect of drugs used in the ICU.

EFFECT OF DRUGS ON NEUROMUSCULAR FUNCTION

The need for neuromuscular blocking agents is controversial.[24,34] Its use in medical and surgical ICUs is limited by the serious potential of disuse muscle atrophy and the complexity of nursing care. Muscle relaxant drugs may also pose a significant danger to the patient if the ventilator inadvertently becomes disconnected. Neurologic examination is limited to examination of pupils that remain normal in size because nicotinic receptors are absent (in many patients, miosis is seen because of additional use of narcotics). In ICU practice, muscle relaxation is considered in patients with high airway pressures and decreased pulmonary compliance during mechanical ventilation, patients with tetanus, patients with tenuous surgical repairs, and patients with severe hypothermia to eliminate intense shivering that increases oxygen consumption and myocardial work.[24,26]

Nondepolarizing muscle relaxants

3

are used in medical and surgical ICUs. Recovery from paralysis is seen within 1 hour when the drug is withdrawn, but prolonged paralysis may occur when drugs that may potentiate neuromuscular blockade are administered. Clindamycin, metronidazole, tetracycline, furosemide, corticosteroids, anticholinesterase drugs, local anesthetics, and most antiarrhythmic agents are well known to produce interactions with nondepolarizing agents. Respiratory acidosis, metabolic alkalosis, and electrolyte disorders may increase the blocking effect of nondepolarizing drugs on the neuromuscular junction as well, but the clinical significance in all these circumstances is less clear. Aminoglycosides, but not penicillin and cephalosporin, prolong neuromuscular blockade, probably by inhibition of presynaptic acetylcholine release.[75] Under these conditions, weaning from neuromuscular blockade may take additional hours. In contrast, antiepileptic drugs and aminophylline may diminish the effects of muscle relaxants.

Most reports of prolonged muscle weakness are linked to pancuronium and vecuronium.[21,34] Pancuronium produces a consistent tachycardia, which makes it less favorable for use, although the cost is considerably lower than that of vecuronium or atracurium. Table 1–1 shows commonly used doses and duration of clinical effect for four nondepolarizing muscle relaxants. Duration of action after a single bolus is usually 90 minutes. Therefore, 25% of the initial dose is usually repeated every 45 to 90 minutes. Others favor infusion of vecuronium at a rate of 1 μg/kg per minute.

Nondepolarizing drugs should be monitored in the ICU with the use of peripheral nerve stimulators[3,40,60] (Fig. 1–1). As with many procedures and monitoring devices, the peripheral nerve stimulator was introduced in ICUs after being used for years in the operating room. This technique of estimating the neuromuscular transmission is easily applied at the bedside and is becoming standard care. The response of the twitching thumb is manually assessed after the median nerve is stimulated supramaximally at the wrist through cutaneous electrodes. Depth of neuromuscular blockade can be assessed by objective criteria, such as post-tetanic potentiation, but the train-of-four method (four twitches every 0.5 second with supramaximal stimuli) is more practical. Frequent use of the peripheral nerve stimulator should guide the infusion rate of neuromuscular blocking agents and the need for an additional bolus. Standard practice is to titrate to one or two twitches. As a rule, ablation of more than three twitches suggests a muscle relaxant overdose.

Recovery from vecuronium or pancuronium has a stereotypical pattern. The diaphragm is relatively more resistant to muscle relaxants.[18] Therefore, restoration of diaphragmatic motion, evident

Table 1–1 NONDEPOLARIZING MUSCLE RELAXANTS

Agent	Initial Dose, mg/kg	Initial Drip Rate, mg/kg/h	Duration, min
Metocurine	0.3	0.1	60–90
Pancuronium	0.1	0.025	60–90
Atracurium	0.4	0.7	30–60
Vecuronium	0.08	0.07	30–60

From Coyle, JP and Cullen, DJ: Anesthetic pharmacology and critical care. In Chernow, B (ed): The Pharmacologic Approach to the Critically Ill Patient, ed 2. Williams & Wilkins, Baltimore, 1988, pp 241–253, with permission of the publisher.

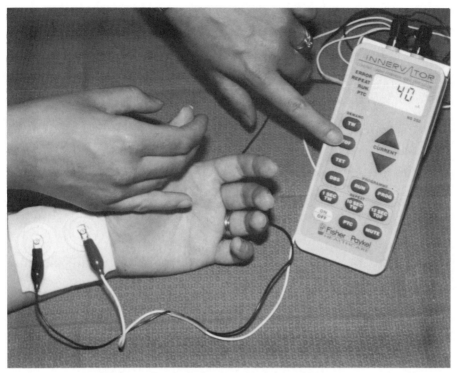

Figure 1–1. Peripheral nerve stimulator.

by triggering of the ventilator, usually comes first and is soon followed, in decreasing order, by improved head lift and recovery of bulbar, proximal, and distal muscles. Without the ability to routinely measure plasma levels of vecuronium or pancuronium and the dangerous side effects of physostigmine used to counteract blockade in ICU patients, it may be difficult to know whether active metabolites have blocked the neuromuscular junction. In 1990, Segredo and colleagues[69] found that metabolites of vecuronium may accumulate in patients with renal failure, metabolic acidosis, and hypermagnesemia. This may superficially indicate that metabolites would prolong its effect, but electrophysiologic data were not available in this study.[69] However, it is very likely that before control of neuromuscular blockade with bedside peripheral nerve stimulators, overdose may have significantly prolonged paralysis in many patients. For example, in one patient who had no administration of pancuronium 6 days before death, large doses of the drug were found in muscles at autopsy.[78]

Therefore, persistent muscle paralysis after discontinuation of muscle relaxants usually implies overdose or enhancement from other drugs, in most patients immediately evident by persistence of train-of-four abnormalities after withdrawal of the paralytic agent.

Nonetheless, pancuronium and vecuronium have been associated with weakness lasting for weeks to months after administration has stopped.[33,46,59,64,69,79] Carefully documented electrophysiologic studies are not available in patients with prolonged muscle weakness. An axonal polyneuropathy may develop in some of these patients, whereas others eventually recover completely (see Fig. 3-1). Prolonged muscle paralysis has also recently been linked to atracurium, but no verified published cases have yet appeared. Fewer problems can be expected with use of atracurium. Atracurium is very expensive, however, and a propensity to increasing doses during use results in formidable total costs. Prolonged use of neuromuscular agents without measures that protect peripheral nerves from compression may also cause multiple entrapment neuropathies. Bilateral peroneal and ulnar palsies from prolonged immobilization and insufficient protection at compression points may occur, but no study of prevalence in the ICU is available. A comprehensive discussion of causes of generalized weakness can be found in Chapter 3.

EFFECT OF DRUGS ON PUPILS

In many ICUs, the initial neurologic examination is limited to assessment of pupillary response, and, as alluded to previously, changes in pupil diameter may be the only indication of neurologic deterioration in critically ill patients receiving muscle relaxants. Pupil size may vary considerably in mechanically ventilated patients. Hippus is often exaggerated, particularly in patients with large tidal volume settings.[56] Any anisocoria should be taken seriously and not be attributed to physiologic fluctuations or, worse, to interobserver variability among critical care nursing staff. A recent study with experienced nursing personnel found that interobserver agreement with simple pupil measurements at bedside was excellent; only agreement on pupillary reaction to light was poor.[85] Anisocoria, defined as difference in pupil size of more than 1 mm, should be further evaluated. A simplified flow chart for bedside testing is given in Figure 1-2.

In most patients, acute pupillary abnormalities are associated with an acute brain injury that complicates critical illness. Effects of pharmacologic agents, however, may mimic structural brain or brain stem damage. It is virtually impossible to categorize all pharmacologic agents that may potentially cause pupillary abnormalities. Fraumfelder[27] provides an excellent monograph devoted to this subject.

Causes of Miosis in the ICU

Bilateral miosis with preserved light reflex is frequently encountered in critically ill patients. Small pupils are often present in patients with severe respiratory distress who are hypercapnic and tachypneic. Miosis may also be additional evidence for metabolic encephalopathy, but systematic studies are not available. Pinpoint pupils were reported in a patient with nonketotic hyperglycemia.[10] However, a large proportion of patients in the ICU have miosis from treatment with narcotic agents. The miotic action of morphine or morphine-like agents has been well documented; this action can be antagonized with naloxone.[5,13,54,62]

Pinpoint pupils are traditionally seen in patients with large pontine hemorrhages, but the additional presence of skew deviation, intranuclear ophthalmoplegia, or ipsilateral conjugate gaze paresis is more diagnostic. Unilateral miosis almost always represents Horner's syndrome. Unilateral miosis can be exaggerated by examination in the dark or after loud noise. Anisocoria therefore may become less apparent in brightly illuminated ICU rooms. Fluctuations in anisocoria may simply result from changes in light exposure. Horner's syndrome may have causes at any level of the sympathetic pathway, but in medical and surgical ICUs, internal jugular vein catheterization (see Chapter 4), acute brachial plexopathies, and extensive thoracic surgery are the most frequent associated conditions. The positive predictive value of cocaine

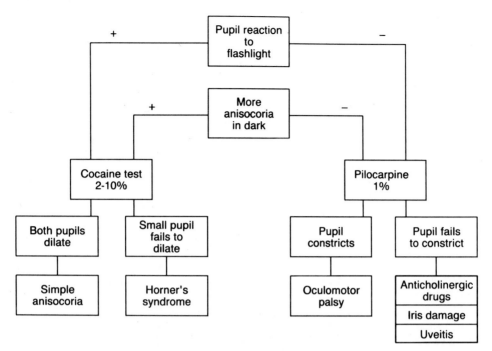

Figure 1–2. Bedside test for anisocoria in the ICU. (Further localization of Horner's syndrome can be done with the use of 1% hydroxyamphetamine. Adie's [tonic] pupil, common in the general population but rare in the ICU, should be considered if no cause is found; it can be investigated by slit-lamp examination [sector palsy of sphincter], or its supersensitivity can be examined with diluted pilocarpine 0.1%.) (Modified from Thompson, HS and Pilley, SFJ: Unequal pupils: A flow chart for sorting out the anisocorias. Surv Ophthalmol 21:45–48, 1976.)

for Horner's syndrome is high, but its use in clinical practice is seldom needed.

Causes of Mydriasis in the ICU

Pharmacologic agents are frequent causes of bilateral mydriasis but do not result in unresponsiveness to bright light. Extreme cases of fixed, dilated pupils have been reported in patients with antibiotic-induced paralysis. In every patient in respiratory failure who has additional bulbar symptoms, botulism should be considered, but the condition is very rare.[39,77,86] Systemically administered atropine in standard doses (0.03 mg/kg) may cause some pupillary dilatation, but its effect is often too small to be appreciated clinically.[29,31] In cardiac resuscitation, bilat-

eral mydriasis may have its origin in large doses of atropine and dopamine and in the adrenergic stress response. Excessive doses of dopamine in four patients were reported to dilate and fix the pupils, but more often, pupillary reactions remain normal in patients treated with dopamine no matter what dose is used.

Patients with bilateral mydriasis receiving neuromuscular blockade may signal anxiety or have a florid delirium. When associated with tachycardia, mydriasis may signal inadequate sedation. When unrecognized, this condition in pharmacologically paralyzed patients is similar to a locked-in syndrome and is one of the most terrifying experiences. In critical illness, sudden unilateral fixed, dilated pupil is often evidence of third nerve dysfunction through direct compression or from brain stem distortion caused by a rapidly expanding intracranial mass.

However, accidental unilateral pupillary dilatation has been reported in several cases in association with aerosolized anticholinergics,[38] or it may occur with accidental spilling of atropine droplets during preparation of the syringe. Unilateral or bilateral fixed pupils may transiently occur during focal seizures or as part of a petit mal seizure.[28,41]

Figure 1 – 3 summarizes pupillary abnormalities and potential causes in critically ill patients.

EFFECT OF DRUGS ON LEVEL OF CONSCIOUSNESS

Many patients need sedation to achieve a desired level of relaxation, but the metabolism of drugs in critically ill patients is uncertain and patient response may vary.

Narcotic Agents

Narcotic agents may effectively relieve pain (Table 1 – 2). Epidural administration of narcotics has recently been introduced as a pain-relieving measure in patients with major thoracic surgery. Narcotic analgesia is very helpful in surgical ICUs and additionally may mute stress-related cardiac ischemia.[19] To overcome prolonged awaking times with benzodiazepines, short-acting opioids have also been used to induce sedation, but depression of the level of consciousness is not particularly pronounced with standard doses.

Most patients in the ICU are treated with intermittent doses of morphine. Intravenous morphine drips of 1 to 3 mg/h produce minimal side effects. Alternative narcotic drugs, such as alfentanil and sufentanil, are generally used to induce anesthesia.[68,87]

Seizures or seizure-like movements have been observed after induction with opioids. Anesthesiologists more often

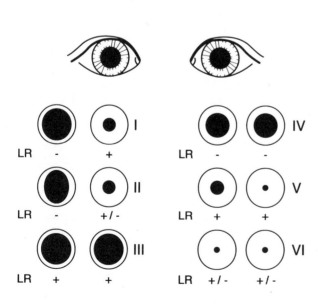

Figure 1 – 3. Pupillary signs in the intensive care unit. LR, light response. *I*, Oculomotor palsy from acute intracranial mass; contusion of bulbus oculi (late phenomenon, aerosolized anticholinergics); *II*, Oval pupil (often transitory appearance of pupils in brain death); *III*, Mydriasis (anxiety, delirium, pain, seizures, botulism, atropine, aerosolized albuterol, amyl nitrite, magnesium excess, norepinephrine, dopamine, aminoglycoside, polypeptide, and tetracycline overdose); *IV*, Pupils fixed in midposition, typical of brain death after, for example, major stroke, fulminant hepatic failure, or postanoxic encephalopathy; *V*, Horner's syndrome (traumatic carotid dissection, brachial plexopathy, internal jugular vein catheter, excessive thoracic surgery); spastic miosis (in acute corneal penetration); *VI*, Miosis (narcotic agents, any metabolic encephalopathy, acute pontine lesion, nonketotic hyperglycemia, hypercapnia); light response should be present but may be very difficult to appreciate, even with the use of a magnifying glass.

Table 1–2 OPIOID AGENTS COMMONLY USED IN THE INTENSIVE CARE UNIT

Agent	Elimination Half-Life, h
Morphine	1.5–4
Fentanyl	2–5
Sufentanil	2–3
Alfentanil	1.5–3.5
Phenoperidine	1.5–4
Pethidine	3–6.5
Nalbuphine	3.5–4

than neurologists are aware of these movements induced by opioids. Many patients experience sudden onset of rigidity of abdominal and chest wall muscles,[8] flexion in the neck, and myoclonic jerks in the upper and lower limbs, at times associated with flexion at the elbows and fingers and extension at the hips and knees.[11,58]

The time course of these "convulsions" may strongly resemble that of generalized tonic-clonic seizures, but electroencephalographic recordings during these manifestations never reveal specific epileptiform activity.[67,74] The risk of tonic-clonic seizures after opioid administration is low in patients with no history of epilepsy. However, as noted in Chapter 2, narcotic agents may be associated with new-onset seizures after sudden withdrawal.

Midazolam

Patients requiring mechanical ventilation need adequate sedation to overcome the distress of being in an ICU environment.[81] Benzodiazepines are widely used in ICUs, but pharmacokinetics are changed in critical illness. Claims of short elimination half-life for some of the recently introduced benzodiazepines may not always apply in this category of patients.

Midazolam, a water-soluble imidazole benzodiazepine, is twice as potent as diazepam. After a single dose of midazolam, an elimination half-life of 1 to 4 hours can be expected. Mechanically ventilated patients with multiorgan failure, however, have reduced clearance,[70] causing midazolam to accumulate. Shelly and colleagues[71,72] found that the elimination half-life was greater than 12 hours in half of their patients despite the claim of rapid clearance from the circulation. A 1989 randomized study that compared propofol with midazolam found more realistic data.[1] Patients receiving mechanical ventilation had a return of spontaneous ventilation and adequate response to command 405 minutes after administration of midazolam was discontinued. Isolated reports of extremely prolonged recovery time (up to 3 days) may be related to associated liver disease. Pentobarbital and thiopental enhance the effects of midazolam. Small doses of opioids and cimetidine, frequently used in the ICU, may increase the plasma concentration of midazolam. Use of midazolam infusions is increasing in surgical ICUs. If the drug is given by continuous infusion for prolonged periods without intermittent assessment of the level of consciousness, cumulation may occur,[72] but others have presented contradictory data.[52]

The effects of midazolam can be transiently reversed by the benzodiazepine antagonist flumazenil. The short half-life of flumazenil necessitates intravenous infusion (usually at a rate of 4 mL/h) for at least a few hours. Flumazenil is a competitive antagonist at the benzodiazepine receptor.[61] After administration, onset of reversal is very rapid, within 1 to 2 minutes, and usually a dose of 0.4 to 1.0 mg produces complete antagonism. The duration is dose dependent and ranges from 15 minutes to 2.5 hours. Flumazenil may be given in doses of up to 1 mg at 20-minute intervals, but in patients with suspected benzodiazepine overdose, a continuous infusion of 1 mg/h may be used. Seizures have been reported and tend to occur in patients who have been receiving benzodiazepines for long-term sedation. Use of flumazenil in reversal of hepatic encephalopathy is controversial (see Chapter 9).

Propofol

Propofol, a new agent frequently used for induction of anesthesia, has been introduced in ICUs.[25,35] It may become a preferred drug for sedation but is already accepted as a suitable agent for short procedures, such as endotracheal intubation. Neurologic examination in patients who have received propofol is unreliable, and most brain-stem reflexes may disappear except for pupillary light response.

As mentioned previously, a randomized study of propofol (1 to 3 mg/kg per hour) and midazolam (0.1 to 0.2 mg/kg per hour) showed that propofol had important advantages over midazolam in many respects.[1] The half-life of propofol, even in mechanically ventilated patients,[7] is short, and many patients awaken almost immediately after discontinuation of the intravenous infusion. In general, patients awaken within 30 minutes (longest time, 105 minutes).[2] Clinical experience in the ICU population is limited. Side effects are green discoloration of urine and adrenocortical suppression, although only at extremely high doses, and acid-base abnormalities have been noted in children. It may also decrease cerebral perfusion pressure from hypotension when used in closed head injury (see Chapter 15). A recent cost-benefit analysis of patients admitted to the ICU who needed mechanical ventilation found that propofol had a better cost-benefit ratio than midazolam in continuous sedation. Mean recovery time for short-term sedation with propofol was 0.3 hour compared with 2.5 hours for midazolam recovery; for medium-term sedation, 0.4 hour for propofol and 13.5 hours for midazolam; and for long-term sedation, 0.8 hour compared with 36.6 hours.[16]

Lorazepam

Giving large doses of lorazepam in combination with haloperidol is perhaps the method of choice for sedation of patients with delirium in the ICU.

Lorazepam should be considered a short-acting benzodiazepine, but its half-life is still 10 to 20 hours, making it unsuitable for use other than treatment of delirium. Withdrawal of lorazepam may induce seizures or, as it would with any other benzodiazepine, nonconvulsive status epilepticus.

Failure to Awaken After Drug Withdrawal

Failure to awaken after discontinuation of sedative, narcotic, or neuromuscular agent administration frequently prompts neurologic consultation in the ICU. The reason for unresponsiveness or failure to fully awaken is often clear by focal neurologic signs and abnormal computed tomography (CT) scan findings, but in some patients the cause of bilateral hemispheric dysfunction remains puzzling and challenging, particularly when results of the initial CT scan are normal. The most common conditions that should be considered are listed in Table 1–3.

Very often, neurologists are vexed by the inability of critically ill patients to awaken fully after the critical illness has been controlled. Two recent prospective surveys suggest a high prevalence of metabolic encephalopathy in the ICU.[9,43] Drowsiness and inability to comply with weaning protocols may prevent discontinuation of the mechanical ventilator (phrenic nerve damage from cardiopulmonary bypass or associated with critical illness polyneuropathy may contribute as well). Generally, metabolic encephalopathy in these patients is imprecisely defined, and neurologists are often unable to document a cause. In most patients, decreased oxygen delivery or hypotension may have induced a global hypoxia that prolongs recovery or the patient remains stunned for a long time after the initial severe metabolic insult. Whether a blend of multiple causative factors exists is not clear, and causes of failure to awaken in the ICU require further scrutiny.

Table 1-3 CAUSES OF ALTERATION IN CONSCIOUSNESS AND COMA IN CRITICALLY ILL PATIENTS WITH NORMAL INITIAL COMPUTED TOMOGRAPHY SCAN

Drug overdose
Anoxic-ischemic encephalopathy
Diffuse axonal brain injury
Bilateral isodense subdural hematomas*
Fat embolization
Cholesterol embolization
Diffuse intravascular coagulation†
Thrombotic thrombocytopenic purpura
Connective tissue disease with vasculitis
Prolonged hypoglycemia
Acute severe hyponatremia
Acute severe hypercalcemia
Acute nonketotic hyperglycemia
Metabolic alkalosis
Acute hypercapnia with hypoxemia
Adrenal crisis
Myxomatous coma
Thyrotoxic coma‡
Acute uremia
Acute increase in arterial ammonia
Hypothermia
Acute bacterial, viral, or fungal meningitis
Nonconvulsive status epilepticus
Central pontine myelinolysis
Acute brain-stem stroke§
Hyperpyretic-hyperkinetic syndromes¶
Wernicke's encephalopathy

*More often in patients with multitrauma who have low hematocrit measurements.
†Occasionally multiple intracerebral hemorrhages.
‡Elderly patients.
§May be locked-in syndrome.
¶Catatonia more prominent.

COMMONLY USED DRUGS WITH DIRECT NEUROTOXIC EFFECTS

The neurologic manifestations of drugs frequently used in the ICU are listed in Table 1-4. Many drugs used in the ICU do not contribute to neurologic manifestations, and some of the reported associations may be coincidental. Drug intoxication may occur in patients with multiorgan failure or multiple drug regimens. The most common neurologic manifestations are seizures, decreased level of response, and prolonged blockade of the neuromuscular function or myopathy.

Acute Steroid Myopathy

A well-recognized complication of intravenously administered corticosteroids is acute myopathy.[6,15,80,84] The possibility of an acute myopathy must be considered seriously in a patient with status asthmaticus treated intravenously with pancuronium and large doses of corticosteroids (usually up to 1 g/d), in whom severe muscle weakness and markedly increased creatine kinase levels develop.[45,47,49,57,76] Complete ophthalmoplegia and severe proximal limb weakness have been described as

Table 1-4 NEUROLOGIC MANIFESTATIONS OF DRUGS FREQUENTLY USED IN THE INTENSIVE CARE UNIT

Agent	Neurologic Manifestations
Amiodarone[17,20,50]	Optic neuropathy, tremor, gait ataxia, peripheral neuropathy (4 or more months of treatment)
Amphotericin B[82]	Headache, tremor, confusion, akinetic mutism
Aminophylline[58]	Seizures, headache, insomnia
Cimetidine[51]	Myokymias, seizures, dysarthria, drowsiness, hallucinations
Hydralazine[12]	Distal axonopathy
Hydrocortisone	Acute myopathy
Ketamine	Myoclonus
Lidocaine	Myokymias, myoclonus, paresthesias
Local anesthetics[22,53]	Seizures
Metoclopramide[23]	Oculogyric crises, torticollis, trismus, parkinsonism
Metronidazole	Distal axonopathy, bizzare psychotic episodes, and visual hallucinations
Neuroleptic agents	Malignant neuroleptic syndrome
Penicillin derivatives	Multiple myoclonus, asterixis, coma
Sodium nitroprusside	Muscle spasm, convulsions
Succinylcholine	Malignant hyperthermia

part of a corticosteroid and pancuronium myopathy.[73] Acute steroid myopathy does not involve respiratory muscles. Muscle biopsy may show necrotic changes and vacuolar changes in all fiber types, which also reflect the increased creatine kinase values and occasional myoglobinuria in these patients (for a comprehensive discussion, see Chapter 3).

Malignant Hyperthermia

Malignant hyperthermia is not an exclusively anesthesiologic disorder. The consulting neurologist can assess subtle changes in the neurologic condition and, more important, is familiar with associated myopathies.[14] Malignant hyperthermia frequently occurs in the operating room, and the anesthesiologist determines whether further action (particularly dantrolene infusion) should be undertaken.

The classic clinical presentation (Table 1–5) of malignant hyperthermia is a combination of metabolic change and abnormal muscle activity.[32,48] The most common muscle manifestation is masseter muscle rigidity or trismus.[48,63] Very often, flaccidity, caused by succinylcholine, occurs, but generalized muscle rigidity may soon follow.[48,63] Masseter spasm is dramatic in presentation and may be associated with cyanosis, labile blood pressure, and marked tachycardia. Fasciculations are frequently seen, and masseter trismus seriously hampers intubation. Masseter

Table 1–5 CLINICAL FEATURES OF MALIGNANT HYPERTHERMIA

Fever (≥41°C)
Masseter trismus and skeletal muscle rigidity
Metabolic and respiratory acidosis
Cardiac arrhythmias
Marked hyperkalemia
Marked increase in creatine kinase
  concentration (>20,000 IU/L)
Myglobinuria
Hypercalcemia (fulminant form)
Intravascular coagulopathy (fulminant forms)

Data from Rosenberg.[63]

muscle rigidity subsides within minutes after discontinuation of the triggering anesthetic.

Interpretation of masseter muscle rigidity may be difficult, especially because many patients, if not all, given halothane and succinylcholine have a slight increase in jaw muscle tone.[66] Masseter spasm, more common in children, occurs in 1 in 12,000 anesthetic procedures in which suxamethonium is administered. Whether anesthesia should be continued in patients with rigid masseter muscles is a persistent dilemma, especially in emergency surgery. Progression to fulminant malignant hyperthermia rarely occurs with discontinuation, and treatment with dantrolene may prevent further exacerbation. Masseter spasm is often associated with an increased serum creatine kinase value and myoglobinuria, but the increased concentration of creatine kinase may also be related to an underlying myopathy.

Fulminant malignant hyperthermia is clinically characterized by rapid development of metabolic acidosis and hyperthermia. Myoglobinuria from rhabdomyolysis is an almost obligatory finding. In a significant number of patients, an early sign is tachycardia, often accompanied by labile blood pressure. As a consequence of increased carbon dioxide production, tachypnea occurs but may be considerably hampered by rigidity of chest wall muscles. Laboratory findings include respiratory and metabolic acidosis; increased serum concentrations of creatine kinase, potassium, calcium, and magnesium; and hyperglycemia.[37] A massive potassium flux from the sarcoplasm may cause heart block and ultimately cardiac arrest.

Malignant hyperthermia has been associated with congenital myopathies, most often Duchenne's muscular dystrophy, central core disease, and myotonia congenita.[14] This association has resulted in an as yet unsuccessful search for a malignant hyperthermia gene at the identical locus of the abnormal myopathy gene.

Several skeletal muscle relaxants (e.g., succinylcholine chloride, decamethonium, gallamine) and inhalation anesthetics (e.g., halothane, enflurane, isoflurane) are capable of inducing hyperthermic reactions. New anesthetics have not been adequately tested; propofol probably is harmless. Recently, desflurane, a potential new inhalation anesthetic, appeared to trigger malignant hyperthermia in susceptible swine.[83]

The pathophysiologic mechanism in malignant hyperthermia is complex.[32] In brief, the most impressive biochemical disturbance is an abrupt increase in the intracellular ionized calcium concentration in muscles followed by extreme depletion of adenosine triphosphate reserves that results in rigor and dysfunction of cell membranes. Many experts consider malignant hyperthermia a myopathy in which an impaired calcium regulation mechanism exists.[32] Increased intracellular calcium results in uncoupling of oxidative phosphorylation and enhanced glycolysis. The net effect is increase in oxygen consumption, marked decrease in high-energy phosphate metabolites, and production of large amounts of lactate and heat.

Treatment is summarized in Table 1–6. Hyperventilation with 100% oxygen and discontinuation of inhalational anesthesia are immediately followed by dantrolene infusion.[36] Administration of sodium bicarbonate should be guided by arterial blood gas analysis. Cooling the patient is an essential part of treatment, and vaporization with fans is very effective.

Table 1–6 DRUG TREATMENT OF MALIGNANT HYPERTHERMIA

Dantrolene, 2 mg/kg every 5 min to total dose of 10 mg/kg
Bicarbonate, 2 to 4 mEq/kg
Glucose and insulin IV (if hyperkalemia)
Heparin IV (if disseminated intravascular coagulation)

Data from Harrison.[36]

Neuroleptic Malignant Syndrome

Neuroleptic malignant syndrome is associated with use of neuroleptic agents and closely parallels clinically malignant hyperthermia and lethal catatonia (most likely an identical disorder without the association with neuroleptic agents). The exact neurochemical changes are unclear, but multiple neurotransmitter systems are involved. Hyperthermia and autonomic instability herald the abrupt onset of rapidly progressive deterioration.[4,30,42,44,55] Autonomic dysfunction is characterized by tachycardia, wide swings in blood pressure, tachypnea, and diaphoresis. The typical increasing rigidity may take some days. Mutism is characteristic. Rigidity is reflected by increased creatine kinase levels, but these levels can be extremely variable and normal at the time of fever. Management consists of discontinuing administration of any neuroleptic agent, reinstitution of a dopa agonist if recently withdrawn (particularly in parkinsonian patients), cooling, and liberal amounts of fluid to minimize kidney damage.[65] Bromocriptine and amantadine have been used in addition to dantrolene. Clear benefit has also been noted with high doses of benzodiazepines (lorazepam, clonazepam). Electroconvulsive therapy is a last resort treatment. A large retrospective review of 734 previously reported cases found that amantadine, bromocriptine, and dantrolene, alone or in combination, resulted in improvement and decreased rates of relapse and that use of bromocriptine or dantrolene or both led to a significant decrease in mortality.[65]

CONCLUSIONS

It is common to find that patients in the ICU have numerous drugs listed on their daily medication chart. Extensive use of drugs is almost a part of the definition of critical illness. Neuromuscular blocking agents, often used, have generated controversy. Specifically, neuromuscular weakness months after weaning from the drug has been described. Peripheral nerve stimulators have been introduced for use at the bedside, and close monitoring may indeed substantially decrease the frequency of prolonged muscle paralysis, but mechanical ventilatory practices vary widely.

Familiarity with currently used medication in the ICU is crucial for further evaluation of patients who fail to fully recover their level of consciousness. Fortunately, newer pharmacologic agents are short-acting, and awakening can be expected in a matter of minutes. Nonetheless, the most common cause of alteration of consciousness in critically ill patients is related to previous administration of sedative drugs that accumulate over days because of diminished clearance or pharmacologic interactions. In many other patients, an anoxic-ischemic insult from brief but considerable hypoxemia or hypotension produces a diffuse encephalopathy that may linger for weeks. Recent invasive studies with difficult manipulation may have triggered a cholesterol embolization syndrome, an increasingly recognized clinical entity. For patients in whom the cause is unclear, evaluation should include at least recent arterial blood gas analysis, arterial ammonia determination, endocrine evaluation, electroencephalogram, cerebrospinal fluid examination with cultures, and magnetic resonance imaging whenever transport can be tolerated.

REFERENCES

1. Aitkenhead, AR, Pepperman, ML, Willatts SM, et al: Comparison of propofol and midazolam for sedation in critically ill patients. Lancet 2:704–709, 1989.
2. Albanese, J, Martin, C, Lacarelle, B, et al: Pharmacokinetics of long-term propofol infusion used for ICU patients. Anesthesiology 73:214–217, 1990.
3. Ali, HH and Savarese, JJ: Monitoring of neuromuscular function. Anesthesiology 45:216–249, 1976.
4. Anderson, WH: Lethal catatonia and the neuroleptic malignant sydrome. Crit Care Med 19:1333–1334, 1991.
5. Asbury, AJ: Pupil response to alfentanil and fentanyl: A study in patients anaesthetised with halothane. Anaesthesia 41:717–720, 1986.
6. Bachmann, P, Gaussorgues, Ph, Piperno, D, et al: Myopathie aiguë au décours de l'état de mal asthmatique. Presse Med 16:1486, 1987.
7. Beller, JP, Pottecher, T, Lugnier, A, et al: Prolonged sedation with propofol in ICU patients: Recovery and blood concentration changes during periodic interruptions in infusion. Br J Anaesth 61:583–588, 1988.
8. Benthuysen, JL, Smith, NT, Sanford, TJ, et al: Physiology of alfentanil-induced rigidity. Anesthesiology 64:440–446, 1986.
9. Bleck, TP, Smith, MC, Pierre-Louis, SJ-C, et al: Neurologic complications of critical medical illnesses. Crit Care Med 21:98–103, 1993.
10. Boutros, G and Insler, MS: Reversible pupillary miosis during a hyperglycaemic episode: Case report. Diabetologia 27:50–51, 1984.
11. Bowdle, TA: Myoclonus following sufentanil without EEG seizure activity. Anesthesiology 67:593–595, 1987.
12. Bradley, WG, Karlsson, IJ, and Rassol, CG: Metronidazole neuropathy. Br Med J 2:610–611, 1977.
13. Bromage, PR, Camporesi, EM, Durant, PAC, and Nielsen, CH: Nonrespiratory side effects of epidural morphine. Anesth Analg 61:490–495, 1982.
14. Brownell, AKW: Malignant hyperthermia: Relationship to other diseases. Br J Anaesth 60:303–308, 1988.
15. Brun-Buisson, C and Gherardi, R: Hydrocortisone and pancuronium bromide: Acute myopathy during status asthmaticus (letter). Crit Care Med 16:731–732, 1988.
16. Carrasco, G, Molina, R, Costa, J, et al: Propofol vs midazolam in short-, medium-, and long-term sedation of critically ill patients: A cost-benefit analysis. Chest 103:557–564, 1993.
17. Charness, ME, Morady, F, and Scheinman, MM: Frequent neurologic toxicity

associated with amiodarone therapy. Neurology 34:669–671, 1984.

18. Chauvin, M, Lebrault, C, and Duvaldestin, P: The neuromuscular blocking effect of vecuronium on the human diaphragm. Anesth Analg 66:117–122, 1987.

19. Clemensen, SE, Thayssen, P, and Hole, P: Epidural morphine for outpatients with severe anginal pain. Br Med J 294:475–476, 1987.

20. Coxon, A and Pallis, CA: Metronidazole neuropathy. J Neurol Neurosurg Psychiatry 39:403–405, 1976.

21. Darrah, WC, Johnston, JR, and Mirakhur, RK: Vecuronium infusions for prolonged muscle relaxation in the intensive care unit. Crit Care Med 17:1297–1300, 1989.

22. Davison, R, Parker, M, and Atkinson, AJ Jr: Excessive serum lidocaine levels during maintenance infusions: Mechanisms and prevention. Am Heart J 104:203–208, 1982.

23. Dingwall, AE: Oculogyric crisis after day care anaesthesia (letter). Anaesthesia 42:565, 1987.

24. Durbin, CG Jr: Neuromuscular blocking agents and sedative drugs: Clinical uses and toxic effects in the critical care unit. Crit Care Clin 7:489–506, 1991.

25. Farling, PA, Johnston, JR, and Coppel, DL: Propofol infusion for sedation of patients with head injury in intensive care: A preliminary report. Anaesthesia 44:222–226, 1989.

26. Fiamengo, SA and Savarese, JJ: Use of muscle relaxants in intensive care units (editorial). Crit Care Med 19:1457–1459, 1991.

27. Fraumfelder, FT (ed): Drug-Induced Ocular Side Effects and Drug Interactions, ed 3. Lea & Febiger, Philadelphia, 1989.

28. Gadoth, N, Margalith, D, and Bechar, M: Unilateral pupillary dilatation during focal seizures. J Neurol 225:227–230, 1981.

29. Goetting, MG and Contreras, E: Systemic atropine administration during cardiac arrest does not cause fixed and dilated pupils. Ann Emerg Med 20:55–57, 1991.

30. Granner, MA and Wooten, GF: Neuroleptic malignant syndrome or parkin-sonism hyperpyrexia syndrome. Semin Neurol 11:228–235, 1991.

31. Greenan, J and Prasad, J: Comparison of the ocular effects of atropine or glycopyrrolate with two I.V. induction agents. Br J Anaesth 57:180–183, 1985.

32. Gronert, GA, Mott, J, and Lee, J: Aetiology of malignant hyperthermia. Br J Anaesth 60:253–267, 1988.

33. Haas, JL, Shaefer, MS, Miwa, LJ, et al: Prolonged paralysis associated with long-term pancuronium use. Pharmacotherapy 9:154–157, 1989.

34. Hansen-Flaschen, J, Cowen, J, and Raps, EC: Neuromuscular blockade in the intensive care unit: More than we bargained for. Am Rev Respir Dis 147:234–236, 1993.

35. Harris, CE, Grounds, RM, Murray, AM, et al: Propofol for long-term sedation in the intensive care unit: A comparison with papaveretum and midazolam. Anaesthesia 45:366–372, 1990.

36. Harrison, GG: Dantrolene—dynamics and kinetics. Br J Anaesth 60:279–286, 1988.

37. Heffron, JJA: Malignant hyperthermia: Biochemical aspects of the acute episode. Br J Anaesth 60:274–278, 1988.

38. Helprin, GA and Clarke, GM: Unilateral fixed dilated pupil associated with nebulised ipratropium bromide (letter). Lancet 2:1469, 1986.

39. Hughes, JM, Blumenthal, JR, Merson, MH, et al: Clinical features of types A and B food-borne botulism. Ann Intern Med 95:442–445, 1981.

40. Isenstein, DA, Venner, DS, and Duggan, J: Neuromuscular blockade in the intensive care unit. Chest 102:1258–1266, 1992.

41. Jammes, JL: Fixed dilated pupils in petit mal attacks. Neuroophthalmology 1:155–159, 1980.

42. Kellam, AMP: The neuroleptic malignant syndrome, so-called: A survey of the world literature. Br J Psychiatry 150:752–759, 1987.

43. Kelly, BJ and Matthay, MA: Prevalence and severity of neurologic dysfunction in critically ill patients: Influence on need for continued mechanical ventilation. Chest 104:1818–1824, 1993.

44. Keyser, DL and Rodnitzky, RL: Neuro-leptic malignant syndrome in Parkinson's disease after withdrawal or alteration of dopaminergic therapy. Arch Intern Med 151:794–796, 1991.

45. Knox, AJ, Mascie-Taylor, BH, and Muers, MF: Acute hydrocortisone myopathy in acute severe asthma. Thorax 41:411–412, 1986.

46. Kupfer, Y, Namba, T, Kaldawi, E, and Tessler, S: Prolonged weakness after long-term infusion of vecuronium bromide. Ann Intern Med 117:484–486, 1992.

47. Kupfer, Y, Okrent, DG, Twersky, RA, and Tessler, S: Disuse atrophy in a ventilated patient with status asthmaticus receiving neuromuscular blockade. Crit Care Med 15:795–796, 1987.

48. Larach, MG, Rosenberg, H, Larach, DR, and Broennle, AM: Prediction of malignant hyperthermia susceptibility by clinical signs. Anesthesiology 66:547–550, 1987.

49. MacFarlane, IA and Rosenthal, FD: Severe myopathy after status asthmaticus (letter). Lancet 2:615, 1977.

50. Mansour, AM, Puklin, JE, and O'Grady, R: Optic nerve ultrastructure following amiodarone therapy. J Clin Neuro-ophthalmol 8:231–237, 1988.

51. McGuigan, JE: A consideration of the adverse effects of cimetidine. Gastroenterology 80:181–192, 1981.

52. Michalk, S, Moncorge, C, Fichelle, A, et al: Midazolam infusion for basal sedation in intensive care: Absence of accumulation. Intensive Care Med 15:37–41, 1988.

53. Modica, PA, Tempelhoff, R, and White, PF: Pro- and anticonvulsant effects of anesthetics (part I). Anesth Analg 70:303–315, 1990.

54. Murray, RB, Adler, MW, and Korczyn, AD: Minireview: The pupillary effects of opioids. Life Sci 33:495–509, 1983.

55. Nierenberg, D, Disch, M, Manheimer, E, et al: Facilitating prompt diagnosis and treatment of the neuroleptic malignant syndrome. Clin Pharmacol Ther 50:580–586, 1991.

56. Ohtsuka, K, Asakura, K, Kawasaki, H, and Sawa M: Respiratory fluctuations of the human pupil. Exp Brain Res 71:215–217, 1988.

57. Panacek, EA and Sherman, B: Hydrocortisone and pancuronium bromide: Acute myopathy during status asthmaticus (letter). Crit Care Med 16:732, 1988.

58. Parkinson, SK, Bailey, SL, Little, WL, and Mueller, JB: Myoclonic seizure activity with chronic high-dose spinal opioid administration. Anesthesiology 72:743–745, 1990.

59. Partridge, BL, Abrams, JH, Bazemore, C, and Rubin, R: Prolonged neuromuscular blockade after long-term infusion of vecuronium bromide in the intensive care unit. Crit Care Med 18:1177–1179, 1990.

60. Pedersen, T, Viby-Mogensen, J, Bang, U, et al: Does perioperative tactile evaluation of the train-of-four response influence the frequency of postoperative residual neuromuscular blockade? Anesthesiology 73:835–839, 1990.

61. Pepperman, ML: Double-blind study of the reversal of midazolam-induced sedation in the intensive care unit with flumazenil (Ro 15-1788): Effect on weaning from ventilation. Anaesth Intensive Care 18:38–44, 1990.

62. Rabinowitz, R and Korczyn, AD: The specificity of the pupillary actions of morphine and naloxone. J Ocul Pharmacol 3:17–21, 1987.

63. Rosenberg, H: Clinical presentation of malignant hyperthermia. Br J Anaesth 60:268–273, 1988.

64. Rossiter, A, Souney, PF, McGowan, S, and Carvajal, P: Pancuronium-induced prolonged neuromuscular blockade. Crit Care Med 19:1583–1587, 1991.

65. Sakkas, P, Davis, JM, Hua, J, and Wang, Z: Pharmacotherapy of neuroleptic malignant syndrome. Psychiatr Ann 21:157–164, 1991.

66. Schwartz, L, Rockoff, MA, and Koka, BV: Masseter spasm with anesthesia: Incidence and implications. Anesthesiology 61:772–775, 1984.

67. Scott, JC and Sarnquist, FH: Seizure-like movements during a fentanyl infusion with absence of seizure activity in a simultaneous EEG recording. Anesthesiology 62:812–814, 1985.

68. Sear, JW, Fisher, A, and Summerfield, RJ: Is alfentanil by infusion useful for

sedation on the ITU? Eur J Anaesthesiol Suppl 1:55–61, 1987.

69. Segredo, V, Matthay, MA, Sharma, ML, et al: Prolonged neuromuscular blockade after long-term administration of vecuronium in two critically ill patients. Anesthesiology 72:566–570, 1990.

70. Shafer, A, Doze, VA, and White, PF: Pharmacokinetic variability of midazolam infusions in critically ill patients. Crit Care Med 18:1039–1041, 1990.

71. Shelly, MP, Mendel, L, and Park, GR: Failure of critically ill patients to metabolise midazolam. Anaesthesia 42:619–626, 1987.

72. Shelly, MP, Sultan, MA, Bodenham, A, and Park, GR: Midazolam infusions in critically ill patients. Eur J Anaesthesiol 8:21–27, 1991.

73. Sitwell, LD, Weinshenker, BG, Monpetit, V, and Reid, D: Complete ophthalmoplegia as a complication of acute corticosteroid- and pancuronium-associated myopathy. Neurology 41:921–922, 1991.

74. Smith, NT, Benthuysen, JL, Bickford, RG, et al: Seizures during opioid anesthetic induction—are they opioid-induced rigidity? Anesthesiology 71:852–862, 1989.

75. Sokoll, MD and Gergis, SD: Antibiotics and neuromuscular function. Anesthesiology 55:148–159, 1981.

76. Subramony, SH, Carpenter, DE, Raju, S, et al: Myopathy and prolonged neuromuscular blockade after lung transplant. Crit Care Med 19:1580–1582, 1991.

77. Terranovo, W, Palumbo, JN, and Breman, JG: Ocular findings in botulism type B. JAMA 241:475–477, 1979.

78. Vandembrom, RHG and Wierda, JMKH: Pancuronium bromide in the intensive care unit: A case of overdose. Anesthesiology 69:996–997, 1988.

79. Vanderheyden, BA, Reynolds, HN, Gerold, KB, and Emanuele, T: Prolonged paralysis after long-term vecuronium infusion. Crit Care Med 20:304–307, 1992.

80. Van Marle, W and Woods, KL: Acute hydrocortisone myopathy. Br Med J 281:271–272, 1980.

81. Veselis, RA: Sedation and pain management for the critically ill. Crit Care Clin 4:167–181, 1988.

82. Walker, RW and Rosenblum, MK: Amphotericin B-associated leukoencephalopathy. Neurology 42:2005–2010, 1992.

83. Wedel, DJ, Iaizzo, PA, and Milde, JH: Desflurane is a trigger of malignant hyperthermia in susceptible swine. Anesthesiology 74:508–512, 1991.

84. Williams, TJ, O'Hehir, RE, Czarny, D, et al: Acute myopathy in severe acute asthma treated with intravenously administered corticosteroids. Am Rev Respir Dis 137:460–463, 1988.

85. Wilson, SF, Amling, JK, Floyd, SD, and McNair, MD: Determining interrater reliability of nurses' assessments of pupillary size and reaction. J Neurosci Nurs 20:189–192, 1988.

86. Wright, EA and McQuillen, MP: Antibiotic-induced neuromuscular blockade. Ann N Y Acad Sci 183:358–368, 1971.

87. Yate, PM, Thomas, D, and Sebel, PS: Alfentanil infusion for sedation and analgesia in intensive care (letter). Lancet 2:396–397, 1984.

88. Zwillich, CW, Sutton, FD Jr, Neff, TA, et al: Theophylline-induced seizures in adults: Correlation with serum concentrations. Ann Intern Med 82:784–787, 1975.

Chapter 2

SEIZURES IN THE INTENSIVE CARE UNIT

DRUG-INDUCED AND DRUG-
   WITHDRAWAL SEIZURES
SEIZURES AND ACUTE METABOLIC
   DERANGEMENTS
SEIZURES AND STRUCTURAL
   CENTRAL NERVOUS SYSTEM
   ABNORMALITIES
TONIC-CLONIC STATUS
   EPILEPTICUS
NONCONVULSIVE STATUS
   EPILEPTICUS
MANAGEMENT OF SEIZURES AND
   STATUS EPILEPTICUS
OUTCOME

The circumstances that surround critical illness make patients considerably more vulnerable to seizures. Aside from acute metabolic alterations, changed pharmacokinetics and multiple drug regimens may be precipitating factors.[71] Most isolated seizures occur in patients who have a seizure disorder or who had multiple trauma associated with head injury. New-onset seizures, however, are uncommon. At one of the Mayo Clinic hospitals, only 55 patients were identified in a 10-year period,[77] and drug withdrawal or toxicity was a frequent cause (Table 2–1).

Seizures in the intensive care unit (ICU) are observed by nurses who may be less experienced in recognizing the categories of limb movements. Intensive care specialists seldom witness an attack. Therefore, the consulting neurologist has to trust descriptions that may not be accurate. There may also be a tendency to mistake movements such as shivering or single myoclonic jerks for epileptic fits. Shivering or chills are common in patients who become hypothermic or experience sudden overwhelming bacteremia. In others, myoclonic jerks are associated with a sudden decrease in blood pressure or are noted immediately after administration of anesthetic agents (e.g., etomidate) for brief procedures. Tonic-clonic seizures are more easily recognized by sudden gaze preference, a tonic phase followed by rapidly generalized clonic jerks associated with flushing and labored breathing, and, almost always, postictal confusion and slurred, incoherent speech at the end.

The broad categories of causes of seizure in the ICU are discussed in this chapter. Further details can be found in the chapters on cardiac arrest (Chapter 6), electrolyte disorders (Chapter 7), multisystem trauma (Chapter 15), and transplantation (Chapter 16).

DRUG-INDUCED AND DRUG-WITHDRAWAL SEIZURES

Many drugs commonly prescribed in the ICU decrease the threshold for seizures[3,8] (Table 2–2). When seizures occur, a direct effect from the drug is assumed, but in some instances an electrolyte disorder is produced that in turn causes the seizure.

The Boston Collaborative Drug

Table 2–1 CAUSES OF NEW-ONSET SEIZURES IN CRITICAL ILLNESS

Causes	Patients (n)
Drug withdrawal	18
Morphine	11
Propoxyphene	5
Midazolam	1
Meperidine	1
Metabolic abnormalities	18
Hyponatremia	10
Hypocalcemia	4
Acute uremia	2
Hyperglycemia	1
Hypoglycemia	1
Drug toxicity	8
Antibiotics	5
Antiarrhythmics	3
Stroke	5
Unknown	6
Total	55

From Wijdicks and Sharbrough,[77] with permission of Neurology.

Surveillance Program reported that penicillins, hypoglycemic agents, methylxanthines, antipsychotic drugs, and, in particular, lidocaine were the most commonly involved drugs in seizures,

Table 2–2 DRUG-ASSOCIATED SEIZURES IN THE INTENSIVE CARE UNIT*

Antiarrhythmic agents	Lidocaine
	Flecainide
	Esmolol
Antibiotics	Imipenem
	Norfloxacin
	Ciprofloxacin
	Penicillin derivatives
Antidepressants	Amitriptyline
	Doxepin
	Nortriptyline
Antipsychotics	Chlorpromazine
	Haloperidol
	Thioridazine
	Perphenazine
	Trifluoperazine
Bronchodilators	Theophylline
	Aminophylline
	Terbutaline
Immunosuppressive and chemotherapeutic agents	Cyclosporine
	Busulfan
	Cyclophosphamide

*Seen mostly with documented drug toxicity.[2,8,45]

found in 26 of 32,812 (0.08%) patients admitted to various wards, including ICUs.[5] In most instances, renal failure or recent sudden increase in dosage could be identified as precipitating events. In the more recent study at San Francisco General Hospital,[44] drug-associated seizures accounted for 1.7% of seizures in a consecutive series of 3155 admissions, but suicides were included in this study. Isoniazid, bronchodilators, insulin, psychotropic drugs, and lidocaine accounted for most of the seizures.

Even though drug toxicity is a commonly reported cause of seizures, in a recently published series of new-onset seizures in the ICU only 8 of 55 (15%) patients could be identified.[77] Five patients had documented toxicity to antibiotics and three to antiarrhythmic drugs. All five patients with toxic levels of antibiotics had renal failure. Sudden withdrawal of drugs, however, particularly narcotic agents and benzodiazepines, is more significant as a cause of new-onset seizures in the ICU.[77] Repeated intramuscular injections for at least 7 days, with daily doses that range from 12 to 30 mg in patients given morphine, appear to be sufficient to trigger seizures when suddenly withheld.

Benzodiazepines are frequently used for maintenance of sedation in ventilated patients, and sudden withdrawal may sporadically produce single epileptic seizures. As discussed later, sudden withdrawal of benzodiazepines may also be a major precipitant of nonconvulsive status epilepticus.

Withdrawal in drug addicts may be a cause of tonic-clonic seizures, and in most patients dependence is known. However, as in alcohol abuse, seizures during hospital admission may be the first indication of physical dependence.

Alcohol-related seizures occur only in patients with a history of heavy drinking.[46,48,60,74] Delirium tremens may follow but is absent in most patients. A single seizure or, more frequently, a flurry of seizures in hours may strike within 2 days after admission to the hospital. The seizures are self-limited, and status epilepticus is unusual. A clinically significant intracranial lesion was reported in 6.2% of 259 patients with a first alcohol withdrawal seizure, and in half of these patients, a potential neurosurgical lesion (e.g., subdural hematoma) was found.[16] In Rochester, Minn, from 1982 to 1992, 15 patients with new-onset seizures in ICUs had a history of heavy alcohol use. In 8 of these 15 patients, other triggers (antibiotic or aminophylline toxicity) were identified (Wijdicks, EFM, unpublished observations).

Seizures in patients undergoing transplantation are often related to cyclosporine (see Chapter 16). The association is unresolved.[23,80] Although seizures can occur in patients with therapeutic cyclosporine levels without any other precipitating factor, the risk of seizures after transplantation is increased in cyclosporine-treated patients with any of the following features: high-dose methylprednisolone therapy, aluminum overload, hypertension, hypomagnesemia, low serum cholesterol levels, and structural central nervous system lesions.[23,80]

SEIZURES AND ACUTE METABOLIC DERANGEMENTS

Acute metabolic derangements place critically ill patients at risk for seizures. Seizures occur only in overt metabolic derangements. The threshold serum levels in acute metabolic derangement are never absolute, and the case for a relation remains difficult to prove. The rapidity of decrease in serum level is likely decisive.

Hypocalcemia may be caused by neck surgery, including radical neck dissection, and results from parathyroid suppression from extensive burns, sepsis, pancreatitis, aminoglycosides, cimetidine, or changes in serum magnesium. More commonly, hypocalcemic patients complain of muscle cramps and irregular twitching, which should

not be interpreted as focal seizures when present. Seizures occur quite often in patients who have clinical manifestations of hypocalcemia, such as Chvostek's and Trousseau's signs (Chapter 7).

Hypophosphatemia is primarily caused by gram-negative sepsis and less often associated with iatrogenic malnutrition in patients receiving parenteral nutrition. A considerable decrease in the serum level of phosphate must be present to trigger seizures (Chapter 7). Hypoglycemia usually results from insulin overdose in parenterally fed patients and has traditionally been reported as a frequent cause of status epilepticus without much validation. Seizures associated with hypoglycemia may be focal or multifocal and often become generalized tonic-clonic. Prompt treatment in patients thought to have hypoglycemia may raise blood or plasma levels rapidly. Therefore, the finding of low normal levels may nevertheless indicate that hypoglycemia is the main trigger of seizures. In addition, finger stick – reflectance meter determinations are less accurate in the lower end of the reading scale.

Dilutional hyponatremia, a very common electrolyte disturbance in ICUs, is typically seen in the first postoperative days. Seizures occur in patients who have sudden acute decrease in serum sodium concentrations, often to less than 125 mEq/L. Virtually all patients have a decrease in the level of consciousness and may have a prolonged postictal state, particularly if hyponatremia is not immediately corrected. In a recent study of 55 patients with new-onset seizures, hyponatremia was the most frequent metabolic abnormality[77] (Table 2–1). Ten of the 18 patients with a metabolic cause of seizures had severe hyponatremia (range, 114 to 125 mmol/L; median, 121 mmol/L). As expected, postoperative iatrogenic fluid loading was the most frequent cause. Hyponatremia has also been recognized as a potential precipitating factor of seizures after severe burns (Chapter 14) or liver transplantation (Chapter 16), in both conditions generated by massive fluid shifts.

SEIZURES AND STRUCTURAL CENTRAL NERVOUS SYSTEM ABNORMALITIES

Structural central nervous system abnormalities, some of which may have been previously unrecognized, may be a cause of seizures in the ICU. At both Mayo Clinic hospitals, new-onset seizures from structural causes in critically ill patients were seen most often in those with closed head injury and much less often in those with ischemic or hemorrhagic stroke.[77] Other structural central nervous system lesions that may cause seizures in critical illness are fungal or parasitic infection in patients who are immunosuppressed or have AIDS (Chapter 16), air embolism (Chapter 4), bacterial meningitis (Chapter 5), and intracerebral hematoma with severe coagulopathy (Chapter 10). Seizures may also accompany thrombocytopenic thrombotic purpura with or without structural lesions (Chapter 10).

TONIC-CLONIC STATUS EPILEPTICUS

Recurrence of a tonic-clonic seizure in an ICU is frequently encountered despite therapy, and approximately one third of patients with new-onset seizures have a second or third seizure.[77]

It is rare for tonic-clonic status epilepticus (defined as frequently repeated seizures without full recovery of consciousness between episodes that are often present for at least 30 minutes[81]) to appear in patients without a history of epilepsy.[1] In a critical care unit, status epilepticus develops when a well-known precipitating factor (e.g., acute severe hyponatremia) is not immediately recognized or, more likely, the severity of a metabolic abnormality is improperly assessed.

In general, common triggers for tonic-clonic status epilepticus are iatrogenic drug overdose, impaired absorption of antiepileptic drugs in patients with a seizure disorder after major abdominal surgical procedures, and severe acute metabolic derangements. Factors that could potentially contribute are sleep deprivation during long stays in an ICU and fever from any type of infection or sepsis.

Status epilepticus is a medical emergency.[1,3,6,13] The first priority in treatment is to prevent secondary hypoxic-ischemic damage through adequate ventilation. The mechanism by which prolonged status epilepticus produces neuronal necrosis and precludes recovery, shown in animal models, is not known. Nevander and colleagues[47] found abnormalities in central parts of the globus pallidus, amygdala, and thalamic nuclei after 45 minutes of seizures.

Clinical Presentation and Basic Principles of Management

Generalized convulsive status epilepticus is the most common type of status epilepticus in the ICU. Simple or complex partial status epilepticus is rare; if it is present, a structural central nervous system lesion is likely.

As mentioned previously, generalized tonic-clonic seizures are easily recognized by nonneurologists. Occasionally, vigorous shivering occurs after a tonic-clonic seizure, most likely related to the sedative medication used to stop the seizure. An electroencephalographic accompaniment is never seen, and this phenomenon should not be interpreted as a beginning status. Status epilepticus consists of repeated symmetrical contractions of the face and limbs and may have focal onset and begin with adversive movements of the head and eyes, flexion of the ipsilateral arm, and extension of the ipsilateral leg with repeated vocalizations. Over time, both tonic and clonic phases decrease in duration in patients with continuing seizures, and they may even fade into solitary multifocal twitches in all limbs.

Endotracheal intubation is necessary not only to secure airway and to provide adequate oxygenation when large doses of benzodiazepine are anticipated but also to avoid aspiration of gastric contents. It is prudent to start with 10 L of O_2/min through a standard face mask.

Most laboratory abnormalities seen after a cluster of seizures normalize spontaneously. Severe lactic acidosis should be treated only if blood gas values have not improved within 1 hour and if the pH is consistently lower than 7.20 and is associated with cardiovascular collapse. Sodium bicarbonate (100 mEq, intravenously) usually suffices to correct the acidosis. The concerns of lactic acidosis are probably inflated, and indiscriminate use of bicarbonate may result in alkalemia that decreases the seizure threshold.

Blood tests to search for hyperglycemia, hypoglycemia, hyponatremia, hypocalcemia, and hypomagnesemia should be done immediately. Blood samples should be obtained to screen for toxic drug levels. Fever should be corrected, because fever alone may prevent adequate seizure control.

In new-onset status epilepticus, structural lesions should be actively sought but may be absent.[77] Computed tomography (CT) scanning and cerebrospinal fluid examination usually sufficiently exclude an acute new insult to the central nervous system. Often, CT scanning in status epilepticus yields normal findings, but patients with a hypoxemic insult scan may have attenuation changes or evidence of effacement of sulci from edema (Chapter 6). Contrast CT is discouraged because rhabdomyolysis may transiently impair renal function, and additional contrast agent exposure may adversely affect renal function. Magnetic resonance imaging has not been performed systematically but may show transient hyperintensities, predominantly in focal status epilepticus.[12]

Medical Complications

Hypertension and cardiac arrhythmias are common sequels of acute intracranial events.[30,82] At the onset of status epilepticus, a striking increase in systolic blood pressure, generally accompanied by marked sinus tachycardia, is often found. Both responses are the result of increased sympathetic activity. Increase in venous return associated with motor activity during the tonic phase does not contribute, because cardiovascular responses have been demonstrated to be identical in paralyzed animals.[43] After control of the seizures, blood pressure rapidly returns to normal. Cardiac stunning may be an important manifestation after status epilepticus. A decrease in left ventricular contractility has been documented in an experimental study with neonatal pigs in status epilepticus.[82] Lactic acidosis or perhaps an overwhelming catecholamine output with subsequent subendocardial damage has been suggested.

Cardiac arrhythmias are very common during seizures.[42] Any type of tachyarrhythmia may occur, but sinus tachycardia or paroxysmal supraventricular tachycardia is common. A recent case report documented prolonged sinus arrest alternating with episodes of bradycardia at the time of a complex partial seizure.[30] These cardiac arrhythmias are not life-threatening but may become difficult to manage at the time that status epilepticus is terminated with intravenous administration of phenytoin. With normal infusion rates, side effects of phenytoin infusion are unusual, but hypotension may occur if phenytoin is administered to a hypovolemic patient.

A well-recognized complication after status epilepticus is neurogenic pulmonary edema,[11,65] but in general practice, most cases of pulmonary edema after a series of seizures are caused by aspiration of gastric contents. Typically, the patient becomes severely hypoxic and needs full ventilation with increasing doses of positive end-expiratory pressure. Radiographs may be normal in the very early phase but usually demonstrate a typical "whiteout."

In an earlier study, Terrence and colleagues[65] postulated that neurogenic pulmonary edema may be a cause of unexpected death in young epileptic patients. In an autopsy study of eight patients, gross hemorrhagic pulmonary edema without any pathologic findings in the heart was noted.

The onset of pulmonary edema usually coincides with resolution of the seizure and postictal drowsiness. The hallmark of neurogenic pulmonary edema is proteinaceous bloody, foamy sputum with high albumin fluid and plasma ratios. These findings suggest increased pulmonary vascular permeability. Pulmonary wedge pressures are normal. Therapy is directed toward optimal oxygenation, and the use of positive end-expiratory pressure, usually within the range of 10 to 15 cm H_2O, is of major importance. On the basis of a few anecdotal cases, outcome is good with prompt institution of therapy.

Disseminated intravascular coagulation is exceedingly uncommon but has been reported in status epilepticus associated with sustained muscle injury.[22] The pathophysiologic mechanism is unclear. Patients may have signs that reflect the consequences of both diffuse microvascular thrombosis and hemorrhagic diathesis. These signs include acute renal failure, adult respiratory distress syndrome, skin ecchymosis, venipuncture oozing, and gastrointestinal hemorrhage. In most patients, only laboratory abnormalities exist, and these clinical signs are absent. Laboratory abnormalities include thrombocytopenia, afibrinogenemia, schistocytes on peripheral blood smear, increased fibrin degradation products, and abnormal coagulation test results. Usually, all routine reaction times (activated partial thromboplastin, prothrombin, and thrombin) are prolonged.

Acute disseminated coagulation should be treated initially with a bolus of 10,000 U of heparin and then by intermittent intravenous administration of heparin. Transfusion of platelets and fresh frozen plasma to replenish clotting factors should be started immediately.

Tonic-clonic seizures may substantially damage muscle.[18,51,61,63] A slight increase in serum creatine kinase concentration is invariably found after a single seizure, but in rhabdomyolysis, creatine kinase levels may reach enormous proportions within a day. Abnormal laboratory values should point to the diagnosis. Metabolic acidosis not entirely explained by lactate accumulation, hyperkalemia, increased creatine kinase and aldolase values, hypocalcemia, and myoglobinuria are hallmarks of this complication. Most cases associated with status epilepticus reported in the literature are relatively mild.

Several categories of acid-base disorders have been reported.[50,68,78] Metabolic (lactic) acidosis is common after status epilepticus. Excessive muscular contraction results in glycogen depletion and anaerobic glycolysis, which promotes lactic acid formation from pyruvic acid. Metabolic acidosis was not significantly associated with potential life-threatening cardiac arrhythmias in a recent study.[78] Thus, as mentioned previously, the need for sodium bicarbonate administration is very questionable, and treatment-associated alkalosis may lower the seizure threshold. Respiratory acidosis alone or in combination with metabolic acidosis is equally common.[78] The mechanism by which PCO_2 may increase after status epilepticus is shown in Figure 2–1. Causes for hypoventilation are central depression of respiratory control from benzodiazepines, reduced respiratory drive as a consequence of preceding seizure activity on the central respiratory neurons, and diaphragmatic contraction during seizures followed by peripheral respiratory muscle fatigue. Acid-base disorders are transient, and no additional therapeutic procedures are

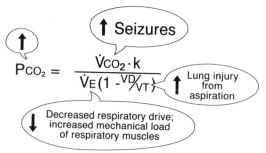

Figure 2–1. Mechanism of respiratory acidosis in status epilepticus. PCO_2 = arterial carbon dioxide tension; k = constant; $\dot{V}CO_2$ = carbon dioxide production; $\dot{V}E$ = expired minute ventilation; VD/VT = anatomic dead space.

necessary if pH values remain above 7.20.

The cerebrospinal fluid may show changes in status epilepticus, and these become important when a lumbar puncture is done to rule out meningitis as a trigger for status epilepticus.[58] A mild increase in erythrocytes and leukocytes with a variable percentage of polymorphonuclear cells may occur after seizures.[58] In a study by Edwards and colleagues,[17] 2 of 98 patients had a transient pleocytosis (up to 65 leukocyte counts) that normalized within 3 days. Although the duration of status epilepticus may be important in the generation of pleocytosis in cerebrospinal fluid, patients with intractable or relapsing status epilepticus may have repeatedly normal cerebrospinal fluid findings. Therefore, an increased cell count should prompt further search for an infectious cause.

Fractures of the long bones and vertebral bodies may occur after status epilepticus, and elderly patients obviously may be more susceptible.[20,21,72] A virtually pathognomonic fracture after seizures is bilateral posterior fracture-dislocation of the humeral head. Excluding patients with associated trauma, Finelli and Cardi[21] found that 7 of 3000 hospital admissions were for seizures and fractures. Vernay and colleagues[72] made the salient point that a compression fracture of the first four lumbar bodies without evidence of com-

pression fractures at other locations is very unusual in osteoporosis. In their study, 2.5% of 227 consecutive hospitalized patients had compression fractures that could be attributed to seizures alone. In a recent series of patients with status epilepticus seen at the Mayo Clinic, one patient had compression fracture[78] (Fig. 2–2).

NONCONVULSIVE STATUS EPILEPTICUS

Confusion, diminished awareness, perseverated speech, and fluctuating responsiveness may signal nonconvulsive status epilepticus.[20,28,34,62] Its incidence in the ICU is not known exactly, but it remains a frequent reason for consultation in patients who do not awaken. Many triggers have been reported, as listed in Table 2–3. Nonconvulsive status epilepticus in critically ill patients is seen after a single generalized tonic-clonic seizure[20] or, more often, after sudden withdrawal of anticonvulsant therapy in patients with known epilepsy undergoing emergency major surgical repairs or after sudden withdrawal of benzodiazepines such as midazolam or propofol.[15,66] In the ICU, nonconvulsive status epilepticus is never a cause of persistent coma. Patients in nonconvulsive status invariably have a fluctuating waxing and

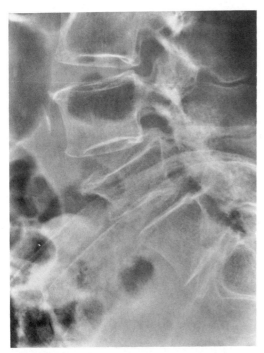

Figure 2–2. Compression fracture of lumbar vertebral body in a patient who recovered from status epilepticus before first noticing back pain.

waning conscious state rather than total unresponsiveness. This cyclic clouding of consciousness is the most apparent clinical expression of nonconvulsive status epilepticus. Total unresponsiveness usually occurs only in episodes of minutes. Trancelike staring

Table 2–3 POTENTIAL TRIGGERS FOR NONCONVULSIVE STATUS EPILEPTICUS IN THE INTENSIVE CARE UNIT

Generalized tonic-clonic seizure
Anticonvulsant withdrawal
Benzodiazepine withdrawal
Psychotropic drugs (lithium carbonate,
  neuroleptics, tricyclic antidepressants)
Metabolic abnormalities (hyponatremia,
  hypocalcemia)
Miscellaneous (metrizamide myelogram,
  cerebral angiogram, electroconvulsive therapy)

Data from references 15, 24, 29, 56, 66, 70, 73, and 75.

has been noted. In some patients, a staring look may be accompanied by a catatonic-like posture, which may come on abruptly.[26] Automatism may appear preferentially in complex partial status epilepticus. These automatisms may include pinching on blankets, face rubbing, stereotypical speech phrases, and verbal perseveration. Many patients, however, are in a twilight state without automatism. Eyelid flutter and myoclonic jerks in jaw muscles are frequently seen and are at times the first clues of nonconvulsive status epilepticus.

Diagnosis of nonconvulsive status epilepticus can be confirmed with an ictal electroencephalographic recording that demonstrates diffuse spike or polyspike and wave complexes at frequencies of 1 to 3 Hz. Frontocentral polyspike waves, however, may occur in bursts of rapid generalized spikes mixed with slow activity.[24]

In most patients, intravenous diazepam in a dose of 2 mg/min up to 20 mg/min aborts the ictus. In occasional cases, phenobarbital is indicated, but in most patients and certainly in those with sudden withdrawal of benzodiazepine therapy, benzodiazepine therapy suffices.

MANAGEMENT OF SEIZURES AND STATUS EPILEPTICUS

Antiepileptic treatment must be considered after a single tonic-clonic seizure. It is very reasonable to administer a loading dose of phenytoin and continue treatment for 1 month in critically ill patients with a flurry of new-onset seizures, in patients with increased intracranial pressure, and in patients in a barely compensated cardiovascular state (e.g., after cardiac transplantation or with cardiogenic shock and arrythmias after myocardial infarction). When seizures result in the removal of central lines, a brief period of phenytoin treatment should be allowed.

The decision to treat a single tonic-clonic seizure is difficult. In patients with a seizure associated with an acute metabolic derangement that can be corrected, it is prudent to withhold anticonvulsant therapy while correcting the metabolic derangement. However, when multiple seizures are seen, a loading dose of phenytoin is warranted to cover this occurrence. Treatment with antiepileptic drugs calls for meticulous attention to changes in the underlying condition of the critically ill patient. Changes in pharmacokinetics occur mainly through drug interactions and may result in subtherapeutic or toxic levels. The most common drug interactions with phenytoin are summarized in Table 2–4. Phenytoin must be administered intravenously because the absorption of phenytoin remains poor with tube feeding.[4]

Equally important, hypoalbuminemia can be expected in critical illness. Therefore, monitoring of total serum phenytoin can be misleading. In addition, the high propensity of phenytoin binding may be altered by drugs, usually antibiotics, and in patients with multiorgan failure, hepatic failure may contribute to a decrease in clearance of the unbound drug. Unfamiliarity with these pharmacologic changes may prompt an increase in the dose of phenytoin in a patient with a normal serum phenytoin level who in fact has an increased free phenytoin level. Severe phenytoin intoxication in four patients as a result of hypoalbuminemia[37] is shown in Figure 2–3. Increased free phenytoin concentration indicates toxicity better than total concentration. Phenytoin toxicity characteristically involves a combination of cerebellar signs, nystagmus, and diplopia, but a gradual decrease in level of consciousness or, paradoxically, an increase in the number of seizures may occur.[52]

Many successful protocols have been designed for the treatment of status epilepticus.[7,39,40,45,55,59,67] It is important to emphasize that a single intravenous bolus injection of diazepam at 0.3 mg/kg terminates status epilepticus in 80% of patients, and a loading dose of phenytoin effectively stops the convulsions in an additional 10% of the patients. The different approaches for refractory status have not been compared in a controlled study.

Benzodiazepines are the first-line drugs, but the choice of one over another is a matter of debate. Clonazepam, lorazepam, and diazepam are equally effective and have similar side effects.[35,36] Many experts consider lorazepam to be one of the first options in the treatment of repeated seizures, but it is not yet approved by the Food and Drug Administration, and comparative trials have not shown lorazepam to be superior to diazepam or phenytoin.[35]

Initial treatment of status epilepticus is probably most effectively managed with intravenously administered diazepam in loading doses of 10 to 20 mg followed by maintenance doses of 4 to 8 mg/h to sustain a therapeutic concentration of the drug. Diazepam is quickly distributed, and the maximal duration of action is 60 minutes. Treatment with intravenously administered phenytoin should begin as rapidly as possible, usually within 5 to 10 minutes after the first

Table 2–4 DRUG INTERACTIONS WITH PHENYTOIN

INCREASE PHENYTOIN SERUM LEVEL
Amiodarone
Chloramphenicol
Chlorpromazine
Cimetidine
Isoniazid
Propoxyphene
Sulfonamide

DECREASE PHENYTOIN SERUM LEVEL
Cyclosporine
Digitoxin
Doxycycline
Glucocorticoids
Oral anticoagulants
Theophylline
Carbamazepine
Clonazepam, diazepam
Valproic acid
Phenobarbital

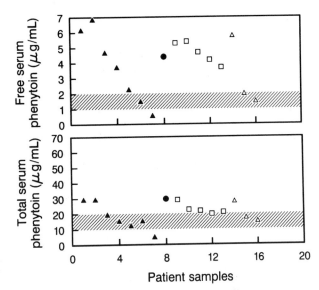

Figure 2–3. Matched pairs of free and total serum phenytoin levels in four critically ill patients with hypoalbuminemia. Each kind of symbol represents one patient. The normal range is shaded. (From Lindow and Wijdicks,[37] with permission of the American College of Chest Physicians.)

intravenous dose of diazepam. Typically, a loading dose of phenytoin of 18 to 20 mg/kg at a rate of 50 mg/min is instituted (Table 2–5). Lower infusion rates should be tried when hypotension or prolongation of the QRS interval occurs. If seizures have not halted at the end of the infusion, an additional one third of the initial loading dose can be given.

Phenobarbital remains a very attractive option as first-line treatment in critically ill patients with a history of cardiac arrhythmias. A 1988 study demonstrated that phenobarbital alone was equally effective in control of status epilepticus.[59] Phenobarbital (initial dose, 10 mg/kg; rate, 100 mg/min) should be considered the drug of choice in patients in the ICU who continue to have seizures after loading doses of benzodiazepine and phenytoin. Aggressive treatment with high doses of phenobarbital (60 mg/kg) may obviate pentobarbital coma, but results of studies in adult patients are not available. An al-

Table 2–5 INTRAVENOUSLY ADMINISTERED DRUGS USED IN THE TREATMENT OF STATUS EPILEPTICUS

Drug	Loading Dose	Rate of Administration	Therapeutic Level
Diazepam	10–20 mg	Push	0.5–0.8 µg/ml
Lorazepam	4–8 mg	Push	Not available
Phenytoin	18–20 mg/kg	50 mg/min	10–20 µg/mL
Phenobarbital	15–60 mg/kg	100 mg/min	10–40 µg/mL
Thiopental	2–4 mg/kg	30 min	BS on EEG
Pentobarbital	10–15 mg/kg	30 min	BS on EEG
Paraldehyde	0.2 mL/kg	0.5 mL/min	>300 µg/mL
Lidocaine	2–3 mg/kg	3–10 mg/kg/hr	Not available
Propofol	1–3 mg/kg	Push	Not available
Midazolam	0.4 mg/kg	Push	Not available

Data from references 9, 10, 31, 32, 35, 36, 38, 41, 49, 54, 57, 69, 76, and 79.
BS = burst suppression; EEG = electroencephalogram.

ternative approach with midazolam has been suggested and may be promising.[33]

A difficult situation arises if seizures do not cease with this management protocol. Immediate intubation, full mechanical ventilation, and intravenously administered pentobarbital or thiopental are appropriate next steps when status epilepticus is not controlled.[53]

Thiopental is administered in a loading dose of 2 to 4 mg/kg per hour followed by continuous intravenous infusion of 3 to 5 mg/kg per hour to produce a pattern of burst suppression on electroencephalography. Additional boluses with 25 mg of thiopental may be needed to achieve a burst-suppression pattern. Therapy is continued for at least 24 hours and can be stopped abruptly. Long-term administration of pentobarbital (5 days or more) is strongly discouraged, because pulmonary edema, skin edema, and ileus may occur. More importantly, the risk of *Pseudomonas* and *Staphylococcus* pneumonia is increased from a direct effect on ciliary function. In many patients, seizures are fully controlled with barbiturates, and alternative treatments are not necessary.

The efficacy of alternative therapies in intractable status epilepticus is derived from a few case reports and small series. Side effects are major, and usually these drugs eventually fail to control the seizures.

A drug rapidly becoming obsolete is paraldehyde. Paraldehyde is infused slowly in a dose of 0.2 mL/kg, and the dose may be repeated every 2 hours. Pulmonary edema is a major toxic side effect, and the safety margin is narrow. Fatal microembolization has been reported. Use of the drug is cumbersome because it decomposes plastic syringes and tubing other than polyethylene. Nevertheless, despite the recent availability of more attractive drugs, paraldehyde may stop status epilepticus.

Lidocaine has recently been reported to be effective in refractory convulsive status epilepticus.[54] Good control was reported with a single intravenous dose of lidocaine of 2 mg/kg followed by a maintenance dose of 3 to 4 mg/kg per hour. Lidocaine may paradoxically produce seizures and, more importantly, life-threatening cardiac arrhythmias. Other recent therapeutic options are propofol and midazolam.[33] Both are short-acting agents requiring continuous infusion, and clinical experience is very limited.

Use of anesthetic agents in the ICU may cause problems because efficient scavenging of volatile agents in the ICU is difficult and environmental pollution is inevitable. Isoflurane (3%) may be tried as a last resort, but the outcome in treated patients is not impressively better.

Patients who continue to have seizures after pentobarbital coma has ended are best served by a second, longer course. However, in many patients, secondary damage may perpetuate status epilepticus.

OUTCOME

Seizures in critically ill patients predict poor outcome only in a very select group of patients with liver transplantation or gram-negative infections.[19,25]

Mortality from a cluster of seizures or status epilepticus varied from 1% to 6% in a large series[27,64] but was much higher (34%) in patients admitted to medical or surgical ICUs. Prognosis for good recovery was guarded in patients with seizures associated with acute metabolic changes, but largely because of the underlying illness (Fig. 2–4). In a 1990 prospective study of 143 patients with epilepsy, status epilepticus rarely had an adverse effect on neuropsychologic function,[14] and if it was present, only subtle abnormalities were found.

Prognostic factors for poor outcome in patients treated with barbiturates were reported in 1993.[81] Among these factors are multiorgan failure, no history of epilepsy, age less than 40 years, and hypotension requiring pressors after barbiturate treatment. These findings suggest that alternative treatments should be tested, and, as mentioned

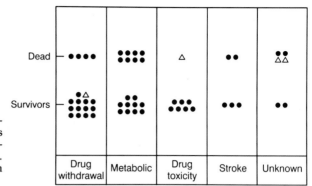

Figure 2-4. Outcome according to etiologic categories in critically ill patients with new-onset seizures. Triangles represent patients with status epilepticus. (From Wijdicks and Sharbrough,[77] with permission of Neurology.)

previously, high doses of midazolam may become a preferred treatment in status epilepticus.[33]

CONCLUSIONS

Many patients in the ICU may become transiently jittery, and some may have seizures. Brief myoclonic jerks are probably more common than epileptic seizures simply because myokymias and myoclonus are well-known side effects of drugs frequently used in the ICU (e.g., ketamine, lidocaine, penicillin derivatives). Probably only occasionally are decorticate or decerebrate responses misinterpreted as seizures by nonneurologists. In generalized convulsive seizures, a history of a seizure disorder is undeniably the strongest risk factor in critically ill patients. New-onset seizures and nonconvulsive generalized seizures are much less commonly observed.

Although it has intuitively been said that in critical illness several interdependent factors are active, new-onset seizures can be classified in major categories of causes.

The diagnostic evaluation of new-onset seizures in critically ill patients depends on the population in which they occur. For example, in transplantation units, immunosuppressive agents such as cyclosporine and OKT3 and antibiotics given prophylactically should be excluded first as major causes. In trauma units, however, a new-onset seizure may signify head injury, alcohol or drug withdrawal that led to the injury, or, less commonly, fat embolization. In medical or surgical ICUs, new-onset seizures are associated with drug toxicity, drug withdrawal, and acute metabolic derangements (most often hyponatremia). Withdrawal of narcotic agents has been found in one third of the patients, for reasons that still have to be clarified. Structural lesions are much less common in critically ill patients. In a few, mostly elderly, patients, the cause of a single tonic-clonic seizure remains unresolved. Although short-term administration of anticonvulsants (e.g., phenytoin) can be considered, the clinical situation is far more complex. Hypoalbuminemia may increase free levels of phenytoin up to toxic levels, and phenytoin may cause changes in other drug levels in both directions. Fortunately, idiosyncratic adverse reactions to anticonvulsant drugs are exceedingly rare, but they may further seriously endanger a critically ill patient. The risk of recurrent seizures is significant, but progression to status epilepticus is rare. Judicious use of anticonvulsants is indicated. It is prudent to defer anticonvulsant medication in a correctable situation (e.g., severe hyponatremia) but to use anticonvulsants when seizures are posing an additional risk to the patient.

Status epilepticus is one of the neurologic emergencies, and every physician should have a prefixed idea of treatment. The sequence is generally benzodiazepines, phenytoin loading, phenobarbital in high doses, and pentobarbital anesthesia. Experimentation with other drugs or, worse, frequent changing of drugs results in an ineffective approach and possible increased risk of sequelae from neuronal dropout. Newer agents (e.g., midazolam) should be rigorously tested in comparative studies before they replace agents with proven efficacy.

REFERENCES

1. Aminoff, MJ and Simon, RP: Status epilepticus: Causes, clinical features and consequences in 98 patients. Am J Med 69:657–666, 1980.
2. Anastasio, GD, Menscer, D, and Little, JM Jr: Norfloxacin and seizures (letter). Ann Intern Med 109:169–170, 1988.
3. Bader, MB: Role of ciprofloxacin in fatal seizures (letter). Chest 101:883–884, 1992.
4. Bauer, LA: Interference of oral phenytoin absorption by continuous nasogastric feedings. Neurology 32:570–572, 1982.
5. Boston Collaborative Drug Surveillance Program: Drug-induced convulsions. Lancet ii:677–679, 1972.
6. Brodie, MJ: Status epilepticus in adults. Lancet 336:551–552, 1990.
7. Browne, TR and Mikati, M: Status epilepticus. In Ropper, AH (ed): Neurological and Neurosurgical Intensive Care, ed 3. Raven Press, New York, 1993, pp 383–410.
8. Chernow, B (ed): Essentials of Critical Care Pharmacology. (Abridged from The Pharmacologic Approach to the Critically Ill, ed 2.) Williams & Wilkins, Baltimore, 1989.
9. Chilvers, CR and Laurie, PS: Successful use of propofol in status epilepticus (letter). Anaesthesia 45:995–996, 1990.
10. Cranford, RE, Leppik, IE, Patrick, B, et al: Intravenous phenytoin in acute treatment of seizures. Neurology 29: 1474–1479, 1979.
11. Darnell, JC and Jay, SJ: Recurrent

12. De Carolis, P, Crisci, M, Laudadio, S, et al: Transient abnormalities on magnetic resonance imaging after partial status epilepticus. Ital J Neurol Sci 13:267–269, 1992.
13. Delgado-Escueta, AV and Swartz, B: Status epilepticus. In Dam, M and Gram, L (eds): Comprehensive Epileptology. Raven Press, New York, 1991, pp 251–270.
14. Dodrill, CB and Wilensky, AJ: Intellectual impairment as an outcome of status epilepticus. Neurology 40(Suppl 2):23–27, 1990.
15. Dunne, JW, Summers, QA, and Stewart-Wynne, EG: Non-convulsive status epilepticus: A prospective study in an adult general hospital. Q J Med 62:117–126, 1987.
16. Earnest, MP, Feldman, H, Marx, JA, et al: Intracranial lesions shown by CT scans in 259 cases of first alcohol-related seizures. Neurology 38:1561–1565, 1988.
17. Edwards, R, Schmidley, JW, and Simon, RP: How often does a CSF pleocytosis follow generalized convulsions? Ann Neurol 13:460–462, 1983.
18. Engel, JN, Mellul, VG, and Goodman, DBP: Phenytoin hypersensitivity: A case of severe acute rhabdomyolysis. Am J Med 81:928–930, 1986.
19. Estol, CJ, Lopez, O, Brenner, RP, and Martinez, AJ: Seizures after liver transplantation: A clinicopathologic study. Neurology 39:1297–1301, 1989.
20. Fagan, KJ and Lee, SI: Prolonged confusion following convulsions due to generalized nonconvulsive status epilepticus. Neurology 40:1689–1694, 1990.
21. Finelli, PF and Cardi, JK: Seizure as a cause of fracture. Neurology 39:858–860, 1989.
22. Fischer, SP, Lee, J, Zatuchni, J, and Greenberg, J: Disseminated intravascular coagulation in status epilepticus. Thromb Haemost 38:909–913, 1977.
23. Gilmore, RL: Seizures and antiepileptic drug use in transplant patients. Neurol Clin 6:279–296, 1988.

postictal pulmonary edema: A case report and review of the literature. Epilepsia 23:71–82, 1982.

24. Guberman, A, Cantu-Reyna, G, Stuss, D, and Broughton, R: Nonconvulsive generalized status epilepticus: Clinical features, neuropsychological testing, and long-term follow-up. Neurology 36: 1284–1291, 1986.

25. Guess, HA, Resseguie, LJ, Melton, LJ III, et al: Factors predictive of seizures among intensive care unit patients with gram-negative infections. Epilepsia 31: 567–573, 1990.

26. Hauser, P, Devinsky, O, de Bellis, M, et al: Benzodiazepine withdrawal delirium with catatonic features: Occurrence in patients with partial seizure disorders. Arch Neurol 46:696–699, 1989.

27. Hauser, WA: Status epilepticus: Epidemiologic considerations. Neurology 40(Suppl 2):9–13, 1990.

28. Hersch, EL and Billings, RF: Acute confusional state with status petit mal as a withdrawal syndrome—five year follow-up. Can J Psychiatry 33:157–159, 1988.

29. Jagoda, A and Riggio, S: Nonconvulsive status epilepticus in adults. Am J Emerg Med 6:250–254, 1988.

30. Kiok, MC, Terrence, CF, Fromm, GH, and Lavine, S: Sinus arrest in epilepsy. Neurology 36:115–116, 1986.

31. Kofke, WA, Snider, MT, Young, RSK, and Ramer, JC: Prolonged low flow isoflurane anesthesia for status epilepticus. Anaesthesiology 62:653–656, 1985.

32. Kofke, WA, Young, RSK, Davis, P, et al: Isoflurane for refractory status epilepticus: A clinical series. Anesthesiology 71:653–659, 1989.

33. Kumar, A and Bleck, TP: Intravenous midazolam for the treatment of refractory status epilepticus. Crit Care Med 20:483–488, 1992.

34. Lee, SI: Nonconvulsive status epilepticus: Ictal confusion in later life. Arch Neurol 42:778–781, 1985.

35. Leppik, IE, Derivan, AT, Homan, RW, et al: Double-blind study of lorazepam and diazepam in status epilepticus. JAMA 249:1452–1454, 1983.

36. Levy, RJ and Krall, RL: Treatment of status epilepticus with lorazepam. Arch Neurol 41:605–611, 1984.

37. Lindow, J and Wijdicks, EFM: Phenytoin toxicity associated with hypoalbuminemia in critically ill patients. Chest 105:602–604, 1994.

38. Lockman, LA: Other antiepileptic drugs: Paraldehyde. In Levy, RH, Dreifuss, FE, Mattson, RH, et al (eds): Antiepileptic Drugs, ed 3. Raven Press, New York, 1989, pp 881–886.

39. Lowenstein, DH and Alldredge, B: Managing status epilepticus (letter). Lancet 336:1451, 1990.

40. Lowenstein, DH, Aminoff, MJ, and Simon, RP: Barbiturate anesthesia in the treatment of status epilepticus: Clinical experience with 14 patients. Neurology 38:395–400, 1988.

41. Mackenzie, SJ, Kapadia, F, and Grant, IS: Propofol infusion for control of status epilepticus. Anaesthesia 45:1043–1045, 1990.

42. Meldrum, BS and Horton, RW: Physiology of status epilepticus in primates. Arch Neurol 28:1–9, 1973.

43. Meldrum, BS, Vigouroux, RA, and Brierly, JB: Systemic factors and epileptic brain damage: Prolonged seizures in paralyzed, artificially ventilated baboons. Arch Neurol 29:82–87, 1973.

44. Messing, RO, Closson, RG, and Simon, RP: Drug-induced seizures: A 10-year experience. Neurology 34:1582–1586, 1984.

45. Modica, PA, Tempelhoff, R, and White, PF: Pro- and anticonvulsant effects of anesthetics. Parts I and II. Anesth Analg 70:303–315, 433–444, 1990.

46. Morris, JC and Victor, M: Alcohol withdrawal seizures. Emerg Med Clin North Am 5:827, 1987.

47. Nevander, G, Ingvar, M, Auer, R, and Siesjö, BK: Status epilepticus in well-oxygenated rats causes neuronal necrosis. Ann Neurol 18:281–290, 1985.

48. Ng, SKC, Hauser, WA, Brust, JCM, and Susser, M: Alcohol consumption and withdrawal in new-onset seizures. N Engl J Med 319:666–673, 1988.

49. Orlowski, JP, Erenberg, G, Lueders, H, and Cruse, RP: Hypothermia and barbiturate coma for refractory status epilepticus. Crit Care Med 12:367–372, 1984.

50. Orringer, CE, Eustace, JC, Wunsch, CD,

and Gardner, LB: Natural history of lactic acidosis after grand-mal seizures: A model for the study of an anion-gap acidosis not associated with hyperkalemia. N Engl J Med 297:796–799, 1977.

51. Os, I and Lyngdal, PT: General convulsions and rhabdomyolysis: Case reports. Acta Neurol Scand 79:246–248, 1989.

52. Osorio, I, Burnstine, TH, Remler, B, et al: Phenytoin-induced seizures: A paradoxical effect at toxic concentrations in epileptic patients. Epilepsia 30:230–234, 1989.

53. Osorio, I and Reed, RC: Treatment of refractory generalized tonic-clonic status epilepticus with pentobarbital anesthesia after high-dose phenytoin. Epilepsia 30:464–470, 1989.

54. Pascual, J, Ciudad, J, and Berciano, J: Role of lidocaine (lignocaine) in managing status epilepticus. J Neurol Neurosurg Psychiatry 55:49–51, 1992.

55. Porter, RJ: Epilepsy: 100 elementary principles. Major Probl Neurol 20:1–186, 1989.

56. Pritchard, PB III and O'Neal, DB: Nonconvulsive status epilepticus following mitrizamide myelography. Ann Neurol 16:252–254, 1984.

57. Rashkin, MC, Youngs, C, and Penovich, P: Pentobarbital treatment of refractory status epilepticus. Neurology 37:500–503, 1987.

58. Schmidley, JW and Simon, RP: Postictal pleocytosis. Ann Neurol 9:81–84, 1981.

59. Shaner, DM, McCurdy, SA, Herring, MO, and Gabor, AJ: Treatment of status epilepticus: A prospective comparison of diazepam and phenytoin versus phenobarbital and optional phenytoin. Neurology 38:202–207, 1988.

60. Simon, RP: Alcohol and seizures (editorial). N Engl J Med 319:715–716, 1988.

61. Singhal, PC, Chugh, KS, and Gulati, DR: Myoglobinuria and renal failure after status epilepticus. Neurology 28:200–201, 1978.

62. Somerville, ER and Bruni, J: Tonic status epilepticus presenting as confusional state. Ann Neurol 13:549–551, 1983.

63. Spengler, RF, Arrowsmith, JB, Kilarski,

DJ, et al: Severe soft-tissue injury following intravenous infusion of phenytoin: Patient and drug administration risk factors. Arch Intern Med 148:1329–1333, 1988.

64. Sung, C-Y and Chu, N-S: Status epilepticus in the elderly: Etiology, seizure type and outcome. Acta Neurol Scand 80:51–56, 1989.

65. Terrence, CF, Rao, GR, and Perper, JA: Neurogenic pulmonary edema in unexpected, unexplained death of epileptic patients. Ann Neurol 9:458–464, 1981.

66. Thomas, P, Beaumanoir, A, Genton, P, et al: 'De novo' absence status of late onset: Report of 11 cases. Neurology 42:104–110, 1992.

67. Treiman, DM: Pharmacokinetics and clinical use of benzodiazepines in the management of status epilepticus. Epilepsia 30 (Suppl 2):S4–S10, 1989.

68. Uthman, BM and Wilder, BJ: Emergency management of seizures: An overview. Epilepsia 30 (Suppl 2):S33–S37, 1989.

69. Van Ness, PC: Pentobarbital and EEG burst suppression in treatment of status epilepticus refractory to benzodiazepines and phenytoin. Epilepsia 31:61–66, 1990.

70. Varma, NK and Lee, SI: Nonconvulsive status epilepticus following electroconvulsive therapy. Neurology 42:263–264, 1992.

71. Vasko, MR and Brater, DC: Drug interactions. In Chernow, B (ed): Essentials of Critical Care Pharmacology. (Abridged from The Pharmacologic Approach to the Critically Ill, ed 2.) Williams & Wilkins, Baltimore, 1989, pp 1–26.

72. Vernay, D, Dubost, JJ, Dordain, G, and Sauvezie, B: Seizures and compression fracture (letter). Neurology 40:725–726, 1990.

73. Vickrey, BG and Bahls, FH: Nonconvulsive status epilepticus following cerebral angiography. Ann Neurol 25:199–201, 1989.

74. Victor, M and Brausch, C: The role of abstinence in the genesis of alcoholic epilepsy. Epilepsia 8:1–20, 1967.

75. Vollmer, ME, Weiss, H, Beanland, C, and Krumholz, A: Prolonged confusion

due to absence status following metrizamide myelography. Arch Neurol 42:
1005–1008, 1985.

76. Walker, JE, Homan, RW, Vasko, MR, et
al: Lorazepam in status epilepticus.
Ann Neurol 6:207–213, 1979.

77. Wijdicks, EFM and Sharbrough, FW:
New-onset seizures in critically ill
patients. Neurology 43:1042–1044,
1993.

78. Wijdicks, EFM and Hubmayr, RD: Acute
acid base disorders following status epilepticus. Mayo Clin Proc (in press).

79. Wood, PR, Browne, GPR, and Pugh, S:
Propofol infusion for the treatment of
status epilepticus (letter). Lancet i:480–
481, 1988.

80. Wszolek, ZK, Aksamit, AJ, Ellingson,
RJ, et al: Epileptiform electroencephalographic abnormalities in liver transplant recipients. Ann Neurol 30:37–41,
1991.

81. Yaffe, K and Lowenstein, DH: Prognostic factors of pentobarbital therapy for
refractory generalized status epilepticus. Neurology 43:895–900, 1993.

82. Young, RS, Fripp, RR, Yagel, SK, et al:
Cardiac dysfunction during status epilepticus in the neonatal pig. Ann Neurol
18:291–297, 1985.

Chapter 3

GENERALIZED WEAKNESS IN THE INTENSIVE CARE UNIT

DISORDERS OF THE SPINAL CORD
DISORDERS OF PERIPHERAL NERVES
DISORDERS OF THE
   NEUROMUSCULAR JUNCTION
DISORDERS OF SKELETAL MUSCLE

Generalized weakness is a diagnostic problem in critically ill patients and more often in those in whom the critical illness has begun to subside. Many patients are too ill to permit adequate assessment of their neuromuscular condition, and for obvious reasons, at that time neurologic consultation often has a low priority. However, it becomes a great concern when patients have marked wasting of muscle and fat and several attempts to wean them from the ventilator have failed.

Whether a debilitated patient in fact has a neuromuscular disorder can be difficult to assess. Results of muscle testing can be misleading in patients with severe sleep deprivation from the fragmented sleep patterns that are very common in intensive care units (ICUs),[2,23] in patients with severe cardiac and respiratory failure resulting in immediate desaturation whenever a movement of limbs is initiated, and in patients who simply are fatigued, underfed, and unwilling to cooperate.

There are large gaps in our knowledge of causes of weakness in ICUs. In all likelihood, one can expect that most patients with generalized weakness in medical or surgical ICUs have so-called critical illness neuropathy, persistent post–paralytic agent weakness, or a previously undiagnosed neurologic disorder that presented with acute respiratory failure. Certainly, a number of neurologic disorders may rapidly progress into involvement of respiratory or bulbar muscles and lead to aspiration pneumonia or mechanical respiratory failure resulting in urgent intubation and mechanical ventilation before a neurologic disorder is entertained.

Moreover, a primary neurologic disorder may not be evident, particularly when the mechanical ventilation strategy includes heavy sedation and paralysis. During examination, attention should be given to severe muscle atrophy, areflexia, fasciculations, myotonia, marked muscle swelling, and skin lesions. This chapter provides an overview of causes of generalized weakness associated with a myelopathy, neuropathy, neuromuscular junction block, or myopathy in the ICU; details can be found in subsequent chapters.

DISORDERS OF THE SPINAL CORD

It is difficult to estimate the frequency of spinal cord damage as a potential cause of generalized limb weakness in critically ill patients. Traumatic spinal cord injury or spinal infarction associated with thoracoabdominal aneurysm repairs is the most frequent consideration, but infectious causes occasionally occur. These patients most likely have been admitted with acute lung injury necessitating mechanical ventilation. Causes of acute lung infection associated with myelitis may include groups A and B coxsackievirus, cytomegalovirus, *Mycoplasma*, and *Legionella*.[29]

In immunosuppressed patients, cytomegalovirus, herpes zoster, and *Aspergillus* infection can involve the spinal cord. *Listeria* may occasionally cause a spinal cord abscess.[19] Bacterial infection of the spinal cord occurs most often after wound infection, but the most common causes of spinal cord damage in surgical ICUs remain ischemic myelopathies associated with major thoracoabdominal vascular repairs. Spinal cord compression from epidural hematoma in coagulopathies has been repeatedly reported, and magnetic resonance imaging is the most useful imaging technique if the suspicion is high (see Chapter 10).

DISORDERS OF PERIPHERAL NERVES

Causes of acute hospital-acquired polyneuropathy are very limited. Systemic illness (e.g., vasculitis, acute porphyria) may concomitantly afflict peripheral nerves, and in very occasional circumstances, a number of drugs may induce a toxic polyneuropathy. Most patients with drug-induced neuropathy have a gradual mode of onset, but several months of treatment may produce a mixed sensorimotor neuropathy.

Drug-induced neuropathies in the ICU are most likely from antineoplastic agents given before the onset of life-threatening illness, but sensorimotor neuropathies after relatively short intervals of treatment (3 months) have been noted with amiodarone and metronidazole, all with nerve biopsy confirmation.[5,21] Metronidazole has been

implicated as a frequent cause of neuropathy, but its role in causing axonal neuropathy in ICUs probably is overestimated. All other drugs used in ICUs produce only transient paresthesias, fleeting numbness, and no diffuse weakness.

Most often, an axonal polyneuropathy occurs in association with sepsis (Chapter 5), but as alluded to earlier, neuromuscular blocking agents alone may result in a polyneuropathy.[13] Guillain-Barré syndrome has been reported to occur after any type of surgery, epidural anesthesia, administration of fibrinolytic agents, and even high doses of methylprednisolone for asthma.[22,24] The clinical features of Guillain-Barré syndrome are distinct from those of critical illness polyneuropathy. Cranial nerve deficits are conspicuously absent in critical illness polyneuropathy, even in patients with complete quadriplegia. Electrodiagnostic tests invariably show evidence for axonal involvement, which has been confirmed at autopsy.[30] The distinction between severe axonal Guillain-Barré syndrome and critical illness polyneuropathy, however, is less clear (see Chapter 5).

In critically ill patients with AIDS, a progressive polyradiculopathy has been described with typical cerebrospinal fluid polymorphonuclear pleocytosis and positive cytomegalovirus cultures; outcome is poor.[11] The incidence of cytomegalovirus radiculopathy may increase because the prevalence of cytomegalovirus-related infections has increased in patients who have had *Pneumocystis carinii* pneumonia prophylaxis. An AIDS-related polyneuropathy, resulting in progressive quadriplegia with electromyographic characteristics of a demyelinating neuropathy has been described; electron micrography demonstrated viral capsids inside the nerve.[18] In a recent series of patients with acute lumbosacral polyradiculopathy, progression was said to have halted in most patients treated with ganciclovir, although many became paraplegic and lost bladder and bowel control. Patients receiving ganciclovir for systemic cytomegalovirus infection should be treated with foscarnet.[26]

DISORDERS OF THE NEUROMUSCULAR JUNCTION

Neuromuscular blockade used for at least 2 days to facilitate mechanical ventilation may produce prolonged muscular weakness, most likely from accumulation of the metabolic products of pancuronium or vecuronium. The mechanism of profound weakness other than continued blockade of the neuromuscular junction by metabolites is not known. Sepsis and intravenous administration of high doses of corticosteroids are often confounders in this situation, but, as mentioned, vecuronium and probably also pancuronium alone may produce a polyneuropathy. A myasthenic syndrome may occasionally cause generalized weakness in the ICU. The most common are myasthenia gravis and Eaton-Lambert syndrome. Tick paralysis and botulism (see Chapter 5) are rare causes of generalized weakness associated with respiratory failure. In both conditions, bulbar involvement and diplopia are cardinal clinical clues.

Drugs that induce neuromuscular blockade are seldom solely responsible for generalized weakness, and an underlying neuromuscular junction disorder should be suspected. Electromyographic evidence of a neuromuscular junction defect on electrodiagnostic testing must be present before weakness can be attributed to neuromuscular blockade from drugs. Antibiotic-induced paralysis from aminoglycosides and polymyxin antibiotics has been described,[1] but anticholinesterase administration has very often been unsuccessful. Antibiotic-induced paralysis remains an unclear entity, particularly in the critical care setting.

Severe electrolyte disorders (e.g., hypermagnesemia) probably can produce severe weakness, most likely from a block at the neuromuscular junction, but in hypophosphatemia and hypokalemia, the mechanism is less clear[15] (see Chapter 7).

DISORDERS OF SKELETAL MUSCLE

Loss of muscle mass is expected in immobilized critically ill patients. Disuse of skeletal muscle rapidly produces atrophy. Biopsy shows intact architecture, little change in type I muscle fibers, and mostly degeneration of type II fibers.[15]

Prolonged immobilization of limbs in patients with neuromuscular blockade may produce pressure necrosis in dorsally located muscles but probably never as striking as that in compartment syndromes.

Rhabdomyolysis may be a cause of weakness in critically ill patients (Table 3–1). The most common causes probably are trauma and ischemia of large fleshy muscles from arterial occlusion.[15] Myoglobinuria can be found when rhabdomyolysis is massive. Most patients have considerable muscle weakness and pain when tested. Biceps, quadriceps, and gastrocnemius muscles can be tender on palpation and may appear swollen. Rapid resolution of weakness and decrease in creatine kinase level, often from serum levels

Table 3–1 CAUSES OF RHABDOMYOLYSIS IN THE INTENSIVE CARE UNIT

Ischemic (occlusion of brachial or femoral artery)
Infectious (septic shock, influenza A, coxsackievirus)
Environmental and crush (heat stroke, mechanical)
Status epilepticus
Malignant neuroleptic syndrome
Drugs (amphotericin B, epsilon-aminocaproic acid, theophylline*)

*May cause seizures, which are the most likely mechanism.[17,27]

around 10,000 IU, are expected within 2 to 3 days.[15]

Nutritional deficiency may also contribute to loss of muscle bulk, often from a catabolic state that is not balanced by high caloric intake. A catabolic state can be expected in any patient with sepsis, trauma, burns, or previous malnourishment from alcohol or drug abuse. Specific vitamin deficiencies have not consistently shown myopathic changes on biopsy examinations except for vitamin E in malabsorption syndromes.[15]

Most commonly, muscle weakness is associated with intravenous infusions of pancuronium and vecuronium.[9,14,20,25,28] A 1992 prospective study found that generalized atrophy, areflexia, and electromyographic evidence of axonal polyneuropathy developed in 5 of 10 patients with prolonged use of neuromuscular blocking agents.[13] There was a significant association with duration and mean dose of vecuronium bromide infusion. Muscle biopsy data are not available except for a preliminary observation in two patients who had evidence of increased regeneration and immature new folds of neuromuscular junction on intercostal muscle biopsy specimens (intercostal muscle is usually examined because the neuromuscular junction can be better studied there than in any other muscle).[28]

Among the many confounders in prolonged postparalytic weakness is the use of steroids (methylprednisolone or hydrocortisone), usually given in high intravenous doses.[9,14,25] Recovery occurs between 2 weeks and 6 months in most patients (see Chapter 1). Muscle biopsy discloses type IIB fiber atrophy or necrotizing myopathy with selective loss of myosin (thick) filaments,[9] but other investigators have not observed these findings.[14] Whether neuromuscular blocking agents can induce a necrotic myopathy alone is unknown. Although a recent study suggested a link in two cases, it is not clear whether rhabdomyolysis played a major role.[31]

Another group of diseases to be considered in patients with generalized weakness consists of primary myopathies associated with respiratory failure.[7,12] There are many reports of respiratory failure as the initial manifestations of dermatomyositis, polymyositis, mitochondrial myopathy, and myotonic dystrophy.[3,7,10,12]

Endocrine causes of myopathies are discussed in Chapter 7. Progressive muscle weakness can be expected in thyrotoxic myopathy, myxedema myopathy, osteomalacia myopathy, and myopathies associated with adrenal and pancreatic diseases. All these disorders, however, affect a minority of patients with muscle weakness in the ICU.

Along with an expected increase in critically ill patients with AIDS comes generalized weakness. Most admissions to the ICU are related to mechanical ventilation for Pneumocystis carinii pneumonia (PCP). After recovery from respiratory failure, many patients are weak and wasted from undernutrition or from AIDS-wasting syndrome, but muscle weakness can be associated with zidovudine treatment. Zidovudine treatment may cause significant generalized weakness, up to inability to walk unassisted, in 3 to 21 months (mean, 13 months).[8] Serum creatine phosphokinase levels are in the 1000 U/L area, and examination of muscle biopsy specimens may reveal mitochondrial changes suggested by ragged red fibers and endomysial inflammation.[8] Recovery can be expected after administration of zidovudine is discontinued or treatment is begun with nonsteroidal anti-inflammatory drugs or, as a last resort, corticosteroids.[6,8] Zidovudine may also be replaced by another nucleoside, dideoxycytidine (ddC); however, this drug in moderate doses may, in susceptible patients, produce reversible painful, burning paresthesias but no weakness except for slight intrinsic foot muscle weakness.[4] (Central nervous system complications, mostly infectious in origin, can be found in the discussion of neurologic complications of immunosuppression in Chapter 16 and in a recent comprehensive discussion in this series.[16])

CONCLUSIONS

When illness is overwhelming, a debilitated clinical condition in itself is a biologically plausible reason for weakness for most critical care physicians. Despite lack of prospective studies of critically ill patients with prolonged mechanical ventilation and hemodynamic monitoring (with the exception of sepsis as a patient selector), several specific issues can be addressed.

Most patients with generalized weakness have an axonal polyneuropathy associated with sepsis or neuromuscular blocking agents, or both. Prolonged proximal muscle weakness after

neuromuscular blockade may be seen relatively frequently without electromyographic abnormalities and with good recovery within weeks (Fig. 3–1). An occasional patient is seen with respiratory failure from a previously undiagnosed neuromuscular disorder. Antibiotics (e.g., aminoglycosides, erythromycin) can uncover myasthenia gravis. In other patients, gathering historical information strengthens the suspicion of an underlying neuromuscular disorder. Generally, the yield of muscle or nerve biopsy is limited, but biopsy may become more important as additional clinical and laboratory abnormalities are identified. The combination of steroid and pancuronium can cause a necrotic myopathy, and zidovudine can cause a mitochondrial myopathy. Both conditions are reversible. In surgical ICUs, generalized limb weakness may

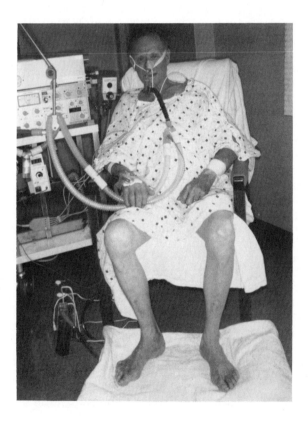

Figure 3–1. A 72-year-old man admitted with severe pulmonary edema received vecuronium for 2 weeks during mechanical ventilation. The patient had generalized muscle weakness (proximal more than distal), and an attempt at weaning had failed. Results of extensive electrophysiologic studies were normal. He had full recovery of muscle strength in 3 weeks.

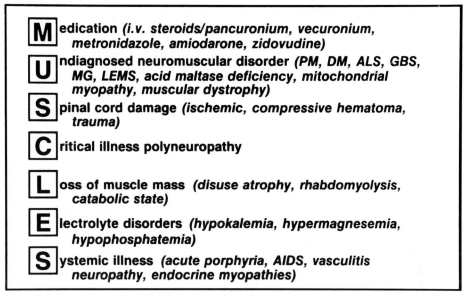

Figure 3–2. Mnemonic for the differential diagnosis of generalized weakness in the intensive care unit. ALS = amyotrophic lateral sclerosis; DM = dermatomyositis; GBS = Guillain-Barré syndrome; LEMS = Lambert-Eaton myasthenic syndrome; MG = myasthenia gravis; PM = polymyositis.

be associated with spinal shock from ischemic damage (i.e., after extensive aortic repairs) or from direct trauma.

A diligent application of the causes outlined in the mnemonic MUSCLES (Fig. 3–2) may help in the diagnostic evaluation. (As prospective data become available, some subcategories may expand and others may become rare.)

REFERENCES

1. Argov, Z and Mastaglia, FL: Disorders of neuromuscular transmission caused by drugs. N Engl J Med 301:409–413, 1979.

2. Aurell, J and Elmqvist, D: Sleep in the surgical intensive care unit: Continuous polygraphic recording of sleep in nine patients receiving postoperative care. Br Med J 290:1029–1032, 1985.

3. Barohn, RJ, Clanton, TL, Sahenk, Z, and Mendell, JR: Recurrent respiratory insufficiency and depressed ventilatory drive complicating mitochondrial myopathies. Neurology 40:103–106, 1990.

4. Berger, AR, Arezzo, JC, Schaumburg, HH, et al: 2′,3′-dideoxycytidine (ddC) toxic neuropathy: A study of 52 patients. Neurology 43:358–362, 1993.

5. Bradley, WG, Karlsson, IJ, and Rassol, CG: Metronidazole neuropathy. Br Med J 2:610–611, 1977.

6. Chalmers, AC, Greco, CM, and Miller, RG: Prognosis in AZT myopathy. Neurology 41:1181–1184, 1991.

7. Cros, D, Palliyath, S, DiMauro, S, et al: Respiratory failure revealing mitochondrial myopathy in adults. Chest 101: 824–828, 1992.

8. Dalakas, MC, Illa, I, Pezeshkpour, GH, et al: Mitochondrial myopathy caused by long-term zidovudine therapy. N Engl J Med 322:1098–1105, 1990.

9. Danon, MJ and Carpenter, S: Myopathy with thick filament (myosin) loss following prolonged paralysis with vecuronium during steroid treatment. Muscle Nerve 14:1131–1139, 1991.

10. DeVere, R and Bradley, WG: Polymyosi-

tis: Its presentation, morbidity and mortality. Brain 98:637–666, 1975.

11. Eidelberg, D, Sotrel, A, Vogel, H, et al: Progressive polyradiculopathy in acquired immune deficiency syndrome. Neurology 36:912–916, 1986.

12. Jammes, Y, Pouget, J, Grimaud, C, and Serratrice, G: Pulmonary function and electromyographic study of respiratory muscles in myotonic dystrophy. Muscle Nerve 8:586–594, 1985.

13. Kupfer, Y, Namba, T, Kaldawi, E, and Tessler, S: Prolonged weakness after long-term infusion of vecuronium bromide. Ann Intern Med 117:484–486, 1992.

14. Lacomis, D, Smith, TW, and Chad, DA: Acute myopathy and neuropathy in status asthmaticus: Case report and literature review. Muscle Nerve 16: 84–90, 1993.

15. Layzer, RB: Neuromuscular Manifestations of Systemic Disease (Contemporary Neurology Series No. 25). FA Davis, Philadelphia, 1985.

16. Levy, RM and Berger, JR: HIV and HTLV infections of the nervous system. In Tyler, KL and Martin, JB (eds): Infectious Diseases of the Central Nervous System (Contemporary Neurology Series No. 41). FA Davis, Philadelphia, 1993, pp 47–75.

17. Lloyd, DM, Payne, SPK, Tomson, CRV, et al: Acute compartment syndrome secondary to theophylline overdose (letter). Lancet 336:312, 1990.

18. Morgello, S and Simpson, DM: Multifocal cytomegalovirus demyelinative polyneuropathy associated with AIDS. Muscle Nerve 17:176–182, 1994.

19. Morrison, RE, Brown, J, and Gooding, RS: Spinal cord abscess caused by *Listeria monocytogenes*. Arch Neurol 37:243–245, 1980.

20. Op de Coul, AAW, Verheul, GAM, Leyten, ACM, et al: Critical illness polyneuromyopathy after artificial respiration. Clin Neurol Neurosurg 93:27–33, 1991.

21. Pellissier, JF, Pouget, J, Cros, D, et al: Peripheral neuropathy induced by amiodarone chlorohydrate: A clinicopathological study. J Neurol Sci 63: 251–266, 1984.

22. Preston, DC and Logigian, EL: Guillain-Barré syndrome during high-dose methylprednisolone therapy. Muscle Nerve 14:378–379, 1991.

23. Richards, KC and Bairnsfather, L: A description of night sleep patterns in the critical care unit. Heart Lung 17:35–42, 1988.

24. Ropper, AH, Wijdicks, EFM, and Truax, BT: Guillain-Barré Syndrome (Contemporary Neurology Series No. 34). FA Davis, Philadelphia, 1991.

25. Shapiro, JM, Condos, R, and Cole, RP: Myopathy in status asthmaticus: Relation to new muscular blockade. J Intensive Care Med 8:144–152, 1993.

26. So, YT and Olney, RK: Acute lumbosacral polyradiculopathy in acquired immunodeficiency syndrome: Experience in 23 patients. Ann Neurol 35:53–58, 1994.

27. Titley, OG and Williams, N: Theophylline toxicity causing rhabdomyolysis and acute compartment syndrome. Intensive Care Med 18:129–130, 1992.

28. Wokke, JHJ, Jennekens, FGI, van den Oord, CJM, et al: Histological investigation of muscle atrophy and end plates in two critically ill patients with generalized weakness. J Neurol Sci 88:95–106, 1988.

29. Woolsey, RM and Young, RR (eds): Disorders of the spinal cord. Neurol Clin 9:503–816, Aug 1991.

30. Zochodne, DW, Bolton, CF, Wells, GA, et al: Critical illness polyneuropathy: A complication of critical illness and multiple organ failure. Brain 110:819–841, 1987.

31. Zochodne, DW, Ramsay, DA, Saly, V, et al: Acute necrotizing myopathy of intensive care: Electrophysiological studies. Muscle Nerve 17:285–292, 1994.

Chapter 4

NEUROLOGIC COMPLICATIONS OF INVASIVE PROCEDURES IN THE INTENSIVE CARE UNIT

GENERAL CONSIDERATIONS
NEUROLOGIC COMPLICATIONS ASSOCIATED WITH SPECIFIC PROCEDURES

On the surface, neurologic complications of invasive procedures in intensive care units (ICUs) are rare. However, the incidence of procedure-related complications in the ICU is probably only a crude estimation, and neurologic complications may be transient, masked by pharmaceutical agents, and remain undetected. Nonetheless, it is unlikely that persistent neurologic deficits are truly unrecognized in sick patients seen by multiple hospital services. In 1986, Moses and Kaden[90] published a study of iatrogenic neurologic conditions from a prospective series of neurologic consultations at Johns Hopkins Hospital. From the study of such data came the awareness that in one third of the cases (22% of patients had angiographic studies), iatrogenic neurologic complications could be attributed to invasive diagnostic procedures.

In recent years, there have been considerable advances in procedure technology. The indications for invasive hemodynamic monitoring have expanded, and consequently the incidence of iatrogenic neurologic complications may increase. Generally, causes of complications of invasive procedures can be best characterized by reaction to injected material (air or contrast medium) or mobilization of intravascular debris. In some procedures, traumatic damage from needle entry itself is the main cause.

GENERAL CONSIDERATIONS

Neurotoxicity of Radiologic Contrast Agents

The pathophysiologic mechanism of neurotoxicity of contrast agents is not known. Adverse reactions to injection of the agents are possibly more commonly caused by inadvertent embolization during manipulation, but there is also some evidence that iodinated radiographic contrast media are directly involved.[19,72] Contrast agents do not enter the brain; therefore, opening of the tight junctions of endothelial cells that maintain the blood-brain barrier is required. A number of investigations have documented that repeated injections of contrast agents within several minutes or a major increase in osmolality may predispose the patient to contrast leaks into the brain.[107,112] This explanation is more likely than diffuse vasospasm, which has been offered as an alternative explanation in patients with acute confusional states but never has been consistently demonstrable. Many complications of contrast studies are related to the hemodynamic condition of the patient, a risk factor that can be avoided. Intensive care physicians typically care for patients who have fever, are in cardiovascular distress, or need chronic hemodialysis, conditions well known to facilitate neurotoxicity (Table 4–1).

The clinical manifestations of neurotoxicity are nonspecific. Combativeness, acute confusional state with many recognizable elements of delirium, and seizures may occur but most likely only in predisposed patients. Transient global amnesia or cortical blindness[68] has also been linked to a direct adverse reaction to the contrast agent. Complete recovery is expected within 1 or 2 days.[52]

Treatment of adverse effects of contrast agents is usually limited to treatment of the allergic manifestations, which include urticaria, angioedema, laryngeal edema, shock, and bronchospasm. Mannitol, 25%, 1 to 2 g/kg, with the aim to osmotically draw contrast material out, and dexamethasone, a 10-mg bolus intravenously followed by 4 mg intravenously every 6 hours, may be used to stabilize the blood-brain barrier. This approach may be appropriate only in patients who have become stuporous or continue to have seizures, but, as alluded to previously, the clinical manifestations exist only for a short time and permanent neurologic deficits are extremely rare.

Drainage of cerebrospinal fluid has

Table 4–1 RISK FACTORS FOR NEUROTOXICITY OF CONTRAST AGENTS IN CRITICALLY ILL PATIENTS

Hyperthermia
Dehydration
Preexisting renal failure
Congestive heart failure
History of seizures
History of recent ischemic stroke

been recommended in patients with spinal cord injury during abdominal aortography, but the value of this intervention remains controversial.

Cholesterol Embolization

Elderly patients with severe atherosclerosis of the aorta are at risk for cholesterol showers. Difficult catheter manipulation and multiple arteriographic procedures may precipitate this often unrecognized entity.[24,25,27,99] One provocative study based on retrospective review of pathologic material from patients who died within 6 months of vascular catheterization reported an unexpectedly high incidence of cholesterol embolization (25%), not found in a control population. Evidence of embolization to the brain was found in 5% of patients who underwent aortography and in 2% of patients with cardiac catheterization.[39] Nonetheless, a recent unselected autopsy series found spontaneous atheroembolism in approximately 2% of the patients.[26]

A universal pathogenesis for cholesterol embolization is not known. Arterial trauma during catheter placement may dislodge cholesterol crystals from atheromatous ulcerated plaques and subsequently result in massive showers of embolic material. Occlusion of many small arterioles and capillaries may result in mononuclear cell infiltration, giant cell formation, and, more characteristically, eosinophilic leukocyte infiltration. The location of these cholesterol crystals may depend on the procedure, but virtually any organ may be affected.

Frequent targets for cholesterol embolization are the skin, kidney, and pancreas.[99] The cutaneous manifestations, such as livedo reticularis and purple toes, are important, if not archetypal, initial clinical findings. Symptoms may occur weeks after the procedure, an interval that suggests an immunologic response to the cholesterol emboli. Neurologic manifestations may also appear after relatively long intervals between the clinical presentation and the invasive procedure. In a 1991 well-documented case from Massachusetts General Hospital, a syndrome characterized by headache, seizure, and encephalopathy occurred 2 months after angiographic examination.[21] Renal failure and hypertension should be a clue to the diagnosis, and renal biopsy may demonstrate typical stacked, needle-shaped crystals. Muscle biopsy, however, is the preferred diagnostic test, with a sensitivity of 92%.[39] Other patients may have only vague complaints of weight loss, headache, myalgias, and fatigue.

Neurologic manifestations of cholesterol embolization are diverse. Muscle weakness masquerading as polymyositis and polyneuropathy have been confirmed by sural nerve or muscle biopsy showing cholesterol clefts that led to arteritis.[63] A polyneuropathy associated with cholesterol embolization has not been previously recognized in critically ill patients and may be a diagnostic consideration in patients with weakness after multiple endovascular procedures.[9] In a recently published, well-documented case report, sural nerve biopsy showed epineural necrotizing arteritis and focal axonal degeneration with cholesterol clefts in vessels of the gastrocnemius muscle.[9] Alternatively, patients may present with clinical signs of a diffuse encephalopathy, retinal hemorrhages, and transient hemiparesis. Cholesterol embolization is found in various parts of the brain but most often in the middle cerebral artery territory, border zone territories, and caudate nuclei. Cholesterol embolus in the fundus is usually pathognomonic in a patient with multiorgan involvement but is difficult to detect.

Several case reports have also mentioned spinal cord injury, usually in relation to abdominal aortography. The lumbosacral part of the spinal cord is frequently involved, but emboli have been found during postmortem examination in patients who remained asymptomatic during life. Slavin and colleagues[105] found that most patients with spinal cord involvement had multiple organ distribution of emboli.

The therapeutic options in patients with disseminated cholesterol emboli are limited, and the overall mortality is high. Management is limited to treatment of hypertension, hemodialysis, and symptomatic treatment of ischemic extremities and ischemic perforation of the small intestine and colon. Anticoagulation is not indicated, is hazardous, and has been implicated as a causative factor. Therapies such as vasodilation, lumbar sympathectomy, emergency surgery of the aorta, and corticosteroid administration are unlikely to be effective.

Air Embolism

The risk of cerebral air embolism in patients in the ICU is very low despite the use of multiple lines. Systemic air embolism has been reported as a complication of central venous pressure catheters, subclavian catheters used for parenteral alimentation,[48] radial catheters, percutaneous aspiration biopsy of the lung,[6] and mechanical ventilation with high levels of positive pressure.[83]

The early clinical presentations of systemic air embolism are sensations of dizziness, fear of death, and substernal chest pain.[66] Air embolism should be strongly considered when cardiovascular collapse, chest pain, severe dyspnea, or cyanosis suddenly develops in a patient with a vascular catheter. A helpful auscultative physical sign is a mill-wheel murmur or sounds resembling a sponge being squeezed. Acute bronchospasm with wheezing may also be heard, and some patients become immediately comatose and have labored breathing. A chest radiograph may demonstrate acute pulmonary edema. Air in the heart is seldom seen, probably because air is dispersed or absorbed.

Symptoms of cerebral air embolism include transient or persistent hemiparesis, generalized tonic-clonic seizures, and, more commonly, sudden onset of coma.[86] A computed tomography (CT) scan within 24 hours of the onset of symptoms may directly visualize air bubbles or areas of gyral enhancement. Most lesions associated with air embolization are seen in the distribution of the middle cerebral artery and the anterior cerebral artery.[60,62,116]

The pathophysiologic mechanism of cerebral air embolism is complex.[16,17] An experimental study of the effect of gas emboli on cerebral blood flow demonstrated that a decline in cerebral blood flow could not be readily explained by bubble trapping in arterioles but was perhaps more likely caused by direct gas-induced changes of blood vessels.[55]

Cerebral air embolism may occur through a retrograde arterial route in patients with radial artery cannulas[23,76] but is prevented by flush rates of solution from 12 to 15 mL/s.[76]

Passage of air may occur through a foramen ovale that is physiologically opened by high atrial pressures, but a patent foramen ovale may not be a necessary factor[84] and air emboli may squeeze through the pulmonary capillaries, particularly during conditions of sudden excessive volumes of air.

Prompt treatment of systemic air emboli may decrease the incidence of neurologic sequelae, but mortality and neurologic morbidity remain high. The patient should receive 100% oxygen immediately and be placed in the Trendelenburg and left lateral decubitus position. The central venous pressure catheter may be advanced to the right ventricle for aspiration. Percutaneous aspiration of the right ventricle with a spinal needle may be tried as a last resort.

NEUROLOGIC COMPLICATIONS ASSOCIATED WITH SPECIFIC PROCEDURES

Although the broad concepts of neurologic complications discussed above apply to many patients, several invasive procedures produce specific neurologic complications, which are reviewed in this section.

Endotracheal Intubation

After extubation, many critically ill patients experience hoarseness, which seldom persists beyond 3 months. Common causes for chronic hoarseness are ulceration and inflammation of the vocal cords, dislocation of the arytenoid cartilages, and vocal polyps, but occasionally direct damage to the recurrent laryngeal nerve produces temporary hoarseness. In a review of the literature, Cavo[22] found that the most likely site of injury determined by a series of anatomic dissections of the larynx was the subglottic region. The anterior branch of the recurrent laryngeal nerve, which supplies the adductors of the larynx, probably is compressed between the endotracheal tube cuff and the thyroid cartilage. Most patients fully recover. Proper tube placement at least 5 cm above the carina is likely to prevent this uncommon complication. Correct placement can easily be achieved by marking the tube 1.5 cm above the upper end of the cuff.

An unusual complication of endotracheal intubation is partial facial paralysis producing weakness of the orbicularis oris muscle only. Forceful and prolonged digital pressure behind the mandible, applied to prevent airway obstruction from retrograde movement of the tongue, may compress the mandibular branch of the facial nerve against the mandibular bone. The reported cases had an excellent outcome.[42]

Internal Jugular Vein Cannulation

The internal jugular vein is a preferred site for central venous cannulation and pulmonary artery catheterization. Carotid artery puncture, the most frequent complication, occurred in 2% of patients in the most recent series of internal jugular vein cannulation alone.[14,15] In one series of 374 internal jugular vein catheterizations, removal of the needle followed by firm pressure over the puncture site did not result in neurologic complications. Ischemic stroke has occasionally been reported after internal jugular vein placement.[3,15] Inadvertent cannulation of the carotid artery for more than 72 hours in one patient resulted in middle cerebral artery stroke despite heparinization.[15] Angiography demonstrated a large catheter-enveloping thrombus in the right common carotid artery. (This report emphasizes that in patients with puncture of the carotid artery with a large dilating cannula, early surgical exploration and repair are advisable.)

Multiple probing attempts may result in peripheral nerve damage. Single case reports have documented Horner's syndrome[96] (Fig. 4–1), damage to cervical nerves, and bilateral vocal cord paralysis.[18] As reported in 1991, in two patients with right ventricular endo-myocardial biopsy after heart transplantation,[1] a procedure usually performed through the internal jugular vein, transient ischemic attacks developed in the vertebrobasilar territory. Brain stem stroke has been reported after inadvertent vertebral artery puncture and use of inappropriate technique.[106]

A recent analysis of a prospective study of internal jugular vein catheterization in critically ill patients revealed no neurologic complications other than Horner's syndrome in 1 of 66 consecutive patients.[45] Many of the patients had coagulopathies and multiple probing attempts, and carotid puncture occasionally occurred. However in the one patient with Horner's syndrome, a large neck hematoma suggested a compartment syndrome rather than direct needle damage; local carotid dissection was another possibility.

In patients with severe coagulopathies or in whom insertion is expected to be difficult, duplex Doppler guidance is

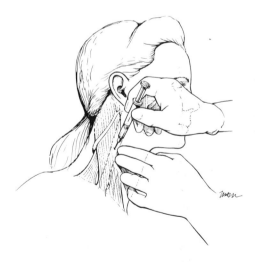
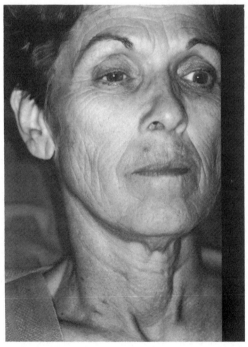

Figure 4–1. Horner's syndrome after internal jugular vein cannulation. *Left,* Drawing of cannulation of internal jugular vein. *Right,* Patient with Horner's syndrome. Note multiple needle-probing attempts in the neck. Two-year follow-up revealed some improvement in ptosis alone.

extremely helpful in localization and may decrease the risk of carotid puncture. After placement of the searching needle or guide wire in the internal jugular vein, the catheter can be connected to a transducer that immediately verifies correct placement. An arterial tracing on the monitor indicates carotid placement and should prompt replacement. This technique decreases the incidence of ischemic complications that are probably related to the introduction of the dilator in the carotid artery before final placement of the catheter.

There is virtually no mention of neurologic complications in patients who require pulmonary artery catheterization.[13,37] In a series of 6245 patients, inadvertent carotid puncture with a 16-gauge catheter in 120 patients (1.9%) did not result in neurologic complications.[103]

Arterial Cannulation

The prevalence of the hazards that are associated with arterial catheters for invasive blood pressure monitoring and blood gas sampling has not been prospectively studied. Radial artery cannulation may be traumatic to peripheral nerves in the vicinity of the puncture site, usually the median nerve. Multiple radial artery punctures, cut-down cannulation, and anticoagulation may predispose the patient to median nerve damage.[8,10] The superficial cutaneous branches of the radial nerve located radially at the wrist lie close to the radial artery but are seldom severed after cannulation. Median nerve compression due to hematoma formation around the cannula with extension over the flexor carpi radialis and compression proximal to the transverse carpal ligament is a possible mechanism.[85] Other studies have suggested compression in the carpal tunnel due to prolonged extension of the wrist at the time of splinting.

Persistent paresthesias or pain in areas innervated by the median nerve indicates compression in the carpal tunnel.[74] Motor weakness of the abductor pollicis brevis muscle may occur early. Even after a few weeks, a change in the contour of the thenar may be seen. Exploration is not indicated, because most cases resolve within 8 weeks. Fortunately, only a minority of patients have some residual sensory loss.

Brachial artery cannulation or, more commonly, puncture in anticoagulated patients may precipitate subfascial hemorrhage leading to a severe median nerve compression syndrome.[77,79] Recognition of this compression neuropathy is much more important, because early treatment decreases the chance of permanent sequelae, but full recovery may occur without specific therapy[28,29] (Fig. 4–2). Compression of the median nerve at the level of the elbow usually causes pain around the elbow and in the forearm region or produces paresthesias in the fingers. The syndrome, often recognized by ecchymosis and swelling in the forearm, is related to compression of the median nerve at the lacertus fibrosus, pronator muscle, or fibrous arch of the flexor digitorum superficialis muscle. Clinically, the pronator syndrome is diagnosed by tenderness over the median nerve, weak and painful pronation, and weakness and pain at selective testing of the flexor digitorum superficialis muscle.

Cardiac Catheterization

Many earlier reports documented central nervous system complications after angiographic procedures[2] (Table 4–2). The overall incidence of central nervous system complications is approximately 0.03% to 0.1% but may increase when a transaxillary approach is used. In the Cleveland Clinic series,[43] many complications were caused by embolization into the posterior cerebral circulation. It has been speculated that the transaxillary approach could easily

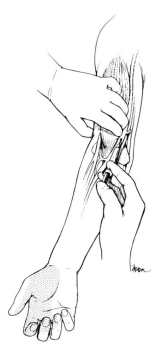

Figure 4–2. Median nerve damage associated with brachial cannulation. Lesion of the median nerve at the elbow produces weakness of the abductor pollicis brevis and flexor digitorum superficialis. Loss of opposition of the thumb may also be seen. As illustrated, sensory loss is indicated in the palm and distal phalanges of the index and middle fingers.

traumatize the vertebral artery, a less likely hazard in femoral catheterization, because the catheter loops around the aortic arch before entering the coronary ostia.[69] Nevertheless, complete blindness has been noted with use of the transfemoral approach.[69]

Cortical blindness during cardiac catheterization is well documented. Patients deny visual loss (Anton's syndrome) and are disoriented or confused. Complete recovery within 24 hours is the rule.[40,56,68,69,113]

Transient amnesia after cardiac catheterization has been anecdotally

noted.[104] The incidence in angiography is low, with no instances in Hodges' series.[58] During injection of contrast medium, patients may become agitated, repeatedly asking the same stereotypical questions. Recall of events over preceding days is patchy, and short-term memory is impaired. In a series reported by Olivecrona,[94] 65 of 3730 patients became "agitated" after catheterization. Perhaps some of the reported patients in whom agitation developed after cardiac catheterization had transient global amnesia. CT-scan findings have always been normal.

We recently reviewed the incidence of ischemic stroke after cardiac catheterization at the Mayo Clinic. In a 15-year period, ischemic stroke was documented in 14 patients (0.04% of the total number of procedures), most often in the anterior cerebral circulation. All patients except one had a ventriculogram to assess ejection fraction and wall motion. Half of the patients had acute Q-wave myocardial infarction, and a mural thrombus was found on

Table 4–2 NEUROLOGIC COMPLICATIONS AFTER CARDIAC CATHETERIZATION

Transient global amnesia
Cortical blindness
Top of the basilar syndrome
Gait ataxia
Migraine with or without aura
Altitudinal hemianopia

echocardiography in two patients. These observations superficially suggest that the stroke arises from a cardioembolic source rather than from manipulation damage in the aortic arch. Whether a ventriculogram in acute myocardial infarction predisposes to stroke after cardiac catheterization is not clear.[5]

Visceral Angiography

Spinal cord damage from visceral angiography has not been reported recently.[12,35,50,67] Paraplegia after abdominal aortography has been carefully detailed by Killen and Foster.[67] Their review showed that most patients had complete paralysis of the legs and loss of sphincter control. Motor function returned in as many as 57% of the patients. Recovery of motor function was detected as early as 2 days after angiography and as late as 6 months after the procedure. High levels of iodine in the cerebrospinal fluid have been repeatedly found in patients with postangiographic neurologic complications, but the nature of the spinal cord injury remains elusive.[87] Lumbar puncture with immediate substitution of isotonic saline has been recommended, but only one report has been published that claims a sustained beneficial effect with this type of cerebrospinal fluid lavage.[89]

Percutaneous Transluminal Coronary Angioplasty

Indications for percutaneous transluminal coronary angioplasty (PTCA) have been expanded and now include multivessel disease. Immediate PTCA and tissue plasminogen activator therapy for myocardial infarction probably are equally effective in preserving myocardium.[46,49]

Major risks of angioplasty are procedure-related myocardial infarction (0.6%) and direct mortality, which can approach 4% in high-risk subsets. The high risks are defined as advanced age, left main coronary artery dilatation, and PTCA for acute myocardial infarction.

Neurologic complications are surprisingly rare.[44] No cerebrovascular complications were mentioned in a series of 6500 PTCA procedures at the Mid America Heart Institute in Kansas City.[54]

Two recent reports of central nervous system complications also indicated a low incidence (approaching 0.2%) of PTCA-associated stroke or spinal cord injury.[31,91] In many patients, neurologic deficits are transitory and suggest rapid embolus migration or air embolus. Fleeting sensory signs, subtle paraphasic errors, or sparse verbal output may not always prompt a neurologic consultation.

The cause of embolization has not been elucidated but is presumably related to atheromatous or cholesterol embolization from ulcerated plaques in the aortic arch.

Intra-aortic Balloon Pump

Established indications for counterpulsation devices are intractable cardiac failure after cardiopulmonary bypass and complications of myocardial infarction refractory to pharmacologic therapy.[78]

Most complications can be attributed to insertion or removal of the device rather than to its being in place. Two cardiologic series[47,64] with a total of approximately 1500 patients mentioned one ischemic stroke and three patients with femoral nerve neuropathy. Leg ischemia is relatively common after placement (5% to 20%),[57] although amputation seldom is needed. Pain in the leg is often reported at the site of insertion, and paresthesias in the cutaneous area of the femoral nerve may also appear transiently. Ischemic neuropathies have been reported in large series and often in patients who required embolectomy after balloon pump removal. Most patients have footdrop and severe pain in the calf, suggesting involvement of branches of the sciatic nerve.

Acute occlusion of a large limb artery may cause an ischemic neuropathy (ischemic monomelic neuropathy).[71,73,92,115] This complication is recognized by severe burning pain despite normal blood flow to the affected limb and absence of signs of a compartment syndrome. The electromyographic findings are consistent with loss of motor and sensory nerve axons in the distal part of the tested extremity. Carbamazepine has been more effective than tricyclic agents or phenytoin.

Misplacement of the balloon may obstruct the left common carotid artery, and any new onset of aphasia or right hemiparesis should prompt relocation of the device. However, in many patients with ischemic stroke associated with balloon pumps, retrograde embolization is a more likely mechanism. Dissection of the descending aorta also may contribute, and extension into the left subclavian artery may cause breakup of embolic fragments that subsequently lodge in the left vertebral artery.

A number of well-documented reports have shown that an anterior spinal artery syndrome can occur suddenly as a result of balloon pump support.[53,98,111] Difficult manipulation on insertion has been implicated, but paraplegia may occur suddenly up to 3 days after removal.[101] Aortic dissection remains the principal causative mechanism in spinal cord infarction in these patients, and occurrence late after insertion may be explained by an expanding hematoma. Alternatively, cholesterol emboli may be responsible for spinal cord infarction after balloon pump insertion. Indeed, cholesterol emboli in radicular arteries were found at autopsy in seven patients with severe atheromatous deposits in the abdominal aorta.[53] As with any other mechanism of spinal cord infarction, outcome is poor.

Ventricular Assist System

Left ventricular assist systems can be expected to become increasingly used to close the gap to cardiac transplantation. The inflow tract of the pump is positioned in the left ventricle and outflow tract in the ascending aorta, with connections to an outside control console. Further technical development may make this console portable.

Neurologic complications have been reported in several series, but the University of Pittsburgh series is the most carefully documented experience.[36] This series of 20 patients with implantation devices clearly demonstrated a risk of transient ischemic attack and ischemic strokes with prolonged duration of the device, although transient ischemic attacks were found as early as 6 days after insertion (average, 3 months). Seven of the 20 patients had transient ischemic attack and ischemic stroke, often in the posterior circulation and frequently more than once in the same territory. One patient had a severely disabling stroke, but all others recovered with mild or no residual deficits and underwent successful cardiac transplantation. Therefore, despite the troubling very high incidence of transient ischemic attack and ischemic strokes, outcome after use of this device and cardiac transplantation seems very satisfactory. Smaller series have documented lower incidences of ischemic stroke but with fewer exposure days.[80] Potential mechanisms for ischemic stroke are abnormalities in blood viscosity or activation of thrombotic pathways, or both.

Epidural Catheterization and Diagnostic Lumbar Puncture

The results of epidural techniques with use of narcotics to relieve pain after thoracotomy are now quite satisfactory, and this mode of therapy is increasingly used in surgical ICUs.

Postoperative analgesia can also be

accomplished with lidocaine or bupivacaine administered by rate-controlling infusion pumps. Anticoagulation during epidural catheterization is a major risk factor for epidural hematoma.[30,32,51,108] Nevertheless, Odoom and Sih[93] reported that there were no neurologic complications in 1000 epidural anesthetic procedures in patients who were anticoagulated, but their follow-up experience was limited to the hospital stay.

No neurologic complications were reported in a recent series of 136 patients who received subcutaneous injection of heparin.[32] In contrast, however, several case reports describe devastating spinal hematoma. Contributing factors are heparinization within 1 hour of needle insertion, particularly if insertion is traumatic; anticoagulant effects outside the therapeutic range; and use of combinations of antithrombotic agents. (In exceptional patients, a cutaneous angioma in the dorsal area may indicate a venous angioma in the epidural space.[34])

The risk of epidural hematoma during epidural catheterization is decreased in anticoagulated patients when heparin infusion is discontinued 4 to 6 hours before insertion[95,100] and not restarted for at least 1 hour after catheter removal, but there are no solid scientific data that support this common practice.[59]

Sudden onset of back pain followed in a few hours by progressive leg weakness is a classic presentation of spinal epidural hematoma, but pain may be absent in patients receiving narcotic agents for postoperative pain control. Emergency laminectomy is not always successful, and paraplegia may remain unchanged even when urgent decompression is done.[97] Patients may have prolonged weakness and sensory loss with a burning, prickling feeling.[63] After epidural anesthesia, these symptoms usually disappear within 5 days. A severe Guillain-Barré syndrome has been reported, but the relation with epidural anesthesia is uncertain and most likely coincidental. A persistent cauda syndrome has been linked to adhesive arachnoiditis, most likely associated with the vehicle of the anesthetic agent. The syndrome of progressive paraparesis is supposedly rare, but occasionally a patient is seen with this complication (Fig. 4–3).

The incidence of epidural infections from catheterization may be higher in critically ill patients treated with steroids or antineoplastic agents. Epidural abscesses have occurred a few days after placement, and intermittent injections and failure to tunnel the catheter have been implicated as potential risks.[110] (The clinical manifestations and outcome of epidural abscess are discussed in Chapter 5.)

Inadvertent puncture of the dura may produce generalized or more frontally located headache on erect position 24 to 72 hours after the procedure. Less common symptoms are nausea, shoulder pain, blurred vision, and abducens palsy, all of which usually resolve within 2 weeks. The incidence of postpuncture headache may indeed be higher in patients who had epidural anesthesia or epidural injections, because larger gauge needles are used than in routine lumbar puncture. A study of 501 patients who had lumbar puncture found that young female patients with low body mass index (weight/height^2) had the highest risk for postlumbar headache.[70] Spontaneous recovery within 1 to 2 weeks is the rule, but in a small percentage, headache is persistently disabling. Meningeal enhancement may be seen on MRI in cerebrospinal fluid hypotension and should not be misinterpreted as evidence of infection.[41,88] Most patients can be effectively treated with epidural blood patch, orally administered caffeine (300 mg), and liberal fluid intake.

Cardioversion

Cardioversion is a frequently used procedure in the ICU. A persistent concern is systemic embolization.[109,114] The risk is remarkably low, even in pa-

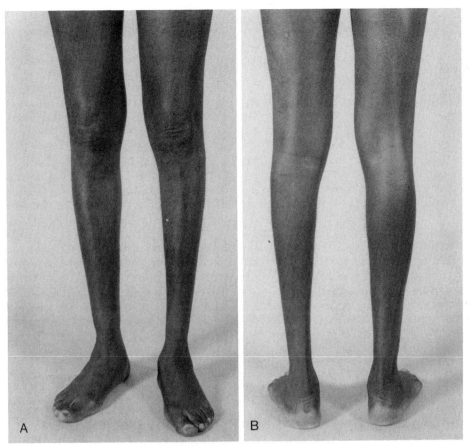

Figure 4–3. *A* and *B*, Partially recovered cauda equina syndrome after epidural anesthesia. Note marked atrophy of both legs.

tients with demonstrated ventricular thrombi. One reported patient tolerated cardioversion without embolization, and echocardiography showed large mobile thrombi.[75] In a study of 454 elective direct-current cardioversions, embolic complications, including peripheral embolism, occurred in 1.3% of the patients. One patient had a fatal ischemic stroke, and the others had "minor visual disturbances."[4] A 1993 study claimed that transesophageal echocardiography may be used to exclude thrombi and obviate anticoagulation,[82] but, not unexpectedly, ischemic stroke in a patient with negative results of transesophageal echocardiographic examination has been reported.[38]

Whether anticoagulation prevents embolization has not been formally addressed in a randomized trial. Anticoagulation beginning at least 2 to 4 weeks before cardioversion is performed is recommended in patients with a history of cardiogenic embolism, mechanical valve prosthesis, mitral stenosis and documented thrombi on echocardiography, and atrial fibrillation for more than 3 days. In many patients in the ICU who have treatment-refractory arrhythmias of short duration, cardioversion is applied without anticoagulation, and the risk of embolization is very low. In a series of 702 patients who had cardioversion for recent arrhythmias in ICUs at a Mayo Clinic hospital, one patient had a pontine infarct immediately after return to sinus rhythm. No peripheral emboli or ocular emboli were noted. Half the patients were receiving anticoagulant therapy (Wijdicks, EFM: Unpublished observations).

Miscellaneous Complications

A malpositioned chest tube after thoracotomy may be attended by brachial plexus injury.[81] The tube may be pushed up through the pleura and compress the brachial plexus at the root or trunk level. Excruciating upper extremity pain may alert the physician, and withdrawal of the tube immediately relieves pain and results in recovery of motor function. Damage to the intercostal nerve and long thoracic nerve was mentioned in a review paper on complications of chest tube placement, but documentation was inadequate. Blunt dissection superior to the rib minimizes damage to the neurovascular bundle that is located under the rib.[61] Inadequate technique may result in radiating truncal pain starting at the insertion site.

An intrascalene brachial plexus block is ordinarily used for selective anesthesia in patients scheduled for arteriovenous grafting, particularly patients who need dialysis.[33] Complications associated with this procedure include Horner's syndrome, recurrent laryngeal nerve block, and a reversible locked-in syndrome caused by inadvertent injection of a local anesthetic into the intravertebral artery.

Selective pulmonary angiography has been limited to spinal cord ischemia. After injection of contrast material into the fifth intercostal artery, complete transverse myelitis may occur.[65]

Transient neurologic deficits or visual field defects, often from carotid sinus stimulation during correction of supraventricular tachycardia, have been documented.[7,20,117] The most impressive case, carefully detailed by Beal and colleagues,[7] showed an embolus in the middle cerebral artery in a patient with severe carotid lesions. The true incidence of this complication is not known.

The procedure is probably contraindicated in patients who have generalized atherosclerosis and carotid bruits.

Nasogastric tubes have been placed in many unwanted locations, and the most spectacular is intracranial placement in patients with basilar skull fracture. Oral insertion, therefore, is the rule in patients with severe head injury and maxillofacial trauma.[11,102]

An unfortunate but probably rare event is ischemic stroke after discontinuation of anticoagulation for ICU procedures associated with a planned biopsy (e.g., bronchoscopy). In two personally observed patients, chronic atrial fibrillation was the clinical indication for anticoagulation. Both patients recovered with only a minimal deficit. Whether transesophageal echocardiography before the procedure can reveal which patients are at risk, as with cardioversion, is not known.

CONCLUSIONS

Performing invasive procedures is thought by many physicians to distinguish critical care medicine, and with the performance come complications. As expected, these complications are associated with misplacement, infection, and dislodging of atheromatous material. Air embolization is uncommon, but when it occurs, it is because of catheters associated with parenteral nutrition and diagnostic lung biopsies.

In most instances, neurologic complications pertaining to invasive procedures and assisting devices are ischemic strokes and isolated peripheral nerve damage. The literature on neurologic iatrogenic complications associated with invasive procedures in the ICU is a collection of anecdotes and may imply oversight by nonneurologists. Neurologic complications indeed may be uncommon, as exemplified by recent prospective clinical data in a large series of critically ill patients with internal jugular vein catheterization. Despite coagulopathy, multiple probing attempts, and inadvertent carotid puncture, only one patient with Horner's syndrome was found. Likewise, in cardioversion, another common procedure in the ICU, the incidence of stroke was low. Data on complications from invasive procedures in the ICU are far too preliminary, and therefore preventive measures are not precisely known. Invariably, a neurologic complication after any invasive procedure is merely an observation without further potential for treatment. Recognition may avoid expensive evaluation in some patients (e.g., those with Horner's syndrome after internal jugular vein cannulation). Fortunately, catastrophic neurologic complications, such as those with cholesterol embolization syndrome, seldom occur.

REFERENCES

1. Adair, JC, Call, GK, and O'Connell, JB: Cerebral ischemia: A complication of right ventricular endomyocardial biopsy. Cathet Cardiovasc Diagn 23: 32–33, 1991.
2. Adams, DF, Fraser, DB, and Abrams, HL: The complications of coronary arteriography. Circulation 48:609–618, 1973.
3. Anagnou, J: Cerebrovascular accident during percutaneous cannulation of internal jugular vein (letter). Lancet ii:377–378, 1982.
4. Arnold, AZ, Mick, MJ, Mazurek, RP, et al: Role of prophylactic anticoagulation for direct current cardioversion in patients with atrial fibrillation or atrial flutter. J Am Coll Cardiol 19: 851–855, 1992.
5. Ayas, N and Wijdicks, EFM: Cardiac catheterization complicated by stroke: The Mayo Clinic experience (submitted).
6. Baker, BK and Awwad, EE: Computed tomography of fatal cerebral air embolism following percutaneous aspiration biopsy of the lung. J Comput Assist Tomogr 12:1082–1083, 1988.
7. Beal, MF, Park, TS, and Fisher, CM: Cerebral atheromatous embolism following carotid sinus pressure. Arch Neurol 38:310–312, 1981.
8. Bedford, RF and Wollman, H: Complications of percutaneous radial-artery cannulation: An objective prospective study in man. Anesthesiology 38:228–236, 1973.
9. Bendixen, BH, Younger, DS, Hain, LS, et al: Cholesterol emboli neuropathy. Neurology 42:428–430, 1992.
10. Bonney, G: Iatrogenic injuries of nerves. J Bone Joint Surg [Br] 68: 9–13, 1986.
11. Bouzarth, WF: Intracranial nasogastric tube insertion (editorial). J Trauma 18:818–819, 1978.
12. Boyarsky, S: Paraplegia following translumbar aortography. JAMA 156: 599–602, 1954.
13. Boyd, KD, Thomas, SJ, Gold, J, and Boyd, AD: A prospective study of complications of pulmonary artery catheterizations in 500 consecutive patients. Chest 84:245–249, 1983.
14. Briscoe, CE, Bushman, JA, and McDonald, WI: Extensive neurological damage after cannulation of internal jugular vein. Br Med J 1:314, 1974.
15. Brown, CQ: Inadvertent prolonged cannulation of the carotid artery. Anesth Analg 61:150–152, 1982.
16. Butler, BD, Bryan-Brown, C, and Hills, BA: Paradoxical air embolism: Transcapillary route (letter). Crit Care Med 11:837, 1983.
17. Butler, BD and Hills, BA: The lung as a filter for microbubbles. J Appl Physiol 47:537–543, 1979.
18. Butsch, JL, Butsch, WL, and Da Rosa, JFT: Bilateral vocal cord paralysis: A complication of percutaneous cannulation of the internal jugular veins. Arch Surg 111:828, 1976.
19. Caillé, JM and Allard, M: Neurotoxicity of hydrosoluble iodine contrast media. Invest Radiol 23 Suppl 1:S210–S212, 1988.
20. Calverley, JR and Millikan, CH: Complications of carotid manipulation. Neurology 11:185–189, 1961.
21. Case records of the Massachusetts General Hospital (Case 2-1991). N Engl J Med 324:113–120, 1991.
22. Cavo, JW Jr: True vocal cord paralysis

following intubation. Laryngoscope 95:1352–1359, 1985.

23. Chang, C, Dughi, J, Shitabata, P, et al: Air embolism and the radial arterial line. Crit Care Med 16:141–143, 1988.

24. Colt, HG, Begg, RJ, Saporito, JJ, et al: Cholesterol emboli after cardiac catheterization: Eight cases and a review of the literature. Medicine (Baltimore) 67:389–400, 1988.

25. Coppeto, JR, Lessell, S, Lessell, IM, et al: Diffuse disseminated atheroembolism: three cases with neuro-ophthalmic manifestation. Arch Ophthalmol 102:225–228, 1984.

26. Cross, SS: How common is cholesterol embolism? J Clin Pathol 44:859–861, 1991.

27. Dahlberg, PJ, Frecentese, DF, and Cogbill, TH: Cholesterol embolism: Experience with 22 histologically proven cases. Surgery 105:737–746, 1989.

28. Dawson, DM and Fischer, EG: Neurologic complications of cardiac catheterization. Neurology 27:496–497, 1977.

29. Dawson, DM and Krarup, C: Perioperative nerve lesions. Arch Neurol 46:1355–1360, 1989.

30. Dean, WM and Woodside, JR: Spinal hematoma compressing cauda equina. Urology 13:575–577, 1979.

31. Detre, K, Holubkov, R, Kelsey, S, et al: Percutaneous transluminal coronary angioplasty in 1985–1986 and 1977–1981: The National Heart, Lung, and Blood Institute registry. N Engl J Med 318:265–270, 1988.

32. Dickman, CA, Shedd, SA, Spetzler, RF, et al: Spinal epidural hematoma associated with epidural anesthesia: Complications of systemic heparinization in patients receiving peripheral vascular thrombolytic therapy. Anesthesiology 72:947–950, 1990.

33. Durrani, Z and Winnie, AP: Brainstem toxicity with reversible locked-in syndrome after intrascalene brachial plexus block. Anesth Analg 72:249–252, 1991.

34. Eastwood, DW: Hematoma after epidural anesthesia: Relationship of skin and spinal angiomas. Anesth Analg 73:352–354, 1991.

35. Efsen, F: Spinal cord lesion as a complication of abdominal aortography: Report of 4 cases. Acta Radiol [Diagn] (Stockh) 4:47–61, 1966.

36. Eidelman, BH, Obrist, WD, Wagner, WR, et al: Cerebrovascular complications associated with the use of artificial circulatory support services. Neurol Clin 11:463–474, May 1993.

37. Elliott, CG, Zimmerman, GA, and Clemmer, TP: Complications of pulmonary artery catheterization in the care of critically ill patients: A prospective study. Chest 76:647–652, 1979.

38. Ewy, GA: Optimal technique for electrical cardioversion of atrial fibrillation. Circulation 86:1645–1647, 1992.

39. Fine, MJ, Kapoor, W, and Falanga, V: Cholesterol crystal embolization: A review of 221 cases in the English literature. Angiology 38:769–784, 1987.

40. Fischer-Williams, M, Gottschalk, PG, and Browell, JN: Transient cortical blindness: An unusual complication of coronary angiography. Neurology 20:353–355, 1970.

41. Fishman, RA and Dillon, WP: Dural enhancement and cerebral displacement secondary to intracranial hypotension. Neurology 43:609–611, 1993.

42. Fuller, JE and Thomas, DV: Facial nerve paralysis after general anesthesia. JAMA 162:645, 1956.

43. Furlan, AJ, Sila, CA, Chimowitz, MI, et al: Neurologic complications of cardiac diagnostic procedures, surgery, and pharmacotherapy. In Goetz, CG, Tanner, CM, and Aminoff, MJ (eds): Handbook of Clinical Neurology, Vol 19 (63). Elsevier Science Publishers B.V., Amsterdam, 1993, pp 175–204.

44. Galbreath, C, Salgado, ED, Furlan, AJ, and Hollman, J: Central nervous system complications of percutaneous transluminal coronary angioplasty. Stroke 17:616–619, 1986.

45. Garcia, EF, Wijdicks, EFM, and Young, BL: Neurologic complications of internal jugular vein catheterization

in critically ill patients. A prospective study in 60 patients. Neurology 44: 951–952, 1994.

46. Gibbons, RJ, Holmes, DR, Reeder, GS, et al: Immediate angioplasty compared with the administration of a thrombolytic agent followed by conservative treatment for myocardial infarction. N Engl J Med 328:685–691, 1993.

47. Grayzel, J: Clinical evaluation of the Percor percutaneous intraaortic balloon: Cooperative study of 722 cases. Circulation 66 Suppl 1:I-223–I-226, 1982.

48. Green, HL and Nemir, P Jr: Air embolism as a complication during parenteral alimentation. Am J Surg 121: 614–616, 1971.

49. Grines, CL, Browne, KF, Marco, J, et al: A comparison of immediate angioplasty with thrombolytic therapy for acute myocardial infarction. N Engl J Med 328:673–679, 1993.

50. Grossman, LA and Kirtley, JA: Paraplegia after translumbar aortography. JAMA 166:1035–1037, 1958.

51. Gustafsson, H, Rutberg, H, and Bengtsson, M: Spinal haematoma following epidural analgesia: Report of a patient with ankylosing spondylitis and a bleeding diathesis. Anaesthesia 43:220–222, 1988.

52. Haley, EC Jr: Encephalopathy following arteriography: A possible toxic effect of contrast agents. Ann Neurol 15:100–102, 1984.

53. Harris, RE, Reimer, KA, Crain, BJ, et al: Spinal cord infarction following intraaortic balloon support. Ann Thorac Surg 42:206–207, 1986.

54. Hartzler, GO, Rutherford, BD, McConahay, DR, et al: "High-risk" percutaneous transluminal coronary angioplasty. Am J Cardiol 61:33G–37G, 1988.

55. Helps, SC, Parsons, DW, Reilly, PL, and Gorman, DF: The effect of gas emboli on rabbit cerebral blood flow. Stroke 21:94–99, 1990.

56. Henzlova, MJ, Coghlan, HC, Dean, LS, and Taylor, JL: Cortical blindness after left internal mammary artery to left anterior descending coronary artery graft angiography. Cathet Cardiovasc Diagn 15:37–39, 1988.

57. Hlonet, JC, Wajszczuk, WJ, Rubenfire, M, et al: Neurological abnormalities in the leg(s) after use of intraaortic balloon pumps: Report of six cases. Arch Phys Med Rehabil 56:346–352, 1975.

58. Hodges, JR: Transient amnesia: Clinical and neuropsychological aspects. Major Probl Neurol 24:1–161, 1991.

59. Horlocker, TT and Wedel, DJ: Anticoagulants, antiplatelet therapy, and neuraxis blockade. Anesthesiol Clin North Am 10:1–11, 1992.

60. Hwang, T-L, Fremaux, R, Sears, ES, et al: Confirmation of cerebral air embolism with computerized tomography. Ann Neurol 13:214–215, 1983.

61. Iberti, TJ and Stern, PM: Chest tube thoracostomy. Crit Care Clin 8:879–895, Oct 1992.

62. Jensen, ME and Lipper, MH: CT in iatrogenic cerebral air embolism. AJNR 7:823–827, 1986.

63. Kane, RE: Neurologic deficits following epidural or spinal anesthesia. Anesth Analg 60:150–161, 1981.

64. Kantrowitz, A, Wasfie, T, Freed, PS, et al: Intraaortic balloon pumping 1967 through 1982: Analysis of complications in 733 patients. Am J Cardiol 57:976–983, 1986.

65. Kardjiev, V, Symeonov, A, and Chankov, I: Etiology, pathogenesis, and prevention of spinal cord lesions in selective angiography of the bronchial and intercostal arteries. Radiology 112: 81–83, 1974.

66. Kashuk, JL and Penn, I: Air embolism after central venous catheterization. Surg Gynecol Obstet 159:249–252, 1984.

67. Killen, DA and Foster, JH: Spinal cord injury as a complication of contrast angiography. Surgery 59:969–981, 1966.

68. Kinn, RM and Breisblatt, WM: Cortical blindness after coronary angiography: A rare but reversible complication. Cathet Cardiovasc Diagn 22:177–179, 1991.

69. Kosmorsky, G, Hanson, MR, and Tomsak, RL: Neuro-ophthalmologic complications of cardiac catheterization. Neurology 38:483–485, 1988.

70. Kuntz, KM, Kokmen, E, Stevens, JC, et al: Post-lumbar puncture headache: Experience in 501 consecutive procedures. Neurology 42:1884–1887, 1992.

71. Lachance, DH and Daube, JR: Acute peripheral arterial occlusion: Electrophysiologic study of 32 cases. Muscle Nerve 14:633–639, 1991.

72. Lantos, G: Cortical blindness due to osmotic disruption of the blood-brain barrier by angiographic contrast material: CT and MRI studies. Neurology 39:567–571, 1989.

73. Levin, KH: AAEE case report #19: Ischemic monomelic neuropathy. Muscle Nerve 12:791–795, 1989.

74. Littler, WA: Median nerve palsy—a complication of brachial artery cannulation. Postgrad Med J 52 Suppl 7:110–111, 1976.

75. Lo, YSA and Swerdlow, CD: Multiple protruding, mobile left ventricular thrombi and risk of embolism after cardioversion (letter). Chest 97:1023, 1990.

76. Lowenstein, E, Little, JW III, and Lo, HH: Prevention of cerebral embolization from flushing radial-artery cannulas. N Engl J Med 285:1414–1415, 1971.

77. Luce, EA, Futrell, JW, Wilgis, EFS, and Hoopes, JE: Compression neuropathy following brachial arterial puncture in anticoagulated patients. J Trauma 16:717–721, 1976.

78. Maccioli, GA, Lucas, WJ, and Norfleet, EA: The intra-aortic balloon pump: A review. J Cardiothorac Anesth 2:365–373, 1988.

79. Macon, WL IV and Futrell, JW: Median-nerve neuropathy after percutaneous puncture of the brachial artery in patients receiving anticoagulants. N Engl J Med 288:1396, 1973.

80. Mandarino, WA, Griffith, BP, Kormos, RL, et al: Novacor left ventricular assist filling and ejection in the presence of device complications. ASAIO Trans 38:M387–M389, 1990.

81. Mangar, D, Kelly, DL, Holder, DO, and Camporesi, EM: Brachial plexus compression from a malpositioned chest tube after thoracotomy. Anesthesiology 74:780–782, 1991.

82. Manning, WJ, Silverman, DI, Gordon, SPF, et al: Cardioversion from atrial fibrillation without prolonged anticoagulation with use of transesophageal echocardiography to exclude the presence of atrial thrombi. N Engl J Med 328:750–755, 1993.

83. Marini, JJ and Culver, BH: Systemic gas embolism complicating mechanical ventilation in the adult respiratory distress syndrome. Ann Intern Med 110:699–703, 1989.

84. Marquez, J, Sladen, A, Gendell, H, et al: Paradoxical cerebral air embolism without an intracardiac septal defect: Case report. J Neurosurg 55:997–1000, 1981.

85. Marshall, G, Edelstein, G, and Hirshman, CA: Median nerve compression following radial arterial puncture. Anesth Analg 59:953–954, 1980.

86. Menkin, M and Schwartzman, RJ: Cerebral air embolism: Report of five cases and review of the literature. Arch Neurol 34:168–170, 1977.

87. Mishkin, MM, Baum, S, and Di Chiro, G: Emergency treatment of angiography-induced paraplegia and tetraplegia (letter). N Engl J Med 288:1184–1185, 1973.

88. Mokri, B, Krueger, BR, Miller, GM, and Piepgras, DG: Meningeal gadolinium enhancement in low pressure headaches (abstr). Ann Neurol 30 Suppl 2:294, 1991.

89. Morariu, MA: Transient spastic paraparesis following abdominal aortography: Management with cerebrospinal fluid lavage (letter). Ann Neurol 3:185, 1978.

90. Moses, H III and Kaden, I: Neurologic consultations in a general hospital: Spectrum of iatrogenic disease. Am J Med 81:955–958, 1986.

91. Murthy, KN, Hubert, G, and Hess, J: Cerebrovascular complications in percutaneous transluminal coronary angioplasty (PTCA) (abstr). Neurology 42 Suppl 3:451, 1992.

92. Nater, B, Kuntzer, Th, and Regli, F: Neuropathie ischémique monomélique par occlusion de l'artère sous-clavière. Rev Neurol 148:232–234, 1992.

93. Odoom, JA and Sih, IL: Epidural analgesia and anticoagulant therapy: Experience with one thousand cases of continuous epidurals. Anaesthesia 38:254–259, 1983.

94. Olivecrona, H: Complications of cerebral angiography. Neuroradiology 14:175–181, 1977.

95. Owens, EL, Kasten, GW, and Hessel, EA II: Spinal subarachnoid hematoma after lumbar puncture and heparinization: A case report, review of the literature, and discussion of anesthetic implications. Anesth Analg 65:1201–1207, 1986.

96. Parikh, RK: Horner's syndrome: A complication of percutaneous catheterisation of internal jugular vein. Anaesthesia 27:327–329, 1972.

97. Rao, TLK and El-Etr, AA: Anticoagulation following placement of epidural and subarachnoid catheters: An evaluation of neurologic sequelae. Anesthesiology 55:618–620, 1981.

98. Rose, DM, Jacobowitz, IJ, Acinapura, AJ, and Cunningham, JN Jr: Paraplegia following percutaneous insertion of an intra-aortic balloon. J Thorac Cardiovasc Surg 87:788–789, 1984.

99. Rosman, HS, Davis, TP, Reddy, D, and Goldstein, S: Cholesterol embolization: Clinical findings and implications. J Am Coll Cardiol 15:1296–1299, 1990.

100. Ruff, RL and Dougherty, JH Jr: Complications of lumbar puncture followed by anticoagulation. Stroke 12:879–881, 1981.

101. Scott, IR and Goiti, JJ: Late paraplegia as a consequence of intraaortic balloon pump support. Ann Thorac Surg 40:300–301, 1985.

102. Seebacher, J, Nozik, D, and Mathieu, A: Inadvertent intracranial introduction of a nasogastric tube, a complication of severe maxillofacial trauma. Anesthesiology 42:100–102, 1975.

103. Shah, KB, Rao, TLK, Laughlin, S, and El-Etr, AA: A review of pulmonary artery catheterization in 6,245 patients. Anesthesiology 61:271–275, 1984.

104. Shuttleworth, EC and Wise, GR: Transient global amnesia due to arterial embolism. Arch Neurol 29:340–342, 1973.

105. Slavin, RE, Gonzalez-Vitale, JC, and Marin, OSM: Atheromatous emboli to the lumbosacral spinal cord. Stroke 6:411–416, 1975.

106. Sloan, MA, Mueller, JD, Adelman, LS, and Caplan, LR: Fatal brainstem stroke following internal jugular vein catheterization. Neurology 41:1092–1095, 1991.

107. Speck, U, Press, W-R, and Mützel, W: Osmolality-related effects of injections into the central nervous system. Invest Radiol 23 Suppl 1:S114–S117, 1988.

108. Spurny, OM, Rubin, S, Wolff, JW, and Wu, WQ: Spinal epidural hematoma during anticoagulant therapy. Arch Intern Med 114:103–107, 1964.

109. Stein, B, Halperin, JL, and Fuster, V: Should patients with atrial fibrillation be anticoagulated prior to and chronically following cardioversion? In Cheitlin, MD (ed): Dilemmas in Clinical Cardiology. FA Davis, Philadelphia, 1990, pp 231–247.

110. Strong, WE: Epidural abscess associated with epidural catheterization: A rare event? Report of two cases with markedly delayed presentation. Anesthesiology 74:943–946, 1991.

111. Tyras, DH and Willman, VL: Paraplegia following intraaortic balloon assistance. Ann Thorac Surg 25:164–166, 1978.

112. Velaj, R, Drayer, B, Albright, R, and Fram, E: Comparative neurotoxicity of angiographic contrast media. Neurology 35:1290–1298, 1985.

113. Vik-Mo, H, Todnem, K, Følling, M, and Rosland, GA: Transient visual disturbance during cardiac catheterization with angiography. Cathet Cardiovasc Diagn 12:1–4, 1986.

114. Weinberg, DM and Mancini, GBJ: Anticoagulation for cardioversion of atrial fibrillation. Am J Cardiol 63:745–746, 1989.

115. Wilbourn, AJ, Furlan, AJ, Hulley, W, and Ruschhaupt, W: Ischemic mono-

melic neuropathy. Neurology 33:447–
451, 1983.

116. Yamaki, T, Ando, S, Ohta, K, et al: CT
demonstration of massive cerebral air
embolism from pulmonary baro-
trauma due to cardiopulmonary resus-

citation. J Comput Assist Tomogr
13:313–315, 1989.

117. Zeman, FD and Siegal, S: Monoplegia
following carotid sinus pressure in the
aged. Am J Med Sci 213:603–607,
1947.

Part II

NEUROLOGIC COMPLICATIONS IN THE MEDICAL INTENSIVE CARE UNIT

Chapter 5

NEUROLOGIC MANIFESTATIONS OF BACTERIAL INFECTION AND SEPSIS

BACTERIAL MENINGITIS
SPINAL EPIDURAL ABSCESS
INFECTIVE ENDOCARDITIS
CLOSTRIDIAL SYNDROMES
SEPSIS

Bacterial infections may either prompt admission to the intensive care unit (ICU) or be a complication of aggressive monitoring in patients with life-threatening disorders. An association between invasive devices and bacterial infections has long been recognized, and these nosocomial infections may result in bacteremia and overt sepsis. Contamination of surgical wounds may also contribute to hospital-acquired bacteremias. However, the most crucial mode of transmission and colonization in the ICU is direct contact with personnel, and this has led to programs to stimulate hand-washing rituals.

Bacterial infections associated with multiorgan failure may damage peripheral nerves. The indirect effect of sepsis on the peripheral nerves was recognized by Bolton and colleagues,[11-13] who have been operating on the frontier of clinical research on polyneuropathy in critical illness. Until recently, virtually no mention of the neurologic complications of sepsis and septic shock appeared in leading textbooks of critical care medicine.

This chapter focuses on selected dis-orders chosen largely because they are potential reasons for consultation in ICU practice. Infections associated with immunosuppression are discussed in Chapter 16. The risk of neurologic involvement in bacterial infections in the ICU is not marginal, and in specific circumstances (e.g., infective endocarditis), neurologic complications determine outcome.

BACTERIAL MENINGITIS

Bacterial meningitis seldom develops as part of a bacteremia or sepsis syndrome. Drowsiness and meningeal signs are common clinical features in critically ill patients with signs of systemic toxicity, but hematogenous dissemination to the meninges is extremely uncommon. The risk of meningitis also remains low in fulminant bacteremias. In Mylotte and colleagues'[90] consecutive study of patients with *Staphylococcus aureus* bacteremia, only 1 of 114 episodes was associated with meningitis, and in this patient staphylococcal endocarditis was found.

Clinical Features

The classic symptoms of bacterial meningitis may remain unrecognized in patients admitted to ICUs. Obviously, neuromuscular blocking drugs can mask the leading clinical signs, such as meningeal irritation and seizures, and most patients in the ICU are not able to signal severe headaches. Bacterial meningitis generally is manifested by high-grade fever of new onset, nuchal rigidity, and positive Kernig's and Brudzinski's signs. Nuchal rigidity may be slightly difficult to appreciate in intubated patients, but the modern flexible endotracheal tubes should not greatly confound assessment of neck flexion. Moreover, meningeal irritation is often demonstrated in the first 30° of passive flexion. Fever and diminished level of consciousness are important initial diagnostic clues in critically ill patients. In a seminal article on clinical features of bacterial meningitis, only 9 (5%) of 191 patients were alert.[21]

Certain skin lesions may designate specific microorganisms. A maculopapular rash may suggest meningitis caused by *Streptococcus pneumoniae* or *Staphylococcus aureus*. Subconjunctival hemorrhages, petechial hemorrhages, and purpura are traditionally linked to meningococcal meningitis. Petechial and hemorrhagic rash over extensive skin surfaces may indicate staphylococcal sepsis and endocarditis.

Focal neurologic signs are not seen in the early stages of purulent meningitis but develop during the clinical course in 10% to 20% of patients. Papilledema is as frequent as focal signs. Both clinical signs may suggest subdural empyema, intracranial abscess, or cavernous sinus thrombosis.

Seizures occur in 20% to 30% of patients with acute bacterial meningitis. Early seizures are not associated with a poor prognosis, but seizures that occur in the course of a few days of antibiotic treatment may indicate an intracranial mass or a venous cerebral infarction.

Purulent meningitis is confirmed by examination and culture of the cerebrospinal fluid (CSF). Frequent sampling of blood is helpful in culturing the organism. Swartz and Dodge[112] demonstrated positive results in 52% of blood cultures but with sensitivity varying by organism (79% in *Haemophilus influenzae* meningitis, 56% in *Streptococcus pneumoniae* meningitis, 33% in *Neisseria meningitidis*, 29% in betahemolytic streptococcal meningitis, and only 17% in *Staphylococcus aureus*). A constant CSF feature of acute purulent meningitis is cloudy, milky, or turbid appearance and increased pressure. Gram's stain frequently demonstrates the microorganism, but the result is negative in approximately 20% of cases, and previous antibiotic treatments can alter the number of positive results on Gram's stains.

Very early CSF samples may fail to demonstrate pleocytosis not only in meningitis but also in specific conditions, such as pneumococcal meningitis in asplenic persons and neutropenia in patients with hematologic malignant disease.

Typically, CSF analysis reveals polymorphonuclear pleocytosis, with leukocyte counts up to 100,000; decreased glucose level, to less than 50% of the serum glucose concentration; and increased protein and lactate values. In traumatic lumbar punctures, the leukocyte count can be estimated by subtracting the leukocytes per 700 erythrocytes, but a ratio of CSF to serum is probably more reliable.[32] (True leukocytes [CSF] = actual leukocytes [CSF] − leukocytes [serum] × erythrocytes [CSF]/erythrocytes [serum].)

A troublesome clinical problem in critically ill patients in whom bacterial meningitis is suspected is whether a computed tomography (CT) scan should precede lumbar puncture. Fear of inducing herniation after lumbar puncture in patients with unrecognized infectious intracranial masses derives from anecdotal reports before the CT scan era. Many neurologists perform lumbar punctures before CT scanning is done, but scanning is warranted in patients with seizures, unequivocal focal signs, or papilledema, or when heavy sedation or paralysis truly hampers neurologic examination. The mortality from delayed antibiotic treatment in bacterial meningitis is 10 to 20 times greater than the risk of complications associated with lumbar puncture.[5]

Delay of antibiotic treatment in a patient with bacterial meningitis results in considerably less potential for complete recovery.[114] On the other hand, bacterial identification and, more important, the validity of antibiotic-sensitivity testing markedly decrease after the first intravenous treatment. Culturing and identification of the infective organism are unlikely to be influenced if CSF is obtained within 2 hours. In a study of 78 patients with bacterial meningitis, positive CSF cultures of the most frequent bacteria were found in 43% of those treated with ceftriaxone and in 58% of those treated with ampicillin or chloramphenicol when specimens were obtained after 4 to 12 hours of treatment.[41]

Alternative ways to identify bacterial pathogens are available. CSF counterimmunoelectrophoresis, CSF latex agglutination, and coagulation tests may detect common bacterial antigens in from 70% to 100% of patients, and it has been suggested that these tests are useful in patients pretreated with antibiotics.

The yield of CT scan in uncomplicated bacterial meningitis is low. In occasional patients, a subdural empyema collection or dural sinus thrombosis is detected, but magnetic resonance imaging (MRI) is a much better modality in these complications. MRI may also detect bacterial meningitis when the meninges are enhanced with gadolinium.[27]

Treatment

Rapid CSF sterilization of pathogens is adequately achieved with one of the new third-generation cephalosporins administered with ampicillin in high doses.[29,104] An empiric regimen pending culture and sensitivity results is proposed in Table 5 – 1. In patients with a fulminant streptococcal pneumonia,

Table 5 – 1 SUGGESTED EMPIRIC THERAPY FOR BACTERIAL MENINGITIS IN UNCOMPROMISED HOSTS

Cefotaxime	2 g IV q4h
or	
Ceftazidime	2 g IV q6h
or	
Ceftriaxone	2 g IV q12h
plus	
Ampicillin	2 g IV q4h

Modified from Cunha, BA: The diagnosis and therapy of acute bacterial meningitis. In Schlossberg, D (ed): Infections of the Nervous System. Springer-Verlag, New York, 1990, pp 3 – 24.

penicillin-resistant organisms may be implicated, which should prompt treatment with vancomycin or third generation cephalosporins. Specific treatment is suggested in Table 5 – 2. Dexamethasone as an adjunctive therapeutic agent is effective in children, reduces mortality, and significantly reduces moderate to severe sensorineural loss, but corresponding data in adults are not yet available.[104,124] Dexamethasone (10-mg intravenous bolus; 4 mg every 6 hours for 4 days) should be strongly considered for use in adult patients with fulminant bacterial meningitis.

Causes in the ICU

Potential sources for bacterial meningitis in the uncompromised host are sinusitis, spinal anesthesia, infective endocarditis, and traumatic CSF fistula. Patients often have central venous catheters, pacing wires, drains, and endotracheal tubes, all of which can become infected but rarely cause meningitis.

Paranasal sinusitis secondary to prolonged nasotracheal intubation is a frequently unrecognized cause of fever. The reported incidence ranges from 2% to 5%, and occurrence may be more common in patients who had emergency intubation.[43,81] *Staphylococcus epidermidis* and nosocomial gram-negative organisms predominate in cultures. Removal of nasotracheal and na-

Table 5-2 ANTIBIOTIC TREATMENT FOR BACTERIAL MENINGITIS

Organism	Antibiotic	Suggested Dose
Streptococcus pneumoniae Neisseria meningitidis	Penicillin G	20-24 million U daily IV in divided doses q4h or by infusion
Gram-negative organisms	Ceftriaxone	4 g/d IV in divided doses q12h
	Ceftazidime	8 g/d IV in divided doses q6h (for Pseudomonas aeruginosa coverage)
Staphylococcus aureus Methicillin-resistant	Nafcillin	9-12 g/d IV in divided doses q4h
Staphylococcus	Vancomycin	1 g IV q12h
Enterobacteriaceae	Ceftriaxone or	4 g/d IV in divided doses q12h
	Cefotaxime	2 g IV q4h

Data from Kim, JH, van der Horst, C, Mulrow, CD, and Corey, GR: *Staphylococcus aureus* meningitis: Review of 28 cases. Rev Infect Dis 11:698-706, 1989, and references 29, 104, and 124.

sogastric tubes leads to clearing of mucopurulent drainage and subsequent disappearance of sinus infiltrates on sinus films or CT scan.[22]

Extension of maxillary sinusitis to the sphenoid sinus has been noted in 25% of cases.[78] Delayed recognition may lead to seeding of the meninges, orbital cellulitis, and cavernous sinus thrombosis resulting in permanent blindness. Patients in whom sphenoid sinusitis develops have severe headache, photophobia, and facial paresthesias. CT scan is the most useful radiographic examination and will almost certainly demonstrate the sinus opacification. The treatment of choice in early sphenoiditis is high-dose administration of penicillinase-resistant penicillin, but surgical drainage is indicated for patients with bacterial meningitis.

The prevalence of meningitis after diagnostic or therapeutic lumbar puncture and spinal anesthesia is very low.[71,73,76,102,115] Bacterial meningitis after spinal anesthesia is a serious condition and is frequently associated with *Pseudomonas aeruginosa* and *Staphylococcus aureus*. The patient's skin is obviously an important source, but contaminated disinfectants, needles, or hands of the physician who performs the procedure increase the risk as well.

Meningitis after basal skull fractures in patients with multitrauma is primarily due to *Streptococcus pneumoniae*, but a trend toward gram-negative organisms has been noted in recent years.[42,47,57,62] It is important to differentiate among nasal secretion, saliva, and perilymph or endolymph. An extra band of transferrin in the beta$_2$ fraction on protein electrophoresis and modestly high levels of glucose (50 to 70 mg/dL) identify a CSF leak (see Chapter 15).

Spontaneous sealing of the CSF fistula is common in basilar fractures but less frequent in mid-face fractures. Prophylaxis with antibiotics promotes selection of resistant organisms and is therefore not recommended.[47,62] In the unfortunate situation when bacterial meningitis is associated with CSF leaks, the infection can be successfully treated in most patients.

Immunocompromised patients in the ICU are a separate population in whom the major bacterial infections include those caused by *Listeria monocytogenes* and *Nocardia asteroides*. The clinical presentation of these central nervous system infections is discussed in Chapter 16.

Drugs can induce aseptic meningitis[54,55,65] (Table 5-3), but symptoms usually resolve within 24 hours after administration is discontinued.

Outcome

Mortality from bacterial meningitis is still considerable, and rates up to 22% with pneumococcal meningitis have

Table 5–3 DRUGS KNOWN TO INDUCE ASEPTIC MENINGITIS

Trimethoprim (sulfamethoxazole)
Ibuprofen
Cytosine arabinoside (high doses)
Carbamazepine
Sulindac
OKT3
Isoniazid

been reported.[53] Elderly patients, as expected, may have higher fatality rates. One study found that mortality (35%) was most frequent in patients with diminished level of consciousness and inadequate initial antibiotic therapy.[8] Mortality is higher with gram-negative meningitis than with gram-positive meningitis. Within the first 3 days after onset, brain swelling is seen in 14% of patients and hydrocephalus in 12%,[98] but these seldom result in herniation and death.

Outcome in meningitis associated with traumatic CSF leak (almost always caused by *Streptococcus pneumoniae*) is good when treatment is with a third-generation cephalosporin, but repair is needed when this complication occurs.

SPINAL EPIDURAL ABSCESS

Any infection may set the stage for spread to the epidural space.[6,35] Possible causes of epidural abscess are decubitus ulcers, operative wounds, psoas abscess, endocarditis, and sinusitis.[31,58,70,128] Cervical epidural abscess may occur in patients with a postintubation retropharyngeal abscess as well.[72] In up to 40% of the patients with a spinal epidural abscess, a source cannot be found, but the common organism isolated from CSF is *Staphylococcus aureus*. Many patients with spinal epidural abscesses have positive results only on blood cultures.

Clinical Features

Many patients are acutely ill, incoherent, and confused. In the acute form of spinal epidural abscess, fever suggests the diagnosis. Many patients complain of spinal tenderness, which can be associated with weakness and paresthesias[74,128] (Table 5–4). The pain is typically unresponsive to conventional narcotics. The primary symptom of pain is usually not localized at physical examination, and spinal tenderness may be felt over several vertebrae. Alternatively, cauda equina compression may produce severe radicular pain.

Although many initial symptoms and signs may be subtle and difficult to appreciate, a fair number of patients present with motor signs or have progression within a few hours to paraplegia with little prospect for later ambulation, even after emergency laminectomy.

Most series report clinical deterioration over days, but the clinical course can be more dramatic, with rapid deterioration to complete paraplegia with no potential for reversal.

Misdiagnosis of epidural abscesses is common, and common misdiagnoses are intra-abdominal abscess, pyelonephritis, and cholecystitis.[6,35]

Additional Studies

Magnetic resonance imaging, probably the best study for identifying epidural abscess, may give false-negative results in patients without osteomye-

Table 5–4 CLINICAL CHARACTERISTICS OF ACUTE SPINAL EPIDURAL ABSCESS

Signs of systemic infection and fever
Severe back pain or radicular pain
Limb weakness
Paraplegia or paraparesis
Impaired bladder control (relatively rare)
Distinctive sensory level (relatively rare)

litis.[4,44,49,115] Epidural pus and CSF may yield similar signals on MRI, and additional gadolinium may be needed to visualize or outline the abscess. Myelography and CT scan can be used when monitoring devices in the ICU preclude MRI. In Danner and Hartman's experience,[35] plain CT scan performed at admission was positive for epidural abscess in only one third of the patients. Myelography or myelography-CT, however, may enable detection in most cases and may even be more sensitive than MRI in patients with small pus collections and little granulation tissue.

Cerebrospinal fluid examination is helpful in patients without muscle weakness, sensory deficits, sphincter disturbances, or abnormal deep tendon reflexes, but any other patient should have imaging studies of the spine first. CSF examination frequently demonstrates increased protein concentration and increased neutrophils, usually more than 80 cells/mm^3. As noted previously, CSF cultures frequently fail to demonstrate the offending microorganism, and more often the results of blood cultures dictate the mode of antibiotic coverage. Because *Staphylococcus aureus* is almost always the pathogen, empiric antibiotic therapy should include a third-generation cephalosporin and a penicillinase-resistant penicillin (vancomycin or nafcillin).

Treatment

Standard therapy for patients with epidural abscess and neurologic deficits is emergency surgery followed by antibiotic therapy for 8 weeks. Neurosurgeons may prefer extensive laminectomy to expose the posteriorly located pockets.

Nonoperative treatment of epidural infection has been suggested in patients without neurologic deficits, and results have been excellent.[80,85] The criteria for conservative medical treatment in patients without neurologic deficiency are debatable. Conservative treatment can be considered in patients with a large

Table 5-5 OUTCOME IN SPINAL EPIDURAL ABSCESS

Outcome	Patients, n (%)
Complete recovery	74 (39)
Weakness	49 (26)
Paralysis	41 (22)
Death	24 (13)
Total	188 (100)

Modified from Danner and Hartman.[35]

epidural abscess involving a considerable length of the vertebral canal.

Most patients with a localized pocket should be managed surgically to avoid rapid deterioration to complete paraplegia. Outcome is related to the extent of neurologic impairment at presentation and to the duration of the neurologic deficit. Complete recovery is possible in patients with paraplegia or quadriplegia when surgical intervention takes place within 24 hours. Outcome in patients with spinal epidural abscess is shown in Table 5-5.

INFECTIVE ENDOCARDITIS

Infective endocarditis should be at the head of the list of differential diagnostic possibilities in a patient who presents with fever and acute onset of focal neurologic signs.[96] Nosocomial endocarditis is an important cause of neurologic morbidity in critically ill patients. Hospital-acquired infective endocarditis is usually caused by *Staphylococcus aureus* or coagulase-negative staphylococci and less commonly by streptococci or *Pseudomonas aeruginosa*.[56,91,99,117] Many patients have no underlying disease, and damage to the endocardium may be produced by intravascular catheters. The consequences of pulmonary artery catheterization were recently addressed in 55 consecutively autopsied patients, of whom 53% had one or more endocardial lesions, including subendocardial hemorrhage and thrombus.[105] These findings were rare in a noncatheterized control population. More frequent iatrogenic portals of entry probably are the genitourinary tract, intratracheal airways, biopsy sites, and surgical wounds.

Central nervous system involvement in endocarditis is a highly complex clinical problem. Both neurologists and cardiologists must expect formidable difficulties in decision-making and management.[39]

Clinical Features and Course

The clinical diagnosis of infective endocarditis requires a high degree of awareness, particularly because the limits of its protean clinical manifestations cannot be defined. Symptoms of infective endocarditis may develop insidiously. The mean duration before hospitalization is usually 2 months for *Streptococcus viridans* and 2 weeks to 1 month for the more virulent and destructive *Staphylococcus aureus* species. The presenting symptoms are typically nonspecific. Musculoskeletal manifestations have been noted in 44% of patients, and when they are present, pain, redness, and tenderness can be found in one or more joints. Patients may complain of diffuse myalgias that are usually localized in both the thighs and calves,[30] but pain in a radicular distribution can be more prominent in other patients.[24,25,60,67,131] Fever occurs in more than 90% of patients.

The presenting symptoms may be different in several age groups. Tachycardia occurs less often in elderly patients, and the febrile response is significantly lower than in the younger population.[116] A new regurgitation murmur or a preexisting murmur changing in intensity may not be prominent and may even be absent, particularly in patients with right-sided endocarditis. It is useful to search under fingernails or toenails for splinter hemorrhages that represent embolic lesions or vasculitis. Other helpful clinical features are conjunctival petechiae in the lower eyelid; tender erythematous nodes in the pads of the fingers or toes (Osler's nodes);

small, flat, nontender erythematous spots that blanch on pressure (Janeway lesions); and splenomegaly (Table 5–6).

Without previous antimicrobial coverage, 95% of blood cultures are positive for the causative microorganism, often already in the first sample. Negative blood cultures in patients with infective endocarditis have been reported in 2% to 31% of the patients,[20,126] often because difficult-to-isolate fungal species are involved. *Legionella* may be the causative agent in prosthetic valve endocarditis; it requires special culture media and can remain undetected in routine studies.[120]

A suggested practical approach is three separate venous blood cultures on the first day, two more venous cultures if these cultures are negative by day 2, and two more venous cultures and one arterial culture if all cultures are negative on day 3.[123] Our practice is comparable with this recommendation but involves not more than two blood cultures each day until plate growth. Laboratory findings may include increased erythrocyte sedimentation rate, increase in neutrophil counts, and normochromic, normocytic, or hemolytic anemia. Red cell blood cast and proteinuria may occur as a result of immune complex glomerulonephritis.

Echocardiography is very useful for demonstrating vegetations.[93] The sensitivity for diagnosing infective endo-

Table 5–6 FREQUENT SYMPTOMS AND SIGNS OF INFECTIVE ENDOCARDITIS

Signs and Symptoms	Incidence, %
Cardiac murmur	97
Malaise	94
Fever	86
Anorexia	75
Weight loss	50
Splenomegaly	31
Rales	30
Splinter hemorrhages	28
Petechiae	20
Osler's nodes and Janeway lesions	21

Modified from Von Reyn, et al.[131]

carditis ranges from 80% to 90%, and the specificity is 98%. Transesophageal two-dimensional echocardiography is superior to transthoracic imaging,[48] particularly in patients with small vegetations. Echocardiography of prosthetic endocarditis may be more cumbersome because dense echoreflections of the prosthetic valve may overshadow reflections from vegetations.

Acute infective endocarditis occurs with *Staphylococcus aureus* bacteremia and has a high propensity for life-threatening complications from extensive valve destruction. Left ventricular failure refractory to treatment, abscesses of the annulus of the infected valve, and multiple systemic emboli are accepted indications for valve replacement.[37,45,133]

The clinical manifestations of prosthetic valve endocarditis differ substantially from those of native valve infective endocarditis.[34,36] The initial presentation is rapid (an indolent clinical course is very unusual). Peripheral vascular collapse and embolic showers are common. Mortality is high.

Prosthetic valve endocarditis may occur early after cardiotomy. Methicillin-resistant *Staphylococcus epidermidis* associated with contaminated operating room equipment, pump-oxygenators, and postoperative wound infections are often implicated. In patients with late-onset prosthetic valve endocarditis, streptococci are the predominant causative agents.

Risk factors for the development of prosthetic valve endocarditis were identified in a series of 2642 patients at Massachusetts General Hospital.[18] Recipients of a mechanical prosthesis had a greater early risk of endocarditis than patients who received porcine valves, but the late risk of endocarditis, defined as occurrence 2 months or more after placement, was greater in porcine valves. A greater risk was also evident in patients with multiple valve replacements.

Theoretically, appropriate antibiotic therapy can eradicate the infection in prosthetic valve endocarditis, but the hemodynamic status usually is greatly compromised. The causes of death are congestive heart failure, septic shock, and cardiac arrest; surgical intervention is often the only option.

Use of anticoagulation in native or prosthetic valve endocarditis is controversial. In general, anticoagulants are not indicated in the standard treatment of infective native valve endocarditis. In prosthetic valve endocarditis, anticoagulation should be continued. Valvular lesions are often not propagating clots, and anticoagulation probably will not prevent pieces of vegetation from breaking off. Control of infection alone decreases the risk of embolization. Most cardiovascular surgeons replace the infected valve when infection is not controlled or when multiple emboli occur.

Infective Aneurysms

Septic emboli may lodge in small distal branches and cause inflammatory erosion of the arterial wall. The evolution of cerebral aneurysms is not clear.[87,88] Molinari and colleagues[87] suggested that pulsation against a necrotic wall produces fusiform aneurysms.

Mycotic aneurysms may develop in multiple arteries. The vessels involved are the aorta, cerebral arteries, superior mesenteric artery and branches, and the vessels of the extremities. In a postmortem study from the preantibiotic era, Stengel and Wolferth[111] found more than one aneurysm in 41 of 217 cases (19%). Multiple mycotic aneurysm formation (one third of the patients) is not unique to certain bacterial species.[50,121]

Mycotic aneurysms of the intracranial circulation are often located at proximal or distal branches of the middle cerebral artery. Posterior circulation sites are less common.

The incidence of ruptured mycotic aneurysm in infective endocarditis varies from 0.6% to 4%.[40,107,108] Size of the aneurysm probably is not relevant to the risk of rupture.[19] Mortality from ruptured bacterial aneurysm is high (50% to 60%).

The clinical presentation of a ruptured mycotic aneurysm is variable.[17,127] Typically, patients present with a lobar intracerebral hematoma.

Cisternal clots, common in saccular aneurysms, are seldom seen on admission CT scans except in ruptured mycotic aneurysms of the posterior circulation.[129]

Rupture 6 months after antibiotic treatment of endocarditis has been reported,[7] but in a 1989 study that added 3 cases to the 67 cases of bacterial aneurysm reported in the literature since 1957, late rupture of mycotic aneurysm was rare.[108]

Mycotic aneurysms are probably more often present in patients with ischemic stroke and infective endocarditis.[107] Fundamental problems in the management of mycotic aneurysm are that the true incidence of mycotic bacterial cerebral aneurysms in patients with treated infective endocarditis is not known, although it may be as high as 15%,[16,66,68] and that no risk factors have been identified that predict rupture.[59,75,77] Also not known is how many patients have complete disappearance of aneurysms after appropriate antibiotic treatment.[89] Resolution of mycotic aneurysm may, however, be as low as 50%, and the aneurysm may even enlarge during antibiotic treatment. At the other extreme, patients may have early rupture with catastrophic consequences.

The incidence of transient ischemic attacks and ischemic strokes ranges from 10% to 30%[100] in patients with bacterial endocarditis and should mandate magnetic resonance angiography or conventional angiography. Large territory strokes are rare; more frequently, septic emboli occlude small penetrating vessels, causing subcortical infarcts. Most ischemic strokes in infective endocarditis occur at presentation, before adequate antimicrobial control. Although both Staphylococcus aureus

and Aspergillus are uncommon causes of endocarditis and difficult to detect, the endocarditis they cause has a high propensity for embolization. Therefore, the threshold for angiography when these agents are implicated should be somewhat lower. Ultrasonographic evidence of infectious emboli in liver and spleen should also strongly influence the decision to proceed with angiography.

Peripheral aneurysms of the middle cerebral artery are usually easily removed with very low morbidity and mortality. Proximal aneurysms are difficult to manage and may necessitate temporary occlusion of the vessel. In some patients, additional intracranial bypass grafting is necessary to supply the ischemic area.[38] Monitoring the aneurysms angiographically and trapping those that enlarge, as suggested by Bohmfalk and colleagues,[10] appear reasonable. Surgical clipping of an infective aneurysm is difficult, and the infectious aneurysmal sac may easily break off.[94] Endovascular occlusion with coils may become a promising alternative treatment (Fig. 5–1).[52]

A suggested guideline for monitoring patients is presented in Figure 5–2. This guideline is based on indirect evidence and ideally should be tested in a new set of patients. A recent study analyzed the need for cerebral angiography in infective endocarditis and concluded that it should not be routinely performed.[125] This study estimated a low mortality from ruptured mycotic aneurysm (25%) and therefore seriously skewed the data toward a conservative approach. In addition, magnetic resonance angiography and thin-section, high-resolution CT with high-dose contrast medium can be used to monitor infectious aneurysms.[2]

This guideline is different in patients who need valve replacement after infective endocarditis. Four-vessel angiograms are indicated in patients with mechanical valves who need lifelong anticoagulation.[110,139]

The management of a ruptured my-

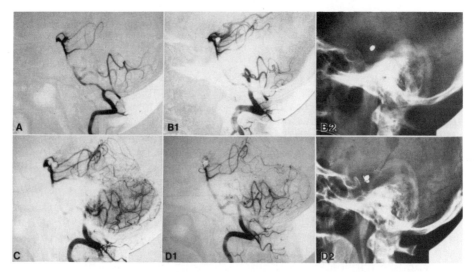

Figure 5–1. In a 45-year-old man with a lobulated mycotic aneurysm involving the distal basilar artery (*A*), platinum coils were inserted in the most worrisome lobule because it was believed to be the source of the bleeding; the other lobule was not amenable to coil occlusion (*B1* and *B2*). A follow-up angiogram 1 week later demonstrated enlargement of the nontreated lobule of the aneurysm (*C*), which was successfully clipped (*D1* and *D2*). The patient did extremely well during both procedures. (Courtesy of Dr. D. A. Nichols, Diagnostic Radiology.)

cotic aneurysm in a patient with a prosthetic valve is extremely complex. Discontinuation of anticoagulation (warfarin) to an international normalized ratio of 2 is preferred, and this is followed by a low dose of heparin (partial thromboplastin time, 40 to 50 seconds) to reduce the risk of embolization. The risk of systemic embolization from a prosthetic valve may also be higher if the patient's heart is in atrial fibrillation rather than sinus rhythm.

CLOSTRIDIAL SYNDROMES

The two most well-known infections with *Clostridium* species are tetanus and botulism. The clinical features of these diseases, caused by their toxins, are diametric to each other, but both diseases are alarming and immediately life-threatening. Medical and neurologic management is difficult because experience in handling these emergencies is typically lacking. ICU stays can be long, and residual psychological disturbances and fatigue are much more common than appreciated.

The following sections may assist in management when one is suddenly faced with these entities in the medical ICU. Details on epidemiology, pathology, and mechanism of infection can be found in infectious disease textbooks or review papers.[9,86] (The clostridial infection associated with gas gangrene is a local muscle infection with signs of vascular collapse and will not be discussed further.)

Botulism

Clostridium botulinum types A, B, and E spores produce a toxin that induces presynaptic inhibition of acetylcholine release. The toxin can be identified in serum or feces by a mouse toxin neutralization test that takes at least 1 to 2 days for completion. The clinical manifestations can be protracted over months but more commonly last for hours to 1 week. Persistent vomiting marks the ingestion of contaminated food (frozen food, undercooked meat, or, more often, home-canned preparations of fruits and vegetables).[28,61,132] Wound botulism after contamination from soft

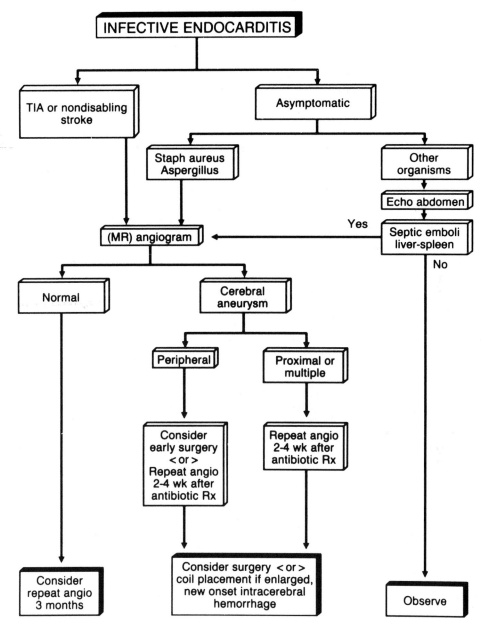

Figure 5–2. Possible guideline for the management of neurologic complications of infective endocarditis. TIA = transient ischemic attack.

tissue injury, compound fractures, or intravenous drug abuse is more easily missed because vomiting, abdominal cramps, and diarrhea are absent and wounds may be clean to the naked eye.

The neurologic manifestations follow each other fairly rapidly (Table 5–7). Initially, difficulty with focusing to a near point or diplopia is seen. Dilated

Table 5–7 CLINICAL FEATURES OF BOTULISM

Dilated (sluggish) pupils
Ptosis
Ophthalmoplegia
Facial diplegia
Absent gag reflex
Limb weakness
Hyporeflexia

pupils with sluggish light response are a sine qua non, often with palsies of nerves VI, IX – X, XII, and III (in decreasing order of frequency).[118] Complete bilateral internal ophthalmoplegia has been reported without any further progression to extremity weakness.[46] Ptosis is usually present, whereas dilated pupils may be absent. A typical progression in botulism is prominent ocular signs, dysphagia, and slurred speech, which are followed by diaphragmatic failure and quadriplegia over days.[101] In addition to the descending pattern, preserved deep tendon reflexes, absent paresthesias, and normal CSF protein concentration may serve to differentiate it from Guillain-Barré syndrome, a condition much more common than botulism.

Autonomic dysfunction is common and has recently been reported in patients subjected to sophisticated tests,[130] but in most patients, constipation, orthostatic hypotension, diminished lacrimation, decreased salivation resulting in dry mouth, and urinary retention are spontaneously mentioned.[64] Rapid, wide swings in blood pressure, such as in tetanus, are not part of the clinical description. Supportive care with mechanical ventilation is often the only option until the manifestations subside. Guanidine hydrochloride may perhaps improve muscle weakness.[69] Polyvalent antitoxin is ineffective once neurologic symptoms are present. Edrophonium, 10 mg intravenously, may improve the ocular manifestations, muscle weakness, and even diaphragmatic function, but its effect is transient. As an additional therapeutic agent 4-aminopyridine may be considered but it has occasionally been associated with seizures. Plasma exchange should be considered, particularly because marked, almost immediate improvement occurred in a patient with wound botulism.[101] Most patients have remarkable improvement within 1 month, but prolonged mechanical ventilation has been necessary up to 11 weeks after the onset.[79] Improvement can be expected within 2 weeks; there-

fore, tracheostomy should not be routinely performed in every patient, and one should allow time for spontaneous improvement in vital capacity.

Tetanus

In developed Third World countries, infection with *Clostridium tetani* remains a considerable health problem. In the United States, the incidence is 0.04 per 100,000, and this infection often occurs in elderly persons who have not received a primary series of tetanus toxoid. The incubation period varies from several days to months. Within days, however, trismus and reflex spasm are seen.

The clinical diagnosis of generalized tetanus is made with relative ease because virtually no other disease produces the set of findings consisting of trismus, risus sardonicus, reflex muscle spasm precipitated by touch, laryngospasm, sympathetic storm, and rapid respiratory failure[9] (Table 5 – 8). Reflex spasm, besides being extraordinarily painful, may result in often unrecognized instances of tendon rupture, fractures, and rhabdomyolysis. Tetanus is the result of the blocking of inhibitory neurons at the level of the synapse with the alpha motor neuron and loss of inhibition by the intermediolateral cells in the spinal cord. This imbalance causes the excitation and sympathetic storm and can be fatal if not appropriately muted by muscle-relaxing agents, sedation, and narcotics.

Table 5 – 8 CLINICAL FEATURES OF TETANUS

Localized or generalized weakness
Stiffness
Difficulty chewing
Trismus (lockjaw)
Risus sardonicus
Reflex spasm
Opisthotonos
Laryngospasm
Sympathetic storm

Basic management consists of tetanus toxoid (500 to 3000 U), human tetanus immune globulin, metronidazole (500 mg every 6 hours), and débridement of the wound, if identified. Spiraling respiratory failure may develop in a patient with evolving tetanus. Underdetection therefore may result in delayed intubation and ventilation, which may contribute to aspiration, an important cause of death.[122] Initial management concentrates on neuromuscular blockade with vecuronium or pancuronium usually guided by a peripheral nerve stimulator (see Chapter 1). Use of the peripheral nerve stimulator is cumbersome in patients with tetanus because a train-of-four stimulus may easily elicit reflex spasm. Its use should be minimized. Intrathecal injections with baclofen (800 to 1000 μg) are effective as well and have prevented mechanical ventilation or reduced the time on the ventilator in preliminary studies.[106] Dantrolene as an intravenous bolus of 1 mg/kg resolved muscle spasm in a case report, and manifestations of the infection with tetanus were milder.[119] Both adjuvant therapies can be useful when long-term ventilation and paralyzing become necessary, particularly to reduce the risk of postparalytic weakness (see Chapter 3). Adequate sedation is achieved with midazolam (5 to 15 mg/hour) or lorazepam (50 mg/hour).

Dysautonomia remains a challenging management problem, and cardiac arrest is the most common cause of death in most large series. A complete spectrum of bradycardia, sweating, salivation, and rapid swings in blood pressure may be seen. Sudden episodes of tachycardia and hypertension are best muted with a morphine bolus (5 to 30 mg intravenously over 30 minutes) (Fig. 5–3). Beta-blockers have been linked to sudden cardiac arrest and should be avoided.[134,142] Intensive care management has remarkably reduced mortality. Time on the ventilator is often at least 3 to 6 weeks, and, therefore, tracheostomy should be considered early in the disease.

Outcome is less favorable in patients who need intubation but is largely determined by fatigue and depression and difficulties in balance and cognitive function.[83]

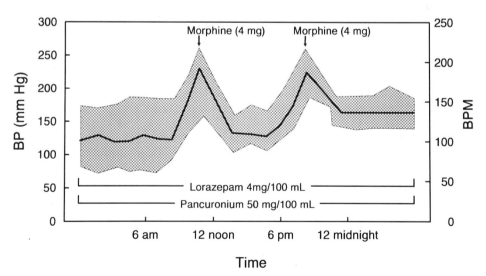

Figure 5–3. Two brief episodes of tachycardia and hypertension in a patient with tetanus are almost immediately muted by intravenous administration of morphine. Inadequate neuromuscular relaxation and sedation or hypovolemia should always be considered as alternative possibilities. Upper boundary of the crosshatched area is systolic pressure; lower boundary is diastolic pressure. Solid line is heart rate. BP = blood pressure; BPM = beats per minute.

SEPSIS

Sepsis can be divided into an identified source of infection and a systemic response to that infection. The genitourinary tract is the most common site of infection, which is often initiated by instrumentation of this area. Other common foci are gastrointestinal and respiratory infections, wound infections, burns, pelvic infections, and contaminated intravenous lines. Septic shock denotes circulatory collapse that develops as a complication of an overwhelming infection, often related to gram-negative enteric bacteria. *Escherichia coli* (followed by the *Klebsiella-Enterobacter-Serratia* group and *Pseudomonas*) remains the predominant pathogen in septic shock.

The systemic response in sepsis is not circulatory collapse but a hyperdynamic and hypermetabolic reaction. Oxidative metabolism is compromised; therefore, lactate in arterial blood is increased. This increase has been considered a sign of global decrease in tissue perfusion and is recognized as an indication of poor prognosis. Urinary output is decreased (output less than 30 mL or 0.5 mL/kg for at least 1 hour). Important clinical manifestations are increased cardiac output with low systemic vascular resistance, proteolysis leading to excessive loss of visceral proteins, and increased urinary secretion of nitrogen.

The leukocyte count increases to levels exceeding 20,000 cells/mm³, with a shift to immature polynuclear cells. Decreased platelet counts may reflect disseminated intravascular clotting. Cultures of material from the septic site may be useful, but only 50% of patients with clinical sepsis have positive blood cultures.

Sepsis may be followed by a sequence of organ failure. An important complication is the adult respiratory distress syndrome, characterized by severe hypoxemia and increased stiffness of the lungs. The pathologic features of adult respiratory distress syndrome consist of pulmonary capillary congestion, endothelial cell swelling, and microatelectasis followed by fluid leakage, fibrin deposition, and hyaline membranes leading to microvascular destruction.

The transition to multiorgan failure has a poor prognosis and a significant risk of mortality (40% to 80%). Hepatic failure is rapidly followed by progressive renal failure, although the sequence of organ failure may vary greatly. Total body protein catabolism is markedly increased, with rapid loss of skeletal muscle mass, often referred to as "autocannibalism."[26] Recently, the American College of Chest Physicians and the Society of Critical Care Medicine Consensus Conference issued a set of definitions[14] (Table 5–9 and Fig. 5–4). The deleterious effects of sepsis on the peripheral and central nervous systems are now well recognized.

Critical Illness Polyneuropathy

Several investigators have reported small series of a severe axonal polyneuropathy in patients with sepsis and multiorgan failure receiving long-term ventilation.[12,13,33,82,84,95,103,138,145]

Critical illness polyneuropathy has been described in all age groups except children. The true prevalence of critical illness polyneuropathy in the ICU is not known, but it probably occurs in 5% to 20% of all patients with severe sepsis and in 50% of all patients remaining in the ICU for more than 2 weeks. Critical illness polyneuropathy is not invariably associated with sepsis, having recently been reported in patients with severe burns.[3,23] In Zochodne and colleagues'[145] original description, 5 patients were seen in a 4-year period and 14 patients in the next 2 years, probably a result of increased recognition. The denominator is not known, although in a 1991 small prospective series from the same group of investigators, 30 of the 43 patients (70%) with multisystem failure had electrophysiologic evidence of critical illness polyneuropathy.[140]

After careful retrospective review of their medical records, no specific cause

Table 5–9 DEFINITIONS OF SEPSIS AND ORGAN FAILURE

Infection: Microbial phenomenon characterized by an inflammatory response to microorganisms or the invasion of normally sterile host tissue by those organisms.

Bacteremia: Viable bacteria in the blood.

Systemic inflammatory response syndrome: The systemic inflammatory response to a variety of severe clinical insults. The response is manifested by two or more of the following conditions: (1) temperature >38°C or <36°C; (2) heart rate >90 beats per minute; (3) respiratory rate >20 breaths per minute or $PaCO_2$ <32 mm Hg; and (4) leukocyte count >12,000/mm³, <4,000/mm³, or >10% immature (band) forms.

Sepsis: The systemic response to infection, manifested by two or more of the following conditions as a result of infection: (1) temperature >38°C or <36°C; (2) heart rate >90 beats per minute; (3) respiratory rate >20 breaths per minute or $PaCO_2$ <32 mm Hg; and (4) leukocyte count >12,000/mm³, <4,000/mm³, or >10% immature (band) forms.

Severe sepsis: Sepsis associated with organ dysfunction, hypoperfusion, or hypotension. Hypoperfusion and perfusion abnormalities may include, but are not limited to, lactic acidosis, oliguria, and an acute alteration in mental status.

Septic shock: Sepsis-induced with hypotension despite adequate fluid resuscitation, along with perfusion abnormalities that may include, but are not limited to, lactic acidosis, oliguria, and an acute alteration in mental status. Patients receiving inotropic or vasopressor agents may not be hypotensive at the time that perfusion abnormalities are measured.

Sepsis-induced hypotension: A systolic blood pressure <90 mm Hg or a reduction of ≥40 mm Hg from baseline in the absence of other causes for hypotension.

Multiple organ dysfunction syndrome: Organ function altered in an acutely ill patient in such a way that homeostasis cannot be maintained without intervention.

From Bone, et al,[14] by permission of the American College of Chest Physicians.

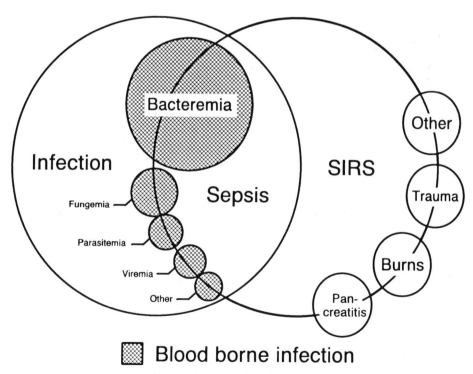

Blood borne infection

Figure 5–4. Relationship of infection, sepsis, and systemic inflammatory response syndrome (SIRS) to one another. (See Table 5–9 for definitions of terms.) (From Bone, et al,[14] with permission of the American College of Chest Physicians.)

has been found. Important findings are decreased albumin and lymphocyte counts, suggestive of a general nutritional deficit, despite adequate nutrition in all patients. Patients with sepsis frequently have a negative energy balance, but the nutritional status in relation to the appearance of critical illness polyneuropathy has not been adequately assessed. A direct toxic effect or effect of a mediator of sepsis on the nerve is mostly speculative. In a prospective study of sepsis-related critical illness polyneuropathy, Witt and colleagues[140] analyzed predictive factors for critical illness polyneuropathy and found that time in the ICU, hypoalbuminemia, and relative hyperglycemia significantly correlated with electrophysiologic findings. A specific bacterial pathogen has not emerged, but it may not have been carefully looked for or cultured. (In one patient with a severe axonal polyneuropathy seen at the Mayo Clinic, cultures for *Campylobacter jejuni* and *Clostridium difficile* were negative.)

Until recently, "failure to wean" marked the first neurologic consultation. Quite often, however, any patient with long-term ventilatory problems is difficult to wean, often from lack of adequate respiratory musculature (disuse atrophy) or more commonly from other contributory factors, such as poor nutrition and chronic lung disease, that may preclude successful weaning. Nevertheless, severe paradoxical breathing indicative of diaphragmatic and intercostal weakness due to axonal degeneration of the phrenic and intercostal nerves has been noted. Recently, five patients were described in whom respiratory failure as the presenting feature of critical illness polyneuropathy was followed by quadriplegia.[140] It is not entirely clear whether phrenic nerve involvement is the main cause of failure to wean in these patients.

On neurologic examination, grimacing may be weak, but other cranial nerves are normal. Ocular signs, swallowing, tongue protrusion, and biting remain normal during the clinical

Table 5–10 CLINICAL FEATURES OF CRITICAL ILLNESS POLYNEUROPATHY

Diaphragmatic and intercostal weakness
Mild facial weakness
Normal ocular signs
Symmetric (usually distal) limb weakness
Reduced or absent tendon reflexes
Variable muscle wasting and fasciculations
Normal autonomic function
Frequent associated drowsiness

course (Table 5–10). Limb weakness is usually severe, worse distally, with prominent wasting. Tendon reflexes are reduced or absent in most patients. Complete quadriplegia is occasionally seen. Clinical dysautonomia is conspicuously absent. Complete recovery in months with return of reflexes has been claimed for patients surviving the systemic illness, including the patients seen by the author[136] at Mayo Clinic–affiliated hospitals. Predictive factors for recovery are not known, but the patient with the most severe quadriplegia may completely recover, to everyone's surprise.

The disorder may resolve in a stereotypical manner. Improvement occurs first in the upper and proximal lower limbs, successful weaning follows, and later the distal portion of the lower limbs improves.

Most electrophysiologic studies have been done at the peak of severity. Characteristic findings are low amplitudes of compound muscle and sensory nerve action potentials, widespread fibrillation potentials, positive sharp waves, and sporadic myotonic or complex repetitive discharges.[11] Results of neuromuscular transmission studies are normal. Phrenic nerve conduction often is bilaterally absent, but this finding may have no significance when cardiac surgery with hypothermic cardiopulmonary bypass has been performed. Needle examination of the external oblique and external intercostal muscles may show evidence of denervation or loss of rhythmic recruitment with breathing.

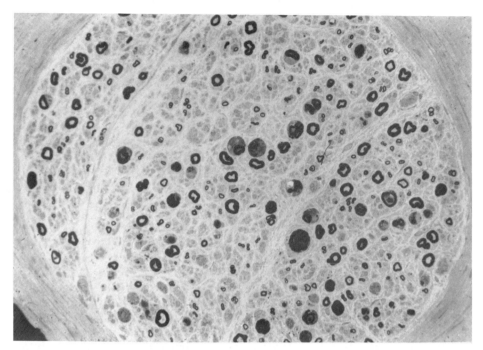

Figure 5-5. Nerve biopsy specimen from patient with critical illness polyneuropathy shows marked axonal loss. Many fibers are undergoing wallerian degeneration.

Autopsy and sural nerve biopsy specimens show severe axonal degeneration of peripheral nerves, mostly in the distal segments (Fig. 5-5). Loss of myelinated fibers may be seen, but significant segmental demyelinization or remyelinization is absent.[145] Phrenic and intercostal nerves have mild axonal degeneration. Muscle biopsy tissue showed muscle fiber necrosis in patients with increased levels of creatine kinase,[144] but type grouping was also found. Some studies showed occasional mononuclear cells and lipid-laden macrophages. Infiltrates were not recognized in muscle and nerve biopsy specimens.[144] Muscle biopsy specimens from the soleus (often taken at the time of sural nerve biopsy) may not be reliable because of pressure necrosis caused by prolonged immobility. In the most severe of 11 cases of axonal polyneuropathy of critical illness seen at the Mayo Clinic by the author, biopsy tissue taken from iliopsoas muscle showed

neurogenic changes but also numerous regenerating fibers of similar age, which suggested a monophasic impact to the muscle. A recent electron microscopy study noted abnormalities at the neuromuscular junction, possibly associated with pharmacologic denervation with muscle relaxants.[141] All these preliminary findings in muscle biopsy specimens need further confirmation.

As mentioned in Chapter 3, the distinction between an axonal form of Guillain-Barré syndrome and critical illness polyneuropathy is difficult. Three patients with critical illness polyneuropathy treated at our institution with intravenously administered gamma globulin did not have improvement in 2 months.[135] Whether this type of axonal neuropathy represents a mixed bag in the critical care setting or a separate entity is not resolved, but as alluded to in Chapter 3, the differential diagnosis of acute hospital-acquired axonal neuropathy is very limited.

Septic Encephalopathy

Septic encephalopathy is a clinical syndrome that probably is one of the diffuse and metabolic brain disorders.[63,137,143] The term "septic encephalopathy" has not gained universal acceptance or credibility, largely because many clinical manifestations of sepsis can produce drowsiness.

The initial clinical manifestations of sepsis are nonspecific. Patients are confused, disoriented, and restless. In the earlier stages, many patients have tachypnea and hyperventilation. These may be a result of circulating immunologic mediators on respiratory drive in the brain stem or a result of early lung injury. Additional manifestations, such as tachycardia, hypotension, and acute lung injury, may follow but can be absent. Therefore, the central nervous system manifestations in early sepsis may be a direct result of hypercapnia, hypoxemia, and hyperthermia. Unless marked hypotension or hypoxia develops from rapidly evolving adult respiratory distress syndrome, confusion generally does not progress into an unresponsive state. Typically, patients are intubated, paralyzed, or sedated and cannot be evaluated properly during management of septic shock and multiple organ failure. Frequently, neurologists are consulted when the acute episode has been mastered and the patient remains unresponsive. At that time, these patients may have survived episodes of severe hypoglycemia, cardiac arrhythmias, diffuse intravascular coagulation, and renal and hepatic failure.

The true incidence and degree of septic encephalopathy are not known exactly. Reasons are lack of systematic studies by neurologists and poor definition of this type of encephalopathy. In a large Veterans Administration study, septic encephalopathy was defined as altered mental status as judged by behavioral or cognitive abnormalities.[109] Young and colleagues[143] defined septic encephalopathy as difficulty with attention, recall, and orientation, but these factors may be very difficult to accurately assess in very sick patients.

In their study, 49 of 69 patients qualified for the diagnosis of septic encephalopathy, 16 of whom were in a coma with less than nonpurposeful movements to pain.[143] In our retrospective study[137] of 84 patients with surgical sepsis, 14 had decrease in level of consciousness beyond drowsiness and half were unresponsive to pain. Myoclonic jerks and seizures occasionally occurred but were rare. Persistent focal signs were absent.

Many patients with septic encephalopathy had severe episodes of hypotension often managed with increasing doses of inotropic medication. The contribution of other elements of organ failure was not significant in a logistic regression and strongly suggested that septic encephalopathy is hypoxic-ischemic in origin.[1,137] Cerebral blood flow is decreased in sepsis, with concordant changes in cerebral oxygen extraction ratios, and severe hypotension may simply augment the decrease in cerebral perfusion.[15]

Other potential mechanisms for septic encephalopathy, not thoroughly explored, are disordered amino acid transport similar to that in hepatic encephalopathy[51,92,113] and primary infection of the central nervous system. Both Jackson and associates[63] and Pendlebury and colleagues[97] found a high frequency of microabscesses in the brains of autopsied patients, but this mechanism in the absence of endocarditis seems highly improbable.

Additional studies, including lumbar puncture, have been noncontributory, but when sepsis is associated with disseminated intravascular coagulation, multiple hemorrhages may occasionally explain coma (see Chapter 10). Until prospective studies are available, aggressive control of hypotension early in the course of sepsis and treatment of marginal systolic blood pressures (120 mm Hg or greater) may improve neurologic outcome.

CONCLUSIONS

Vigorous efforts to define sepsis and systemic inflammatory syndrome continue. Underlying these discussions of definition is the attempt to develop adequate and cost-effective therapies for a frequently fatal disease. Allowing the pathogen to induce a massive inflammatory response greatly decreases the chances of survival, and early recognition and intervention, if possible, are paramount.

The focus, however, has widened, and more insights into neurologic complications of sepsis have been gained. Major deficiencies in our understanding of the two main manifestations, septic encephalopathy and critical illness polyneuropathy, remain. Failure to awaken or considerable change in cognitive function during or after sepsis predicts poor outcome. Because many patients have been hypotensive and hypoxemic, hypoxic-ischemic insult may be a major contender in so-called septic encephalopathy. In other patients who fail to awaken fully, the findings can be caused by the effects of disseminated intravascular coagulation, multiple intracranial hemorrhages (Chapter 10), vertebrobasilar stroke from complicated endocarditis, or, highly unusual, bacterial meningitis.

Critical care physicians also frequently call in neurologists for patients with endocarditis. No data validate one approach over another, but the increased risk of mycotic aneurysm in patients with transient ischemic attacks, nondisabling stroke, or endocarditis from *Staphylococcus aureus* or *Aspergillus* dictates a more aggressive approach. This consists of follow-up with MRI and angiography and possible surgical intervention or coil placement when the aneurysm is still present or enlarged after a course of antibiotics.

REFERENCES

1. Adams, JH, Brierley, JB, Connor, RCR, and Treip, CS: The effects of systemic hypotension upon the human brain; clinical and neuropathological observations in 11 cases. Brain 89: 235–268, 1966.
2. Ahmadi, J, Tung, H, Giannotta, SL, and Destian, S: Monitoring of infectious intracranial aneurysms by sequential computed tomographic/magnetic resonance imaging studies. Neurosurgery 32:45–50, 1993.
3. Anastakis, DJ, Peters, WJ, and Lee, KC: Severe peripheral burn polyneuropathy: A case report. Burns 13:232–235, 1987.
4. Angtuaco, EJC, McConnell, JR, Chadduck, WM, and Flanigan S: MR imaging of spinal epidural sepsis. AJNR Am J Neuroradiol 8:879–933, 1987.
5. Archer, BD: Computed tomography before lumbar puncture in acute meningitis: A review of the risks and benefits. Can Med Assoc J 148:961–965, 1993.
6. Baker, AS, Ojemann, RG, Swartz, MN, and Richardson, EP Jr: Spinal epidural abscess. N Engl J Med 293:463–468, 1975.
7. Bamford, J, Hodges, J, and Warlow, C: Late rupture of a mycotic aneurysm after "cure" of bacterial endocarditis. J Neurol 233:51–53, 1986.
8. Behrman, RE, Meyers, BR, Mendelson, MH, et al: Central nervous system infections in the elderly. Arch Intern Med 149:1596–1599, 1989.
9. Bleck, TP: Tetanus. In Scheld, WM, Whitley, RL, and Durack, DT (eds): Infections of the Central Nervous System. Raven Press, New York, 1991, pp 603–624.
10. Bohmfalk, GL, Story, JL, Wissinger, JP, and Brown, WE Jr: Bacterial intracranial aneurysm. J Neurosurg 48: 369–382, 1978.
11. Bolton, CF: Electrophysiologic studies of critically ill patients. Muscle Nerve 10:129–135, 1987.
12. Bolton, CF, Gilbert, JJ, Hahn, AF, and Sibbald, WJ: Polyneuropathy in critically ill patients. J Neurol Neurosurg Psychiatry 47:1223–1231, 1984.
13. Bolton, CF, Laverty, DA, Brown, JD, et al: Critically ill polyneuropathy: Elec-

trophysiological studies and differentiation from Guillain-Barré syndrome. J Neurol Neurosurg Psychiatry 49: 563–573, 1986.

14. Bone, RC, Balk, RA, Cerra, FB, et al: Definitions for sepsis and organ failure and guidelines for the use of innovative therapies in sepsis. Chest 101:1644–1655, 1992.

15. Bowton, DL, Bertels, NH, Prough, DS, and Stump, DA: Cerebral blood flow is reduced in patients with sepsis syndrome. Crit Care Med 17:399–403, 1989.

16. Brust, JCM, Taylor Dickinson, PC, Hughes, JEO, and Holtzman, RNN: The diagnosis and treatment of cerebral mycotic aneurysms. Ann Neurol 27:238–246, 1990.

17. Bullock, R and Van Dellen, JR: Rupture of bacterial intracranial aneurysms following replacement of cardiac valves. Surg Neurol 17:9–11, 1982.

18. Calderwood, SB, Swinski, LA, Waternaux, CM, et al: Risk factors for the development of prosthetic valve endocarditis. Circulation 72:31–37, 1985.

19. Calopa, M, Rubio, F, Aguilar, M, and Peres, J: Giant basilar aneurysm in the course of subacute bacterial endocarditis. Stroke 21:1625–1627, 1990.

20. Cannady, PB Jr and Sanford, JP: Negative blood cultures in infective endocarditis: A review. South Med J 69: 1420–1424, 1976.

21. Carpenter, RR and Petersdorf, RG: The clinical spectrum of bacterial meningitis. Am J Med 33:262–275, 1962.

22. Carter, BL, Bankoff, MS, and Fisk, JD: Computed tomographic detection of sinusitis responsible for intracranial and extracranial infections. Radiology 147:739–742, 1985.

23. Carver, N and Logan, A: Critically ill polyneuropathy associated with burns: A case report. Burns 15:179–180, 1989.

24. Case records of the Massachusetts General Hospital (Case 7-1988). N Engl J Med 318:427–440, 1988.

25. Case records of the Massachusetts General Hospital (Case 14-1990). N Engl J Med 322:988–999, 1990.

26. Cerra, FB, Siegel, JH, Coleman, B, et al: Septic autocannibalism: A failure of exogenous nutritional support. Ann Surg 192:570–580, 1980.

27. Chang, KH, Han, MH, Roh, JK, et al: Gd-DTPA-enhanced MR imaging of the brain in patients with meningitis: Comparison with CT. AJNR Am J Neuroradiol 11:69–76, 1990.

28. Cherington, M: Botulism: Ten-year experience. Arch Neurol 30:432–437, 1974.

29. Cherubin, CE, Eng, RHK, Norrby, R, et al: Penetration of newer cephalosporins into cerebrospinal fluid. Rev Infect Dis 11:526–548, 1989.

30. Churchill, MA Jr, Geraci, JE, and Hunder, GG: Musculoskeletal manifestations of bacterial endocarditis. Ann Intern Med 87:754–759, 1977.

31. Clark, R, Carlisle, JT, and Valainis, GT: Streptococcus pneumoniae endocarditis presenting as an epidural abscess. Rev Infect Dis 11:338–340, 1989.

32. Conly, JM and Ronald, AR: Cerebrospinal fluid as a diagnostic body fluid. Am J Med 75 Special Issue IB:102–107, 1983.

33. Covert, CR, Brodie, SB, and Zimmerman, JE: Weaning failure due to acute neuromuscular disease. Crit Care Med 14:307–308, 1986.

34. Dalen, JE: Valvular heart disease, infected valves and prosthetic heart valves. Am J Cardiol 65:29C–31C, 1990.

35. Danner, RL and Hartman, BJ: Update on spinal epidural abscess: 35 cases and review of the literature. Rev Infect Dis 9:265–274, 1987.

36. Davenport, J and Hart, RG: Prosthetic valve endocarditis 1976–1987. Antibiotics, anticoagulation, and stroke. Stroke 21:993–999, 1990.

37. David, TE, Bos, J, Christakis, GT, et al: Heart valve operations in patients with active infective endocarditis. Ann Thorac Surg 49:701–705, 1990.

38. Day AL: Extracranial-intracranial bypass grafting in the surgical treatment of bacterial aneurysms: Report of two

cases.   Neurosurgery   9:583–588, 1981.

39. Dean, RH, Meacham, PW, Weaver, FA, et al: Mycotic embolism and embolo-mycotic aneurysms: Neglected lesions of the past. Ann Surg 204:300–307, 1986.

40. Delahaye, JP, Poncet, PH, Malquarti, V, et al: Cerebrovascular accidents in infective endocarditis: Role of antico-agulation. Eur Heart J 11:1074–1078, 1990.

41. Del Rio, M, Chrane, D, Shelton, S, et al: Ceftriaxone versus ampicillin and chloramphenicol for treatment of bac-terial meningitis in children. Lancet i:1241–1244, 1983.

42. Denning, DW and Gill, SS: *Neisseria lactamica* meningitis following skull trauma. Rev Infect Dis 13:216–218, 1991.

43. Deutschman, CS, Wilton, P, Sinow, J, et al: Paranasal sinusitis associated with nasotracheal intubation: A fre-quently unrecognized and treatable source of sepsis. Crit Care Med 14:111–114, 1986.

44. Donovan Post, MJ, Guencer, RM, Montalvo, BM, et al: Spinal infection: Evaluation with MR imaging and in-traoperative US. Radiology 169:765–771, 1988.

45. Dreyfus, G, Serraf, A, Jebara, VA, et al: Valve repair in acute endocar-ditis. Ann Thorac Surg 49:706–713, 1990.

46. Ehrenreich, H, Garner, CG, and Witt, TN: Complete bilateral internal oph-thalmoplegia as a sole clinical sign of botulism: Confirmation of diagnosis by single fibre electromyography. J Neurol 236:243–245, 1989.

47. Eljamel, MS and Foy, PM: Acute trau-matic CSF fistulae: The risk of intra-cranial infection. Br J Neurosurg 4:381–385, 1990.

48. Erbel, R, Rohmann, S, Drexler, M, et al: Improved diagnostic value of echo-cardiography in patients with infec-tive endocarditis by transoesophageal approach: A prospective study. Eur Heart J 9:43–53, 1988.

49. Erntell, M, Holtaś, S, Norlin, K, et al: Magnetic resonance imaging in the diagnosis of spinal epidural abscess. Scand J Infect Dis 20:323–327, 1988.

50. Frazee, JG, Cahan, LD, and Winter, J: Bacterial intracranial aneurysms. J Neurosurg 53:633–641, 1980.

51. Freund, HR, Ryan, JA Jr, and Fischer, JE: Amino acid derangements in pa-tients with sepsis: Treatment with branched chain amino acid rich infu-sions. Ann Surg 188:423–430, 1978.

52. Frizzell, RT, Vitek, JJ, Hill, DL, and Fisher, WS III: Treatment of a bacterial (mycotic) intracranial aneurysm using an endovascular approach. Neurosur-gery 32:852–854, 1993.

53. Geiseler, PJ, Nelson, KE, Levin, S, et al: Community-acquired purulent meningitis: A review of 1,316 cases during the antibiotic era, 1954–1976. Rev Infect Dis 2:725–745, 1980.

54. Gordon, MF, Allon, M, and Coyle, PK: Drug-induced meningitis. Neurology 40:163–164, 1990.

55. Gorson, KC and Ropper, AH: Acute respiratory failure neuropathy: A var-iant of critical illness polyneuropathy. Crit Care Med 21:267–271, 1993.

56. Griffin, MR, Wilson, WR, Edwards, WD, et al: Infective endocarditis: Olmsted County, Minnesota, 1950 through 1981. JAMA 254:1199–1202, 1985.

57. Hand, WL and Sanford, JP: Post-trau-matic bacterial meningitis. Ann Intern Med 72:869–874, 1970.

58. Harries-Jones, R, Hernandez-Bron-chud, M, Panslow, P, and Davies, CJ: Meningitis and spinal subdural em-pyema as a complication of sinusitis (letter). J Neurol Neurosurg Psychiatry 53:441, 1990.

59. Hart, RG, Kagan-Hallet, K, and Joerns, SE: Mechanisms of intracra-nial hemorrhage in infective endocar-ditis. Stroke 18:1048–1056, 1987.

60. Hermans, PE: The clinical manifesta-tions of infective endocarditis. Mayo Clin Proc 57:15–21, 1982.

61. Hughes, JM, Blumenthal, JR, Merson, MH, et al: Clinical features of types A and B food-borne botulism. Ann Intern Med 95:442–445, 1981.

62. Ignelzi, RJ and VanderArk, GD: Anal-ysis of the treatment of basilar skull

fractures with and without antibiotics. J Neurosurg 43:721–726, 1975.

63. Jackson, AC, Gilbert, JJ, Young, GB, and Bolton, CF: The encephalopathy of sepsis. Can J Neurol Sci 12:303–307, 1985.

64. Jenzer, G, Mumenthaler, M, Ludin, HP, and Robert, F: Autonomic dysfunction in botulism B: A clinical report. Neurology 25:150–153, 1975.

65. Joffe, AM, Farley, JD, Linden, D, and Goldsand, G: Trimethoprim-sulfamethoxazole-associated aseptic meningitis: Case reports and review of the literature. Am J Med 87:332–338, 1989.

66. Jones, HR Jr and Siekert, RG: Neurological manifestations of infective endocarditis: Review of clinical and therapeutic challenges. Brain 112:1295–1315, 1989.

67. Jones, HR Jr, Siekert, RG, and Geraci, JE: Neurologic manifestations of bacterial endocarditis. Ann Intern Med 71:21–28, 1969.

68. Kanter, MC and Hart, RG: Cerebral mycotic aneurysms are rare in infective endocarditis (letter). Ann Neurol 28:590, 1990.

69. Kaplan, JE, Davis, LE, Narayan, V, et al: Botulism, type A, and treatment with guanidine. Ann Neurol 6:69–71, 1979.

70. Kaufman, DM, Kaplan, JG, and Litman, N: Infectious agents in spinal epidural abscesses. Neurology 30:844–850, 1980.

71. Kilpatrick, ME and Girgis, NI: Meningitis—a comparison of spinal anesthesia. Anesth Analg 62:513–515, 1983.

72. Kricun, R, Shoemaker, EI, Chovanes, GI, and Stephens, HW: Epidural abscess of the cervical spine: MR findings in five cases. AJR Am J Neuroradiol 158:1145–1149, 1992.

73. Lanska, DJ, Lanska, MJ, and Selman, WR: Meningitis following spinal puncture in a patient with a CSF leak (letter). Neurology 39:306–307, 1989.

74. Lasker, BR and Harter, DH: Cervical epidural abscess. Neurology 37:1747–1753, 1987.

75. Le Cam, B, Guivarch, G, Boles, JM, et al: Neurologic complications in a group of 86 bacterial endocarditis. Eur Heart J 5 Suppl C:97–100, 1984.

76. Lee, JJ and Parry, H: Bacterial meningitis following spinal anaesthesia for caesarean section. Br J Anaesth 66:383–386, 1991.

77. Leipzig, TJ and Brown, FD: Treatment of mycotic aneurysms. Surg Neurol 23:403–407, 1985.

78. Lew, D, Southwick, FS, Montgomery, WW, et al: Sphenoid sinusitis: A review of 30 cases. N Engl J Med 309:1149–1154, 1983.

79. Lewis, SW, Pierson, DJ, Cary, JM, and Hudson, LD: Prolonged respiratory paralysis in wound botulism. Chest 75:59–61, 1979.

80. Leys, D, Lesoin, F, Viaud, C, et al: Decreased morbidity from acute bacterial spinal epidural abscesses using computed tomography and nonsurgical treatment in selected patients. Ann Neurol 17:350–355, 1985.

81. Linden, BE, Aguilar, EA, and Allen, SJ: Sinusitis in the nasotracheally intubated patient. Arch Otolaryngol Head Neck Surg 114:860–861, 1988.

82. Lopez Messa, JB and Garcia, A: Acute polyneuropathy in critically ill patients. Intensive Care Med 16:159–162, 1990.

83. Luisto, M: Outcome and neurological sequelae of patients after tetanus. Acta Neurol Scand 80:504–511, 1989.

84. Lycklama, À, Nijeholt, J and Troost, J: Critical illness polyneuropathy. In Vinken, PJ, Bruyn, GW, and Klawans, HL (eds): Handbook of Clinical Neurology. Vol 51: Neuropathies. Elsevier Science Publishers, Amsterdam, 1987, pp 575–585.

85. Mampalam, TJ, Rosegay, H, Andrews, BT, et al: Nonoperative treatment of spinal epidural infections. J Neurosurg 71:208–210, 1989.

86. Mandell, GL, Douglas, RG Jr, and Benniff, JE: Principles and Practice of Infectious Diseases, ed 3. Churchill Livingstone, New York, 1990.

87. Molinari, GF, Smith, L, Goldstein, MN, and Satran R: Pathogenesis of cerebral

mycotic aneurysms. Neurology 23: 325–332, 1973.

88. Morawetz, RB and Karp, RB: Evolution and resolution of intracranial bacterial (mycotic) aneurysms. Neurosurgery 15:43–49, 1984.

89. Moskowitz, MA, Rosenbaum, AE, and Tyler, HR: Angiographically monitored resolution of cerebral mycotic aneurysms. Neurology 24:1103–1108, 1974.

90. Mylotte, JM, McDermott, C, and Spooner, JA: Prospective study of 114 consecutive episodes of *Staphylococcus aureus* bacteremia. Rev Infect Dis 9:891–907, 1987.

91. Naggar, CZ and Forgacs, P: Infective endocarditis: A challenging disease. Med Clin North Am 70:1279–1294, Nov 1986.

92. Naylor, CD, O'Rourke, K, Detsky, AS, and Baker, JP: Parenteral nutrition with branched-chain amino acids in hepatic encephalopathy: A meta-analysis. Gastroenterology 97:1033–1042, 1989.

93. O'Brien, JT and Geiser, EA: Infective endocarditis and echocardiography. Am Heart J 108:386–394, 1984.

94. Ojemann, RG, Heros, RC, and Crowell, RM: Surgical management of cerebrovascular disease, ed 2. Williams & Wilkins, Baltimore, 1988, pp 337–346.

95. Op de Coul, AAW, Lambregts, PCLA, Koeman, J, et al: Neuromuscular complications in patients given Pavulon (pancuronium bromide) during artificial ventilation. Clin Neurol Neurosurg 87:17–22, 1985.

96. Osler, W: Gulstonian lectures on malignant endocarditis. Lancet i:415–418, 459–464, 505–508, 1885.

97. Pendlebury, WW, Perl, DP, Karibo, RM, and McQuillen, JB: Disseminated microabscesses of the central nervous system (abstr). Neurology 33 Suppl 2:223, 1983.

98. Pfister, HW, Feiden, W, and Einhäupl, K-M: Spectrum of complications during bacterial meningitis in adults: Results of a prospective clinical study. Arch Neurol 50:575–581, 1993.

99. Powderly, WG, Stanley, SL Jr, and Medoff, G: Pneumococcal endocarditis: Report of a series and review of the literature. Rev Infect Dis 8:786–791, 1986.

100. Pruitt, AA, Rubin, RH, Karchmer, AW, and Duncan, GW: Neurologic complications of bacterial endocarditis. Medicine (Baltimore) 57:329–343, 1978.

101. Rapoport, S and Watkins, PB: Descending paralysis resulting from occult wound botulism. Ann Neurol 16:359–361, 1984.

102. Roberts, SP and Petts, HV: Meningitis after obstetric spinal anaesthesia. Anaesthesia 45:376–377, 1990.

103. Roelofs, RI, Cerra, F, Bielka, N, et al: Prolonged respiratory insufficiency due to acute motor neuropathy; a new syndrome? (abstr) Neurology 33 Suppl 2:240, 1983.

104. Roos, KL, Tunkel, AR, and Scheld, WM: Acute bacterial meningitis in children and adults. In Scheld, WM, Whitley, RJ, and Durack, DT (eds): Infections of the Central Nervous System. Raven Press, New York, 1991, pp 335–409.

105. Rowley, KM, Clubb, KS, Walker Smith, GJ, and Cabin, HS: Right-sided infective endocarditis as a consequence of flow-directed pulmonary-artery catheterization: A clinicopathological study of 55 autopsied patients. N Engl J Med 311:1152–1156, 1984.

106. Saissy, JM, Demazière, J, Vitris, M, et al: Treatment of severe tetanus by intrathecal injections of baclofen without artificial ventilation. Intensive Care Med 18:241–244, 1992.

107. Salgado, AV, Furlan, AJ, and Keys, TF: Mycotic aneurysm, subarachnoid hemorrhage, and indications for cerebral angiography in infective endocarditis. Stroke 18:1057–1060, 1987.

108. Salgado, AV, Furlan, AJ, Keys, TF, et al: Neurologic complications of endocarditis: A 12-year experience. Neurology 39:173–178, 1989.

109. Sprung, CL, Peduzzi, PN, Shatney, CH, et al: Impact of encephalopathy on mortality in the sepsis syndrome. Crit Care Med 18:801–806, 1990.

110. Stein, PD and Kantrowitz, A: Antithrombotic therapy in mechanical and biological prosthetic heart valves

and saphenous vein bypass grafts. Chest 95 Suppl:S107–S117, 1989.

111. Stengel, A and Wolferth, CC: Mycotic (bacterial) aneurysms of intravascular origin. Arch Intern Med 31:527–554, 1923.

112. Swartz, MN and Dodge, PK: Bacterial meningitis: A review of selected aspects. 1. General clinical features, special problems and unusual meningeal reactions mimicking bacterial meningitis. N Engl J Med 272:779–787, 1965.

113. Takezawa, J, Taenaka, N, Nishijima, MK, et al: Amino acids and thiobarbituric acid reactive substances in cerebrospinal fluid and plasma of patients with septic encephalopathy. Crit Care Med 11:876–879, 1983.

114. Talan, DA, Hoffman, JR, Yoshikawa, TT, and Overturf, GD: Role of empiric parenteral antibiotics prior to lumbar puncture in suspected bacterial meningitis: State of the art. Rev Infect Dis 10:365–376, 1988.

115. Teman, AJ: Spinal epidural abscess: Early detection with gadolinium magnetic resonance imaging. Arch Neurol 49:743–746, 1992.

116. Terpenning, MS, Buggy, BP, and Kauffman, CA: Infective endocarditis: Clinical features in young and elderly patients. Am J Med 83:626–634, 1987.

117. Terpenning, MS, Buggy, BP, and Kauffman, CA: Hospital-acquired infective endocarditis. Arch Intern Med 148:1601–1603, 1988.

118. Terranova, W, Palumbo, JN, and Breman, JG: Ocular findings in botulism type B. JAMA 241:475–477, 1979.

119. Tidyman, M, Prichard, JG, Deamer, RL, and Mac, N: Adjunctive use of dantrolene in severe tetanus. Anesth Analg 64:538–540, 1985.

120. Tompkins, LS, Roessler, BJ, Redd, SC, et al: Legionella prosthetic-valve endocarditis. N Engl J Med 318:530–535, 1988.

121. Trevisani, MF, Ricci, MA, Michaels, RM, and Meyer, KK: Multiple mesenteric aneurysms complicating subacute bacterial endocarditis. Arch Surg 122:823–824, 1987.

122. Trujillo, MJ, Castillo, A, España, JV, et al: Tetanus in the adult: Intensive care and management experience with 233 cases. Crit Care Med 8:419–423, 1980.

123. Tunkel, AR and Kaye, D: Endocarditis with negative blood cultures (editorial). N Engl J Med 326:1215–1217, 1992.

124. Tunkel, AR, Wispelwey, B, and Scheld, WM: Bacterial meningitis: Recent advances in pathophysiology and treatment. Ann Intern Med 112:610–623, 1990.

125. Van der Meulen, JHP, Weststrate, W, van Gijn, J, and Habbema, JDF: Is cerebral angiography indicated in infective endocarditis? Stroke 23:1662–1667, 1992.

126. Van Scoy, RE: Culture-negative endocarditis. Mayo Clin Proc 57:149–154, 1982.

127. Venger, BH and Aldama, AE: Mycotic vasculitis with repeated intracranial aneurysmal hemorrhage: Case report. J Neurosurg 69:775–779, 1988.

128. Verner, EF and Musher, DM: Spinal epidural abscess. Med Clin North Am 69:375–384, March 1985.

129. Vincent, FM, Zimmerman, JE, Auer, TC, and Martin, DB: Subarachnoid hemorrhage—the initial manifestation of bacterial endocarditis: Report of a case with negative arteriography and computed tomography. Neurosurgery 7:488–490, 1980.

130. Vita, G, Gilanda, P, Puglisi, RM, et al: Cardiovascular-reflex testing and single-fiber electromyography in botulism: A longitudinal study. Arch Neurol 44:202–206, 1987.

131. Von Reyn, CF, Levy, BS, Arbeit, RD, et al: Infective endocarditis: An analysis based on strict case definitions. Ann Intern Med 94:505–518, 1981.

132. Wainwright, RB, Heyward, WL, Middaugh, JP, et al: Food-borne botulism in Alaska, 1947–1985: Epidemiology and clinical findings. J Infect Dis 157:1158–1162, 1988.

133. Weinstein, L: Life-threatening complications of infective endocarditis and their management. Arch Intern Med 146:953–957, 1986.

134. Wesley, AG, Hariparsad, D, Pather, M, and Rocke, DA: Labetalol in tetanus. The treatment of sympathetic nervous system overactivity. Anaesthesia 38: 243–249, 1983.

135. Wijdicks, EFM and Fulgham, J: Failure of IVIG to alter the clinical course of critical illness polyneuropathy (submitted).

136. Wijdicks, EFM, Litchey, WJ, Harrison, BA, and Gracey, D: The clinical spectrum of critical illness polyneuropathy. Mayo Clin Proc (in press).

137. Wijdicks, EFM and Stevens, M: The role of hypotension in septic encephalopathy following surgical procedures. Arch Neurol 49:653–656, 1992.

138. Williams, AC, Sturman, S, Kelsey, S, et al: The neuropathy of the critically ill. Br Med J 293:790–791, 1986.

139. Wilson, WR, Geraci, JE, Danielson, GK, et al: Anticoagulant therapy and central nervous system complications in patients with prosthetic valve endocarditis. Circulation 57:1004–1007, 1978.

140. Witt, NJ, Zochodne, DW, Bolton, CF, et al: Peripheral nerve function in sepsis and multiple organ failure. Chest 99:176–184, 1991.

141. Wokke, JHJ, Jennekens, FGI, van den Oord, CJM, et al: Histological investigations of muscle atrophy and end plates in two critically ill patients with generalized weakness. J Neurol Sci 88:95–106, 1988.

142. Wright, DK, Lalloo, UG, Nayiager, S, and Govender, P: Autonomic nervous system dysfunction in severe tetanus: Current perspectives. Crit Care Med 17:371–375, 1989.

143. Young, GB, Bolton, CF, Austin, TW, et al: The encephalopathy associated with septic illness. Clin Invest Med 13:297–304, 1990.

144. Zochodne, DW, Bolton, CF, Thompson, RT, et al: Myopathy in critical illness (abstr). Muscle Nerve 9:652, 1986.

145. Zochodne, DW, Bolton, CF, Wells, GA, et al: Critical illness polyneuropathy: A complication of sepsis and multiple organ failure. Brain 110:819–842, 1987.

Chapter 6

NEUROLOGIC COMPLICATIONS OF CARDIAC ARREST

GENERAL CONSIDERATIONS IN
RESUSCITATION MEDICINE
POSTANOXIC ISCHEMIC
ENCEPHALOPATHY
TREATMENT AND SUPPORTIVE CARE

In many patients who arrive in the emergency room after effective cardiopulmonary resuscitation (CPR), hypoxic-ischemic encephalopathy continues to be a major cause of persistent disability. Some patients may indeed have a good chance to recover to their premorbid state, but only if they survive the systemic complications in the first week.[15,16] Outcome from cardiac arrest, whether the event occurs in the field or in the hospital, is poor, and the number of patients who survive is proportionally small[3,6,7,46,47,71] (Fig. 6–1). Outcome in the resuscitated elderly may be even worse.[46] Therefore, any prediction of outcome in comatose patients after successful CPR should be viewed in terms of best possible outcome. Future treatment in these patients could have more emphasis on minimizing the risk of recurrent cardiac arrest and malignant arrhythmias and on preventing cardiogenic shock than on treating hypoxic-ischemic damage, which may largely be immediately permanent. Although pathologic studies have indicated a potential window for reversing ischemia in tissue and salvaging neurons in the first hours after acute disruption of

blood flow, pharmacologic intervention soon after resuscitation in two major randomized trials did not improve outcome.[6,7]

This chapter describes the current knowledge of resuscitation medicine, the clinical course in survivors, and the most common manifestations of postanoxic encephalopathy. Comprehensive discussions of this subject, but with the major focus on anesthesia management, can be found in Kaye and Bircher's monograph[28] on CPR and in panel discussions from a symposium published in 1988.[60]

GENERAL CONSIDERATIONS IN RESUSCITATION MEDICINE

In recent years, the American Heart Association has achieved a consensus that CPR should be divided into two phases: basic life support and advanced cardiac life support. This basic form of standard CPR has been extended by inclusion of a third phase, "cerebral resuscitation," mainly through the pioneering efforts of the Brain Resuscitation Clinical Trial study group.[59] Although the importance of implementation of standard guidelines for cerebral protection is recognized, its effect on outcome is not established. The data from controlled clinical trials comparing the cerebral resuscitation protocol with and without a cerebral protection

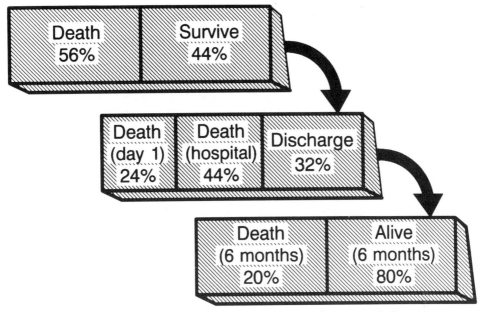

Figure 6–1. Estimated outcome of patients after cardiac resuscitation.

agent did not settle the issue of the best way to additionally manage these patients. Outcome in the placebo group that received aggressive "cerebral resuscitation" was not better than expected in this compromised patient population,[6,7] and this regimen therefore remains unproven.

The steps of basic life support in resuscitation are airway control, breathing, and circulation support. Although there are many unanswered questions about the dynamics of chest compression, the effects on cerebral blood flow have been extensively studied in animal models. Alternative modes of chest compression with additional abdominal compression may increase carotid blood flow, but as yet no clinical studies or animal experiments have demonstrated improved outcome.

The traditional explanation that compression of the heart between the sternum and the vertebral column results in forceful emptying of the cardiac chambers during upstroke is an oversimplification. Angiographic and echocardiographic studies have shown that chest compression sets in motion an increase in intrathoracic pressure that causes blood to flow from the lung passively through the left side of the heart. The marked increase of carotid perfusion pressures to 30% of normal values (rather than the usual 5%) during simultaneous abdominal compression-ventilation CPR also underscores the fact that the thoracic pump is responsible for blood flow during chest compression.[48,78] This finding resulted in the development of alternatives to standard CPR, including the use of circumferential thoracic binders and continuous use of interposed abdominal counterpressure. As expected, only open-chest cardiac massage may correct cerebral blood flow to prearrest levels, and neurologic outcome should theoretically be better than that with any form of closed chest CPR.

The current focus in resuscitation research is use of cardiopulmonary bypass, particularly in patients with severe left ventricular failure. Cardiopulmonary bypass may have a role in the distribution of potential salvaging agents as well. Conversely, cardiopulmonary bypass may increase the risk of air and particulate emboli, which may exacerbate ischemic damage.

After successful cardiac resuscitation, the recognition of postresuscitation multiorgan failure is important.[2] A significant proportion of deaths are caused by recurrent cardiac arrest (approximately 22%), refractory dysrhythmias often ventricular in origin, and irreversible cardiogenic shock. Important prognostic factors for cardiac failure and arrhythmias are a history of remote myocardial infarction, previous congestive heart failure, and previous cardiac arrest from ventricular fibrillation not caused by an acute transmural infarction. The most common deleterious effects of resuscitation are summarized in Table 6-1.

Studies of the neurologic damage in cardiac arrest have focused on reperfusion injury of the brain. This concept has been convincingly demonstrated in animal experiments and is favored by many anesthesiologists expert in reanimation, but data in humans are sparse and conflicting. When ischemia is brief, the brain parenchyma has the ability to recover almost immediately. The exact critical time threshold for reperfusion damage is not known, but injury presumably begins after circulation arrest of more than 5 minutes.

Three phases of cerebral blood flow have been recognized. The first phase after cardiac arrest is probably best characterized by an initial moderate hyperemia during resumption of circulation. This phenomenon lasts for 10 to 20 minutes, most likely is not uniformly distributed in the brain, and is always followed by a considerable decrease in blood flow, up to 50% of normal. This second phase is tentatively explained by vasospasm, glial edema, or microcirculatory plugs. The third phase of cerebral blood flow changes after resuscitation is less well defined. Baseline values may return, or cerebral blood flow may progressively deteriorate to very low levels. This concept is supported by studies[51,52,54] that showed more extensive ischemic neuronal necrosis in comatose patients who survived 24 hours or longer after comparable times of cardiac arrest than in patients who died within 18 hours. Ischemic damage was more severe in these patients with longer survival, a finding suggesting that ischemic injury is not permanent from the outset and may progress in the first hours after resuscitation. If this concept is true, the ideal time to administer pharmacologic agents is in the early hours of the hyperemia episode.

Often clinical investigators have advocated, although again without valid clinical data, the use of hemodilution with dextran, anticoagulation, or blood pressure support to overcome microcirculatory arrest in the phase after hyperemia. In a recent randomized trial, high doses of epinephrine and norepinephrine did not improve neurologic outcome.[11] In addition, a cerebral blood flow study using Xenon 133 showed no marked differences between patients who regained consciousness and patients who remained comatose. Despite adequate blood pressure, postischemic hypoperfusion occurred in all patients immediately after CPR, and perfusion further declined in the subsequent hours.[60] Future research may be more tailored toward restoration of the metabolic changes induced by free radical damage, abnormal calcium shifts, and release of excitatory transmitters. Improvement in field resuscitation and administration of drugs at the site may be

Table 6-1 POSTRESUSCITATION EFFECTS

NEUROLOGIC
Postanoxic ischemic encephalopathy
Ischemic myelopathy
Isolated cerebral infarct in watershed region

CARDIAC
Left ventricular failure
Dysrhythmias
Pulmonary edema and acute respiratory
  distress syndrome

DISTANT
Acute tubular necrosis
Traumatic liver damage
Ischemic colon and sepsis
Fractured ribs, pneumothorax, and bone
  marrow embolus

Data from Kaye and Bircher.[28]

beneficial, but preliminary results are discouraging.

POSTANOXIC ISCHEMIC ENCEPHALOPATHY

The main consequence of hypoperfusion, whether from cardiac arrest, asphyxia, or severe hypovolemic shock, is anoxic ischemic encephalopathy that often produces coma.[1] Cortical laminar necrosis, infarcts in watershed zones, and, rarely, severe white matter lesions characterize the pathologic abnormality. Anoxia from carbon monoxide inhalation may more preferentially affect basal ganglia and white matter areas (for a comprehensive discussion, see Chapter 14). The hallmark of global ischemia is neuronal loss in border zone frontoparietal cortex, insular cortex, putamen, pyramidal layers of the hippocampus, and end folium. In Petito and colleagues' study,[51] microvacuolation and cytoplasmic eosinophilia were noted later than 1 hour after cardiac arrest. The location and degree of damage are unpredictable, and early autopsies may not document hippocampal damage. In severe cases, subcortical gray matter, including thalamus and basal ganglia, cerebellar Purkinje's cells, and even nuclei of the brain stem, may be necrotic. Bilateral boundary zone infarcts are usually hemorrhagic at postmortem examination and are probably related to reperfusion.

Clinical Features

The assessment of postanoxic coma has become a frequent reason for consulting neurologists to be called to the intensive care unit (ICU). Findings in many large cohorts of patients with cardiac arrest who have detailed neurologic assessment show that the initial degree of motor responsiveness may indicate chance of recovery.[35,45]

Outcome is quite favorable when, immediately after CPR, the patient moans and strongly fends off a painful stimulus. On the other hand, lack of a motor response to pain in the first postarrest hours does not necessarily imply that neurologic impairment is inevitable. The chance of good recovery is relatively low, but up to 22% of the patients have recovered in large series (Table 6–2). Patients who awaken on the day of cardiac arrest gradually progress from an amnesic and dazed state to alertness within 12 hours. Some patients may have a profound amnesic syndrome,[76,77] which may persist for months. It has been suggested that focal ischemic hippocampal injury is responsible for this partial memory disorder, which occurs only in patients who have been comatose for at least 24 hours after resuscitation.[76,77]

Long duration of circulatory arrest results in abnormal extensor or flexor response or flaccidity in the arms and legs. The immediate finding of localizing responses is the best evidence that the

Table 6–2 RECOVERY OF INDEPENDENT FUNCTION AFTER INITIAL ABSENCE OF MOTOR RESPONSES

Prospective Series	Patients	No Motor Response to Pain, n (%)	Nonresponding Patients with Independent Recovery, n (%)
Earnest, et al, 1979[15]	117	89 (76)	0 (0)
Snyder, et al, 1980[68]	63	18 (29)	4 (22)
Levy, et al, 1985[35]	210	102 (49)	4 (4)
BRCT I, 1986[6]	262	162 (62)	26 (16)

BRCT = Brain Resuscitation Clinical Trial.

duration of anoxia has been brief.[68] Focal signs are uncommon but may arise from damage in arterial border zones and may have a higher incidence in patients with severe carotid occlusion. Bibrachial paralysis, however, appears to be relatively common in patients who have had cardiac arrest. This syndrome, called *man-in-the-barrel syndrome* by J. P. Mohr, has been reported in up to 32% of patients.[61] This curious clinical finding is probably the result of a bilateral prerolandic lesion sparing the upper limb part of the motor homunculus. This area is supplied by the end branches of the anterior and middle cerebral arteries. Findings on CT scanning are normal, although a recent case report documented the typical bilateral watershed infarctions in the supply areas of anterior and middle cerebral arteries and, after contrast enhancement, in the temporo-occipital areas.[14] A brisk triple flexion response and absent motor response in the arms may be a more likely explanation for the discrepancy of motor response between arms and legs.

Patients with a more severe anoxic-ischemic insult usually remain comatose on the day of resuscitation but recover in the following days. The mean time to awakening (defined as the ability to follow commands or comprehensible speech) was 3 days in a large study that focused primarily on recovery from coma.[38] The longest period before awakening occurred was 100 days. In our series, 17 of 20 patients with postanoxic coma awoke within 24 hours after arrest.[80] The remaining three patients awoke within 5 days.

Deterioration to lower levels of consciousness in the first postarrest days is unusual. Plum and colleagues[53] carefully documented extensive hemispheric white matter demyelination without pathologic evidence of edema in some patients with progression to coma and death after an asymptomatic interval (4 to 14 days). Early ambulation preceded this devastating event, but in a review of this interesting clinical phenomenon, a metabolic derangement (hypoglycemia,

hyponatremia), marked hypoxemia, or labile blood pressure was present and suggested that after an ischemic episode, the white matter is vulnerable to metabolic changes or changes in cerebral perfusion pressure.[19]

Many series have highlighted the dire consequences of abnormal brain stem reflexes.[35,66] Unfortunately, however, either brain stem reflexes have not been systematically examined in large resuscitation series or data acquisition has been incomplete. It remains questionable, however, whether new prospective studies that focus on abnormalities in brain stem reflexes will demonstrate a single powerful indicator of poor outcome. Corneal reflexes are absent in approximately one-third of comatose patients at the initial examination. (In some patients, failure to elicit a corneal reflex may result from an inadequate stimulus such as cotton.[18]) In Levy and colleagues' study,[35] 3 of 71 patients who lacked early corneal reflexes remarkably recovered.

During or immediately after resuscitative efforts, clinicians must be extremely careful in using abnormal eye movements and pupillary light response as signs of a low probability of saving the patient.[22,27] As a rule, the pupil diameter widens and light responses are abolished within a few minutes after cardiac standstill. Initial pupillary dilatation gives way to moderate constriction after return of spontaneous circulation.

A 1988 prospective study of pupil size and light response during CPR pointed out several types of pupil responses.[70] Dilated, fixed pupils were more frequently associated with asystole than with electromechanical dissociation or ventricular fibrillation. Successful cardiac resuscitation with good neurologic recovery more often occurred in patients with persistently contracted pupils from the onset or in patients who had initial dilation of pupils followed by contraction. Not surprisingly, fixed, dilated pupils throughout the resuscitation procedure indicated a poor chance of success. It is questionable whether knowledge of these pupil variables is of importance in clinical practice, and resuscitative efforts should certainly not be gauged by it. Moreover, frequent systemic use of atropine and epinephrine may cause dilated (but not fixed) pupils.[34]

The general clinical impression is that early loss of corneal reflexes together with ophthalmoplegia is a strong predictor of poor or fatal outcome. In addition, there is little hope for patients who have sustained upward gaze.[29] In a study of 15 comatose patients with sustained upward gaze after cardiac arrest or shock, 2 patients regained consciousness, but 1 patient died later in the hospital and the other remained in a vegetative state.[29] Sustained upward gaze can occur immediately after resuscitation and may persist for 2 months, but generally it resolves within 2 weeks. Also, myoclonic facial jerks or generalized myoclonic jerks may produce opening of eyelids with brief repetitive upward jerking of both globes. In patients with sustained upward gaze, horizontal eye movement remains full, although alternating (ping-pong) gaze deviation may occur transiently. Pupillary function is often normal. The neuropathologic counterpart consists of diffuse severe cerebellar and cortical changes, but the upper midbrain is normal. Sustained downward gaze is nonlocalizing and rare. In two comatose patients with downward gaze examined at a Mayo Clinic–affiliated hospital, CT scan findings were normal; clinicopathologic correlations were not available.

A unique eye movement termed *ocular dipping* has been described in postanoxic coma.[31,58] Ocular dipping has been most frequently described in patients with anoxic coma, but it may also occur in other metabolic encephalopathies.

In ocular dipping, both eyes conjugately move downward, sometimes completely obscuring the pupil beneath the lower eyelid, remain in a resting downward position for several seconds, and then rapidly return to their primary position.[58] Pathologic examination in these patients revealed, in addition to diffuse cortical damage, bilateral basal ganglia and thalamic lesions. The prognostic significance of the movement remains uncertain because complete neurologic recovery may occur. (Differentiation of ocular dipping from ocular bobbing may seem ambiguous, but ocular bobbing that is characterized by a conjugate movement with an excursion of only one fourth or one third of the normal voluntary range is strongly associated with intrapontine and cerebellar lesions or transtentorial herniation from a massive hemispheric lesion.[17,18])

Various reports have documented seizures in comatose survivors. The clinical manifestations of seizures are not adequately detailed in all major reports on CPR, in part because they are not directly witnessed by physicians (see Chapter 2). In some patients, spontaneous decerebrate posturing or shivering during or immediately after cardiac massage has likely been interpreted as tonic seizure. The reported frequency of clinical seizures in postanoxic encephalopathy has ranged from 9% to 50%.

Generalized tonic-clonic seizures are infrequent and most often linked to multiple doses of lidocaine during resuscitation. Snyder and colleagues[67] noted that some patients may have frequent rhythmic, rapid, low-amplitude limb movements called *shivering*. The mechanism of these abnormal movements, mostly evident in the immediate aftermath of resuscitation, remains obscure, but the movements are most likely associated with hypothermia, benzodiazepine withdrawal, or use of anesthetic agents. It is perhaps more important, however, to recognize that single tonic-clonic seizures, focal seizures, and shivers are of no prognostic value.

Of greater concern is *myoclonic status*. Myoclonus often involves the limbs as well as the axial muscles.[26,32,81] These rapid and brief jerks may also involve the facial musculature and can often be elicited by hand clap, pressure to the nail beds, insertion of central catheters, or tracheal suctioning. Fre-

SPONTANEOUS AND STIMULUS INDUCED SEIZURES

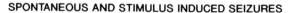

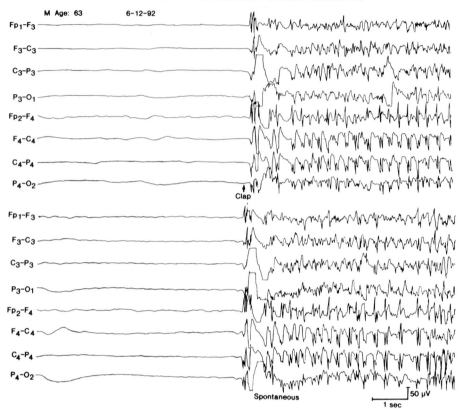

Figure 6–2. Electroencephalographic recording of spontaneous and sound-sensitive burst suppression in a comatose patient with severe generalized myoclonic status.

quently, a burst suppression pattern is found on electroencephalograms, and any loud noise may elicit myoclonic jerks (Fig. 6–2). As alluded to earlier, upward jerking of the globes may occur, often simultaneously with facial jerks and opening of eyelids. Generalized myoclonus is common during resuscitative measures and is very often seen in patients with a sudden drop in blood pressure from decreased cardiac output. (This relationship of myoclonic jerks and hypotension may be similar to that of convulsions during vasovagal collapse, a situation caused by diminished cortical inhibition.)

Myoclonic status strongly indicates severe anoxic cortical damage. A recent pathologic study in comatose patients with therapy-resistant myoclonus dem-

onstrated marked ischemic cell damage in the neocortex and hippocampus dentate nucleus and extensive central gray matter damage in the spinal cord. Myoclonic status in comatose survivors should be considered an agonal phenomenon. The evidence comes from a recent series of 107 comatose survivors of out-of-hospital arrest in which 40 patients had generalized repetitive and often sound-sensitive myoclonus involving the limbs and face.[80] Frequently, mechanical ventilation and gas exchange were hampered by either vigorous movements or involvement of the diaphragm. None of these patients awakened or survived, whereas in a comparable group of comatose patients without myoclonus, one fourth awakened in the first days after resuscitation. Clinical features were not significantly different between both groups, particularly for well-established poor prognosticators such as persistently fixed pupils. Comatose patients with myoclonic status more commonly demonstrate burst-suppression or alpha coma patterns on electroencephalograms, cerebral edema or watershed infarcts on CT scan, and more extensive cortical damage in postmortem histologic sections, all suggesting more severe anoxic damage (Table 6–3). Therefore, aggressive treatment should focus on paralytic agents to assist in mechanical ventilation and to eliminate a dreadful sight to family members; vigorous face twitching may suggest patient discomfort. Use of anticonvulsants has repeatedly failed to influence the frequency of myoclonic jerks. The decision to withdraw support should be strongly influenced by the presence of myoclonic status. Patients with myoclonic status have a very high probability of death. Survivors have been reported, but in this clinical setting none without devastating disability. Myoclonic status should be differentiated from isolated myoclonic jerk, other types of seizures, and an action myoclonus of Lance-Adams, which becomes evident after awakening. Moreover, this syndrome more frequently follows respiratory arrest. Predicting the chance of awakening and, more important, the chance of later disability in a comatose patient can be greatly facilitated when these

Table 6–3 CLINICAL, ELECTROENCEPHALOGRAPHIC, AND COMPUTED TOMOGRAPHIC FINDINGS IN 107 COMATOSE SURVIVORS OF CARDIAC ARREST

Feature	Myoclonic Status, n (%)*	No Myoclonic Status, n (%)†
CRANIAL NERVE DEFICITS		
Fixed pupils	5 (13)	9 (13)
No corneal reflexes	1 (3)	0 (0)
No oculocephalic responses	2 (5)	0 (0)
MOTOR RESPONSE		
None	34 (85)	43 (64)
Posturing	6 (15)	11 (16)
Flexion	0 (0)	13 (19)
EEG FINDINGS		
Burst suppression	33 (83)	5 (7)
Polyspiked waves	3 (8)	2 (3)
PLEDs	0 (0)	4 (6)
Alpha coma	3 (8)	2 (3)
Diffuse slowing	1 (3)	44 (66)
Not done	0 (0)	10 (15)
CT SCAN		
Cerebral infarcts	6 ⎫41	1 ⎫10
Cerebral edema	6 ⎭	3 ⎭
Normal	17	38
Not done	11	25
OUTCOME		
Awakened	0 (0)	20 (30)
Poor outcome or death	40 (100)	52 (78)
Good outcome	0 (0)	15 (22)

From Wijdicks, et al,[80] reprinted with permission from the Annals of Neurology.

*n = 40.

†n = 67.

CT = computed tomography; EEG = electroencephalographic; PLED = periodic lateralized epileptiform discharge.

and other prognosticators of poor outcome are identified. A comprehensive discussion of prognostication rules is found in Chapter 17.

When patients who arrive brain dead in the emergency room are excluded, brain death is seldom encountered after successful restoration of circulation. In our series, 5 of 107 patients fulfilled the clinical criteria of brain death.[80] All these patients were admitted with loss of most brain stem reflexes and ability to trigger the respirator. A marked decrease in blood pressure from cardiogenic shock often preceded loss of these remaining clinical signs. Persistent vegetative state from the outset occurs in approximately 20% of the patients. Patients who survive in a vegetative state have no recognizable emotional or motor response to painful stimulation. All four limbs are flaccid and may at times show a flexion or extension response, but localizing responses are conspicuously absent. Most patients are mute, but some occasionally groan. Generalized paratonia is common. Extraocular motor function is normal, and brisk corneomandibular, palmomental, and snout reflexes are generally seen within a few days. There is no reasonable hope for these patients.

Laboratory Investigations

Many clinicians believe that further diagnostic assessment of acute anoxic ischemic coma provides little benefit for prognostication and adds nothing more to a detailed neurologic examination.

Only a few reports in the literature have reported CT scan descriptions in postanoxic coma, probably because transport to the radiology suite is usually deferred in patients who have frequent arrhythmias, sudden decreases in blood pressure, and need for specific modes of ventilation. The most common early abnormal CT finding in postanoxic coma is effacement of sulci from edema.[43] Decrease in the cortical gray matter density from edema, resulting in loss of contrast difference between gray and white matter and obliteration of basal cisterns, is unusual only in patients who fulfill or almost fulfill the clinical criteria for brain death.[30] (Bird and colleagues[5] convincingly showed that this phenomenon of loss of contrast difference of gray and white matter can be explained by venous distention of the deep white matter veins. Drainage of these veins into subependymal veins is obstructed as a result of a transient increase in intracranial pressure.)

Computed tomography scans of patients in postanoxic coma may also show bilateral watershed infarction, bilateral thalamic hypodensities, and cerebellar infarction, often in patients with other evidence of terminal zone infarction (Fig. 6–3). CT scan findings are usually normal after resuscitation, but these abnormalities may become more apparent in the next days. Brain swelling and cerebral infarcts on CT scan predict a poor outcome, but as mentioned earlier, many patients also have myoclonic status. None of our patients with abnormal findings on CT scan awakened.[80] Laminar necrosis may be demonstrated with high intravenous doses of contrast material, but its value in prognostication is unknown.[36]

Magnetic resonance imaging (MRI) scans have recently been studied. Serial MRI may demonstrate high–signal-intensity lesions in the cortex compatible with laminar necrosis and white matter lesions from watershed infarcts.[63] In a 1993 study of MRI findings in 52 patients with cardiac arrest, 25% had cortical infarcts, 14% had cortical watershed infarcts, 21% had deep cerebral infarcts, and 4% had deep watershed infarcts. One fourth of the patients had normal findings on MRI scans. Comparison with controls showed that only deep cerebral infarcts were significantly more common. Abnormal MRI findings did not predict functional outcome.[56]

The value of electroencephalographic (EEG) recording is unresolved. Many EEG patterns in postanoxic coma have been described, but only some are

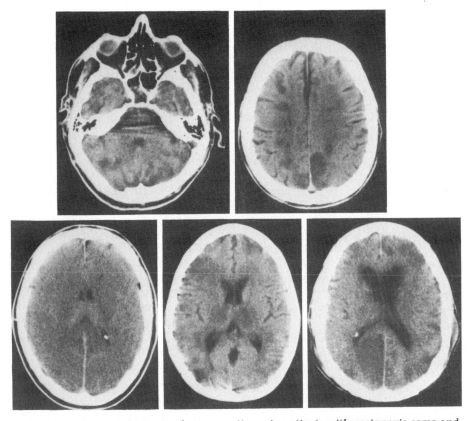

Figure 6–3. Computed tomography scan patterns in patients with postanoxic coma and myoclonic status. *Top row* (one patient): Multiple hypodensities in the cerebellum, cortex, and white matter. *Bottom row* (three patients): *Left*, Cerebral edema evidenced by loss of white-gray matter differentiation and loss of sulci. *Center*, Watershed infarcts with bilateral hypodensities in the thalamus. *Right*, Multiple small and large territory cortical infarcts. (From Wijdicks, et al,[80] reprinted with permission from the Annals of Neurology.)

strong indicators of poor outcome.[4,8,20,23–25,38,44,69,72]

Widespread theta or delta waves, sometimes with clear asymmetries between the activities of both hemispheres, are common findings, and some patients have prominent superimposed isolated sharp waves and spikes. Attention has been drawn to EEG rhythms of alpha frequency (alpha pattern coma).[20,50,75,79] Alpha pattern coma denotes rhythmic activity that emerges more prominently over the anterior or middle regions and is unreactive to auditory, noxious, or photic stimuli. This pattern is seen in the first days after cardiac arrest and is later re-placed by slow delta-theta wave patterns.[20,75,79] Occasionally, this alpha pattern changes into low-voltage theta and beta waves and electro-oculographic potentials indicative of slow, pendular eye movements resembling the first stages of sleep. Alpha coma may also alternate with burst suppression patterns.[80] Generally, it has been accepted that outcome is poor in patients with EEG characteristics of alpha coma, but one report pointed out that the prognosis of patients with alpha coma was not worse than that of other patients with similar depths of coma.[79]

Other well-organized postanoxic EEG patterns are spindle coma (activity resembling slow-wave sleep), burst suppression patterns (common in myoclonus), and rhythmic discharges of synchronous sharp waves (often remarkably similar to the periodic discharges seen in certain stages of Jakob-Creutzfeldt disease).[49] Status epilepticus patterns may be found on EEG in postanoxic coma. Close observation may reveal subtle jerking of jaw and eyelids accompanied by continuous or episodic spike-and-wave activity with occasional sharp transients. These patterns may occur without any clinical signs of seizures. Status epilepticus on EEG in postanoxic coma is resistant to therapy[40,65] and like myoclonic status most likely should be considered a marker of anoxic damage. Convincing series of patients after cardiac arrest in whom treatment with anticonvulsants has improved the level of consciousness or caused awakening are not available.

The difficulties of interpreting conventional EEGs have been overcome by the introduction of compressed spectral array, but this technique may not be available to everyone.[12] A preliminary study in 18 survivors of cardiopulmonary arrest classified the taped data into four groups and found that virtually all patients survived with patterns consisting of predominance of delta frequency with various amounts of theta activity and theta and alpha frequencies with various amounts of delta activity.[42]

A much more promising modality is the use of somatosensory evoked potentials (Fig. 6–4). Somatosensory evoked potentials are not influenced by medication, particularly sedatives. A consistent prognostic rule seems to emerge when tracings of somatosensory evoked potentials are analyzed. Brunko and Zegers de Beyl[10] showed in 50 consecutive patients that lack of cortical bilat-

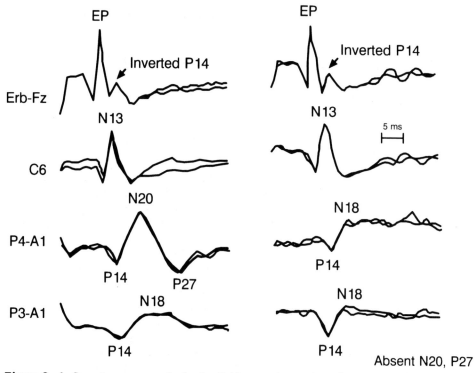

Figure 6–4. Somatosensory evoked potential in comatose patient (best motor response on admission was extension to pain) with absent cortical responses (N_{20} and P_{27}). *Left*, Normal. *Right*, Postanoxic coma. EP = somatosensory evoked potential.

eral short-term $N_{19}-P_{22}$ waves along with retention of identifiable cervical response was associated with a persistent vegetative state or death. All patients were studied within 8 hours after arrest, and serial studies did not show recovery of any cortical component in the first 2 weeks. Widespread anoxic-ischemic damage of cortex, thalamus, and cerebellum has been found at autopsy in patients without cortical responses. Patients with preserved cortical somatosensory evoked potentials have the potential to recover (cortical response is present in approximately two thirds of the patients), and prediction of outcome is not clear. These findings were confirmed in a more recent study that also claimed that long-latency evoked potentials (the third negative cortical peak N_{70}, seen after changing the band-pass filter) may have additional prognostic value in patients with retained cortical (short latency) response.[41] These long-latency sensory evoked potentials probably are generated by thalamocortical and intercortical connections and may disappear in a stepwise fashion while the short-term potentials remain visible. Lack of the N_{70} peak or significant delay differentiated favorable from poor outcome, but recognition of this peak (and its delay) may be very difficult.[41] Moreover, there is considerable disagreement whether this long-delay N_{70} peak has any meaning at all. Motor-evoked responses may, however, have additional prognostic value, particularly in patients with preserved cortical somatosensory evoked potential responses. At present, a negative bilateral cortical somatosensory evoked potential response strongly indicates a persistent, severe disabling deficit.

There has also been considerable interest in finding a useful chemical marker that discriminates between patients who will recover and patients who will never wake up and will remain vegetative.[57,64]

After an ischemic global insult to the brain, the cytosolic enzymes abundantly present in the brain leak into the cerebrospinal fluid. Peaks in brain-type creatine kinase isoenzyme (CK-BB) levels in the cerebrospinal fluid may suggest massive ischemic tissue injury.[57,74]

A preliminary study found a significant association between an increase in CK-BB in the cerebrospinal fluid and histologic damage at autopsy.[74] In a recent study, measurement of CK-BB in the cerebrospinal fluid had a positive predictive value of 93% for persistent coma.[73] Serum CK-BB levels did not correlate with outcome.

Analysis of gamma-enolase, known as a neuron-specific enolase, measured in the cerebrospinal fluid within 24 hours after cardiac arrest was also highly specific in detecting patients who remained comatose. All patients with neuron-specific enolase values greater than 24 ng/mL (controls, 6.4 ± 0.5 ng/mL) remained unconscious and died (positive predictive value of 100% and negative predictive value of 89%).[57]

Whether these tests are superior to clinical assessment and somatosensory evoked potentials remains to be determined.

TREATMENT AND SUPPORTIVE CARE

Very little is known about the merits of current management strategies of cerebral protection in resuscitation survivors. The emphasis has shifted to neuroprotective therapy, and several treatment trials have been performed with no[6] or extremely meager[7] benefit. There are no definitive guidelines in basic management in comatose survivors.

Basic Management

In the absence of drugs that effectively reduce the impact of anoxia and ischemia to the brain, management is tailored to minimize secondary brain damage. Many patients have underlying myocardial infarction with arrhythmias and hypotension. Conversely, transient increases in systolic arterial blood pressure are common after resuscitation. Hypertension is not a reflection of increased intracranial pressure but more often is associated with administration of epinephrine during CPR. In time, blood pressures level off, and aggressive treatment with agents that have a relatively long duration of action may decrease cerebral perfusion pressure in areas devoid of autoregulation.

Safar and Bircher's guidelines[59] consist of induction of mild hypertension (mean arterial pressure, 120 to 140 mm Hg) for 1 to 5 minutes with or without plasma volume expansion with Ringer's solution or dextran 40 in doses of 40 mL/kg. These guidelines have a certain relevance because they reflect the observations in animal models, but their clinical value has not been proven in randomized studies. (A 1992 study of high doses of epinephrine used in out-of-hospital arrest did not show improved neurologic outcome.[9])

Whether maintaining normoglycemia attenuates the anoxic-ischemic damage after resuscitation is unknown.[33,39]

It has been the understanding that dextrose solutions should not be used, because they may greatly increase blood glucose levels after resuscitation. More importantly, dextrose solutions may profoundly increase morbidity and mortality, as they did in a CPR canine study.[13] However, in a randomized study of 5% dextrose in water or 0.5 N saline infused in cardiac arrest by paramedics in Seattle, no significant differences in outcome were found.[37] The significance of hyperglycemia in postanoxic brain damage needs further investigation.

Intracranial Pressure Monitoring

The use of intracranial pressure monitoring after CPR is not well established.[62] It is reasonable to assume that after a considerable ischemic-anoxic insult, brain swelling may occur and may increase intracranial pressure. Frequent suctioning for pulmonary secretions, agitation in patients who are fighting the respirator, and positive end-expiratory pressure greater than 10 cm H_2O are additional factors that may further increase intracranial pressure. It is usually prudent to use muscle relaxants and sedatives in these agitated patients.

The practice of monitoring intracranial pressure in postanoxic coma may have very little justification. Although continuously measured in only a limited number of patients in the reported studies, intracranial pressure did not appear to be of primary importance. A study of six patients with intracranial pressure monitoring showed that none with Glasgow coma scale score of 3 or 4 had values above 20 mm Hg, except one who had seizures.[62] At Saint Marys Hospital in Rochester, Minn., we have occasionally used fiberoptic intracranial monitors in young comatose patients with progressive sulcal effacement on CT scan after severe anoxic insults but have never found significant increased intracranial pressure readings or, more important, a decrease in cerebral perfusion pressure. The similar dilemma of intracranial pressure monitoring in drowning is discussed in Chapter 14.

Specific Treatment

Many enthusiastic reports of possibly effective treatments in animal studies have been published, but the results of clinical controlled trials have been disappointing thus far. A prospective investigator will readily recognize that one of the major drawbacks in controlled randomized trials in this category of patients is that mortality within the first month is very high in comatose survivors, and a marked effect may be difficult to demonstrate. Nevertheless, most randomized studies conducted thus far had sufficient power to detect improvement in disability of at least 20%.[6,7]

The efficacy of thiopental loading has been studied in a randomized, blinded clinical trial. The mechanism of action for thiopental in postanoxic coma has not been satisfactorily clarified but probably is derived from a decrease in cerebral metabolic rate or a decrease in cerebral edema. Patients who had no purposeful motor response to pain after adequate systemic circulation was reestablished were randomly allocated to a thiopental loading dose of 30 mg/kg given intravenously within 10 to 50 minutes. A large percentage of the patients had cardiac arrest outside the hospital. Thiopental loading had no benefit.[59] Use of thiopental in high doses resulted in severe hypotension, and many patients needed vasopressors.

Steroids have not been formally tested in clinical trials of CPR, but in a post hoc analysis of the Brain Resuscitation Clinical Trial I, glucosteroid administration in the first 8 hours after arrest had no effect.[21] (In this study, use of steroids was left to the clinician in charge, and as a result, approximately 70% of enrolled patients received steroids.)

To circumvent the long delay between out-of-hospital cardiac arrest and treatment, intravenous administration of nimodipine was begun in ambulances.[55] Unfortunately, immediate treatment with calcium channel blockers did not significantly change the prognosis for victims of out-of-hospital ventricular fibrillation. However, there was an important trend toward higher 1-year survival and good recovery rates in patients treated after a delay of at least 10 minutes from the time of cardiac arrest — a marginal benefit. In addition, recurrent ventricular fibrillation was significantly lower in the nimodipine-treated group. It is not clear whether calcium channel blockers are promising drugs in CPR. Unfortunately a recent analysis of the Brain Resuscitation Clinical Trial II (lidoflazine intravenously) did not show marked differences in outcome.[7]

CONCLUSIONS

At one end of the spectrum of events after CPR is the devastation of postanoxic ischemic coma. All too often, one is forced to conclude that recovery cannot be expected.

Detailed examination of the comatose patient after successful resuscitation remains the mainstay of assessment. Fixed pupils and myoclonus status on the first day invariably predict very poor outcome (death in most cases). Approximately one third of patients have one or both of these distinguishing features. Additional examination of somatosensory evoked potentials may demonstrate that cortical responses are absent, a finding that may place another 10% to 20% of patients in the grim-outcome category. CT scan of the brain, which may show multiple cerebral infarcts or cerebral edema in an occasional patient, is less likely to add additional prognostic value, because most of these patients have myoclonic status, an early agonal phenomenon. The value of EEG has remained unconvincing, except perhaps in patients with burst-suppression patterns. When these poor prognostic signs are combined (in roughly 40% of patients), one may make a strong case for do-not-resuscitate orders or withdrawal of life-prolonging treatment after extensive discussion with family members. In others, a marked improvement in motor response (more than 2 points on the motor part of the Glasgow coma scale) should occur in the first 72 hours after arrest for the outcome to be potentially good.

Supportive care consists of adequate volume replacement and blood pressure stabilization. Intracranial pressure monitoring should be discouraged. Specific drugs, such as thiopental, nimodipine, lidoflazine, and corticosteroids, have shown no objective benefit.

REFERENCES

1. Adams, JH, Brierley, JB, Connor, RCR, and Treip, CS: The effects of systemic

hypotension upon the human brain, clinical and neuropathological observations in 11 cases. Brain 89:235–268, 1966.

2. Bass, E: Cardiopulmonary arrest: Pathophysiology and neurologic complications. Ann Intern Med 103:920–927, 1985.

3. Bedell, SE, Delbanco, TL, Cook, EF, and Epstein, FH: Survival after cardiopulmonary resuscitation in the hospital. N Engl J Med 309:569–576, 1983.

4. Binnie, CD, Prior, PF, Lloyd, DSL, et al: Electroencephalographic prediction of fatal anoxic brain damage after resuscitation from cardiac arrest. Br Med J [Clin Res] 4:265–268, 1970.

5. Bird, CR, Drayer, BP, and Gilles, FH: Pathophysiology of "reverse" edema in global cerebral ischemia. AJNR Am J Neuroradiol 10:95–98, 1989.

6. Brain Resuscitation Clinical Trial I Study Group: Randomized clinical study of thiopental loading in comatose survivors of cardiac arrest. N Engl J Med 314:397–403, 1986.

7. Brain Resuscitation Clinical Trial II Study Group: A randomized clinical study of calcium-entry blocker (lidoflazine) in the treatment of comatose survivors of cardiac arrest. N Engl J Med 324:1225–1231, 1991.

8. Britt, CW Jr: Nontraumatic "spindle coma": Clinical, EEG, and prognostic features. Neurology 31:393–397, 1981.

9. Brown, CG, Martin, DR, Pepe, PE, et al: A comparison of standard-dose and high-dose epinephrine in cardiac arrest outside the hospital. N Engl J Med 327:1051–1055, 1992.

10. Brunko, E and Zegers de Beyl, D: Prognostic value of early cortical somatosensory evoked potentials after resuscitation from cardiac arrest. Electroencephalogr Clin Neurophysiol 66:15–24, 1987.

11. Callaham, M, Madsen, CD, Barton, CW, et al: A randomized clinical trial of high-dose epinephrine and norepinephrine vs standard-dose epinephrine in prehospital cardiac arrest. JAMA 268:2667–2672, 1992.

12. Cant, BR and Shaw NA: Monitoring by compressed spectral array in prolonged coma. Neurology 34:35–39, 1984.

13. D'Alecy, LG, Lundy, EF, Barton, KJ, and Zelenock, GB: Dextrose containing intravenous fluid impairs outcome and increases death after eight minutes of cardiac arrest and resuscitation in dogs. Surgery 100:505–511, 1986.

14. Delavelle, J, Lalanne, B, and Megret, M: Man-in-the-barrel syndrome: First CT images. Neuroradiology 29:501, 1987.

15. Earnest, MP, Breckinridge, JC, Yarnell, PR, and Oliva, PB: Quality of survival after out-of-hospital cardiac arrest: Predictive value of early neurologic evaluation. Neurology 29:56–60, 1979.

16. Earnest, MP, Yarnell, PR, Merrill, SL, and Knapp, GL: Long-term survival and neurologic status after resuscitation from out-of-hospital cardiac arrest. Neurology 30:1298–1302, 1980.

17. Fisher, CM: Ocular bobbing. Arch Neurol 11:543–546, 1964.

18. Fisher, CM: The neurological examination of the comatose patient. Acta Neurol Scand Suppl 36:1–56, 1969.

19. Ginsberg, MD: Delayed neurological deterioration following hypoxia. Adv Neurol 26:21–47, 1979.

20. Grindal, AB, Suter, C, and Martinez, AJ: Alpha-pattern coma: 24 cases with 9 survivors. Ann Neurol 1:371–377, 1977.

21. Jastremski, M, Sutton-Tyrrell, K, Vaagenes, P, et al: Glucocorticoid treatment does not improve neurological recovery following cardiac arrest. JAMA 262:3427–3430, 1989.

22. Jordanov, J and Ruben, H: Reliability of pupillary changes as a clinical sign of hypoxia. Lancet ii:915–917, 1967.

23. Jørgensen, EO and Malchow-Møller, A: Natural history of global and critical brain ischaemia: Part I: EEG and neurological signs during the first year after cardiopulmonary resuscitation in patients subsequently regaining consciousness. Resuscitation 9:133–153, 1981.

24. Jørgensen, EO and Malchow-Møller, A: Natural history of global and critical brain ischaemia: Part II: EEG and neurological signs in patients remaining

unconscious after cardiopulmonary resuscitation. Resuscitation 9:155–174, 1981.

25. Jørgensen, EO and Malchow-Møller, A: Natural history of global and critical brain ischaemia: Part III: Cerebral prognostic signs after cardiopulmonary resuscitation. Cerebral recovery course and rate during the first year after global and critical ischaemia monitored and predicted by EEG and neurological signs. Resuscitation 9:175–188, 1981.

26. Jumao-as, A and Brenner, RP: Myoclonic status epilepticus: A clinical and electroencephalographic study. Neurology 40:1199–1202, 1990.

27. Kapp, J and Paulson, G: Pupillary changes induced by circulatory arrest. Neurology 16:225–229, 1966.

28. Kaye, W and Bircher, NG (eds): Cardiopulmonary Resuscitation. Clinics in Critical Care Medicine, Vol 16. Churchill Livingstone, New York, 1989.

29. Keane, JR: Sustained upgaze in coma. Ann Neurol 9:409–412, 1981.

30. Kjos, BO, Brant-Zawadzki, M, and Young, RG: Early CT findings of global central nervous system hypoperfusion. AJNR Am J Neuroradiol 4:1043–1048, 1983.

31. Knobler, RL, Somasundaram, M, and Schutta, HS: Inverse ocular bobbing. Ann Neurol 9:194–197, 1981.

32. Krumholz, A, Stern, BJ, and Weiss, HD: Outcome from coma after cardiopulmonary resuscitation: Relation to seizures and myoclonus. Neurology 38:401–405, 1988.

33. Kushner, M, Nencini, P, Reivich, M, et al: Relation of hyperglycemia early in ischemic brain infarction to cerebral anatomy, metabolism, and clinical outcome. Ann Neurol 28:129–135, 1990.

34. Larson, MD: Dilation of the pupil in human subjects after intravenous thiopental. Anesthesiology 54:246–249, 1981.

35. Levy, DE, Caronna, JJ, Singer, BH, et al: Predicting outcome from hypoxic-ischemic coma. JAMA 253:1420–1426, 1985.

36. Liwnicz, BH, Mouradian, MD, and Ball, JB Jr: Intense brain cortical enhancement on CT in laminar necrosis verified by biopsy. AJNR Am J Neuroradiol 8:157–159, 1987.

37. Longstreth, WT Jr, Dennis, LK, Copass, MK, and Cobb, LA: Intravenous glucose after out-of-hospital cardiac arrest: Results from a population-based randomized trial (abstr). Neurology 43 (Suppl):343A, 1993.

38. Longstreth, WT Jr, Diehr, P, and Inui, TS: Prediction of awakening after out-of-hospital cardiac arrest. N Engl J Med 308:1378–1382, 1983.

39. Longstreth, WT Jr and Inui, TS: High blood glucose level on hospital admission and poor neurological recovery after cardiac arrest. Ann Neurol 15:59–63, 1984.

40. Lowenstein, DH and Aminoff, MJ: Clinical and EEG features of status epilepticus in comatose patients. Neurology 42:100–104, 1992.

41. Madl, C, Grimm, G, Kramer, L, et al: Early prediction of individual outcome after cardiopulmonary resuscitation. Lancet 341:855–858, 1993.

42. Morillo, LE, Tulloch, JW, Gumnit, RJ, and Snyder, BD: Compressed spectral array patterns following cardiopulmonary arrest: A preliminary report. Arch Neurol 40:287–289, 1983.

43. Morimoto, Y, Kemmotsu, O, Kitami, K, et al: Acute brain swelling after out-of-hospital cardiac arrest: Pathogenesis and outcome. Crit Care Med 21:104–110, 1993.

44. Moss, J and Rockoff, M: EEG monitoring during cardiac arrest and resuscitation. JAMA 244:2750–2751, 1980.

45. Mullie, A, Buylaert, W, and Michem, N, et al: Predictive value of Glasgow coma score for awakening after out-of-hospital cardiac arrest: Cerebral Resuscitation Study Group of the Belgian Society for Intensive Care. Lancet i:137–140, 1988.

46. Murphy, DJ, Murray, AM, Robinson, BE, and Campion, EW: Outcomes of cardiopulmonary resuscitation in the elderly. Ann Intern Med 111:199–205, 1989.

47. Myerburg, RJ, Conde, CA, Sung, RJ, et al: Clinical, electrophysiologic and he-

modynamic profile of patients resuscitated from prehospital cardiac arrest. Am J Med 68:568–576, 1980.

48. Niemann, JT, Rosborough, JP, Hausknecht, M, et al: Pressure-synchronized cineangiography during experimental cardiopulmonary resuscitation. Circulation 64:985–991, 1981.

49. Nilsson, BY, Olsson, Y, and Sourander, P: Electroencephalographic and histopathological changes resembling Jakob-Creutzfeldt disease after transient cerebral ischemia due to cardiac arrest. Acta Neurol Scand 48:416–426, 1972.

50. Obeso, JA, Iragui, MI, Marti-Masso, JF, et al: Neurophysiological assessment of alpha pattern coma. J Neurol Neurosurg Psychiatry 43:63–67, 1980.

51. Petito, CK, Feldmann, E, Pulsinelli, WA, and Plum, F: Delayed hippocampal damage in humans following cardiorespiratory arrest. Neurology 37:1281–1286, 1987.

52. Petito, CK and Pulsinelli, WA: Sequential development of reversible and irreversible neuronal damage following cerebral ischemia. J Neuropathol Exp Neurol 43:141–153, 1984.

53. Plum, F, Posner, JB, and Hain, RF: Delayed neurological deterioration after anoxia. Arch Intern Med 110:56–63, 1962.

54. Pulsinelli, WA, Brierley, JB, and Plum, F: Temporal profile of neuronal damage in a model of transient forebrain ischemia. Ann Neurol 11:491–498, 1982.

55. Roine, RO, Kaste, M, Kinnunen, A, et al: Nimodipine after resuscitation from out-of-hospital ventricular fibrillation: A placebo-controlled, double-blind, randomized trial. JAMA 264:3171–3177, 1990.

56. Roine, RO, Raininko, R, Erkinjuntti, T, et al: Magnetic resonance imaging findings associated with cardiac arrest. Stroke 24:1005–1014, 1993.

57. Roine, RO, Somer, H, Kaste, M, et al: Neurological outcome after out-of-hospital cardiac arrest: Prediction by cerebrospinal fluid enzyme analysis. Arch Neurol 46:753–756, 1989.

58. Ropper, AH: Ocular dipping in anoxic coma. Arch Neurol 38:297–299, 1981.

59. Safar, P and Bircher, NG: Cardiopulmonary Cerebral Resuscitation: Basic and Advanced Cardiac and Trauma Life Support: An Introduction to Resuscitation Medicine, ed 3. WB Saunders Company, London, 1988.

60. Safar, P, Grenvik, A, Abramson, NS, and Bircher, NG (eds): Reversibility of clinical death: Symposium on resuscitation research. Crit Care Med 16:919–1084, 1988.

61. Sage, JI and Van Uitert, RL: Man-in-the-barrel syndrome. Neurology 36:1102–1103, 1986.

62. Sakabe, T, Tateishi, A, Miyauchi, Y, et al: Intracranial pressure following cardiopulmonary resuscitation. Intensive Care Med 13:256–259, 1987.

63. Sawada, H, Udaka, F, Seriu, N, et al: MRI demonstration of cortical laminar necrosis and delayed white matter injury in anoxic encephalopathy. Neuroradiology 32:319–321, 1990.

64. Scarna, H, Delafosse, B, Steinberg, R, et al: Neuron-specific enolase as a marker of neuronal lesions during various comas in man. Neurochem Int 4:405–411, 1982.

65. Simon, RP and Aminoff, MJ: Electrographic status epilepticus in fatal anoxic coma. Ann Neurol 20:351–355, 1986.

66. Snyder, BD, Gumnit, RJ, Leppik, IE, et al: Neurologic prognosis after cardiopulmonary arrest: IV. Brainstem reflexes. Neurology 31:1092–1097, 1981.

67. Snyder, BD, Hauser, WA, Loewenson, RB, et al: Neurologic prognosis after cardiopulmonary arrest: III. Seizure activity. Neurology 30:1292–1297, 1980.

68. Snyder, BD, Loewenson, RB, Gumnit, RJ, et al: Neurologic prognosis after cardiopulmonary arrest: II. Level of consciousness. Neurology 30:52–58, 1980.

69. Sørensen, K, Thomassen, A, and Wernberg, M: Prognostic significance of alpha frequency EEG rhythm in coma after cardiac arrest. J Neurol Neurosurg Psychiatry 41:840–842, 1978.

70. Steen-Hansen, JE, Hansen, NN, Vaagenes, P, and Schreiner, B: Pupil size and light reactivity during cardiopulmonary resuscitation: A clinical study. Crit Care Med 16:69–70, 1988.

71. Taffet, GE, Teasdale, TA, and Luchi, RJ: In-hospital cardiopulmonary resuscitation. JAMA 260:2069–2072, 1988.

72. Thomassen, A, Sørensen, K, and Wernberg, M: The prognostic value of EEG in coma survivors after cardiac arrest. Acta Anaesthesiol Scand 22:483–490, 1978.

73. Vaagenes, P, Kjekshus, J, and Torvik, A: The relationship between cerebrospinal fluid creatine kinase and morphologic changes in the brain after transient cardiac arrest. Circulation 61:1194–1199, 1980.

74. Vaagenes, P, Safar, P, Diven, W, et al: Brain enzyme levels in CSF after cardiac arrest and resuscitation in dogs: Markers of damage and predictors of outcome. J Cereb Blood Flow Metab 8:262–275, 1988.

75. Vignaendra, V, Wilkus, RJ, Copass, MK, and Chantrian, GE: Electroencephalographic rhythms of alpha frequency in comatose patients after cardiopulmonary arrest. Neurology 24:582–588, 1974.

76. Volpe, BT, Herscovitch, P, and Raichle, ME: PET evaluation of patients with amnesia after cardiac arrest (abstr). Stroke 15:196, 1984.

77. Volpe, BT, Holtzman, JD, and Hirst, W: Further characterization of patients with amnesia after cardiac arrest: Preserved recognition memory. Neurology 36:408–411, 1986.

78. Werner, JA, Greene, HL, Janko, CL, and Cobb, LA: Visualization of cardiac valve motion in man during external chest compression using two-dimensional echocardiography. Circulation 63:1417–1421, 1981.

79. Westmoreland, BF, Klass, DW, Sharbrough, FW, and Reagan, TJ: Alpha-coma: Electroencephalographic, clinical, pathologic, and etiologic correlations. Arch Neurol 32:713–718, 1975.

80. Wijdicks, EFM, Parisi, JE, and Sharbrough, FW: Prognostic value of myoclonus status in comatose survivors of cardiac arrest. Ann Neurol 35:239–243, 1994.

81. Young, GB, Gilbert, JJ, and Zochodne, DW: The significance of myoclonic status epilepticus in postanoxic coma. Neurology 40:1843–1848, 1990.

Chapter 7

NEUROLOGIC MANIFESTATIONS OF ACID-BASE DERANGEMENTS, ELECTROLYTE DISORDERS, AND ENDOCRINE CRISES

ACID-BASE DISORDERS
ELECTROLYTE DISORDERS
ENDOCRINE EMERGENCIES

The spectrum of disorders associated with acute metabolic or endocrine derangements ranges from transient and subtle neurologic manifestations to severe, irreversible damage to the central nervous system. Several electrolyte and acid-base abnormalities are encountered so regularly that they deserve specific discussion. What the ultimate physiologic response will be in any given patient with any acute metabolic crisis is virtually impossible to predict. Rather than irritate the intensive care specialist with terms such as *multifactorial* and *toxic-metabolic*, one must have a clear idea of how each of the various disturbances may produce an effect on the nervous system. In many situations, these neurologic manifestations should be rapidly recognized in order to avoid further metabolic insult to the brain.

ACID-BASE DISORDERS

Acid-base disorders are common in the intensive care unit (ICU), but unless there is an acute change in arterial pH, neurologic manifestations are absent.

Many buffer systems in the body assist in maintaining a constant pH, but arterial blood pH is kept constant primarily as a result of a balance between carbon dioxide (PCO_2) and serum bicarbonate. Either component can become abnormal, resulting in a compensatory response by respiratory or renal control systems. The characteristic features of primary acid-base disturbances are presented in Table 7–1. The interpretation of mixed acid-base conditions is complex and beyond the scope of this chapter.

The cerebrospinal fluid (CSF) acid-base status changes significantly as well, but not always in a similar direction.[9,112] As a rule, the acute changes in serum pH and PCO_2 are similar in CSF, but whether changes in CSF in acid-base disorders reflect clinical signs is unknown. Experimental studies have clearly demonstrated that changes in

**Table 7–1 CHARACTERISTIC FEATURES OF
PRIMARY ACID-BASE DISTURBANCES**

pH	PCO$_2$		
	<36 mm Hg	*36–44 mm Hg*	*>44 mm Hg*
<7.36	Metabolic acidosis	Metabolic acidosis	Respiratory acidosis
>7.44	Respiratory alkalosis	Metabolic alkalosis	Metabolic alkalosis

intracellular brain pH are probably more relevant,[6,9] although the complex mechanisms of the buffering capacity of the brain have not been completely understood.

In acute respiratory acidosis with persistent hypercapnia, CSF pH returns to normal within several hours after the insult.[6,9] In respiratory alkalosis, identical compensation occurs but probably also as a result of cerebral vasoconstriction leading to increased anaerobic metabolism and lactate production, which may in turn produce an effective decrease in CSF bicarbonate.

Counterbalancing changes can also be expected in metabolic acidosis and alkalosis. Even paradoxical reduction of CSF pH from bicarbonate treatment in these patients may occur and is caused by equilibration of carbon dioxide between blood and CSF and poor diffusion of bicarbonate from blood to CSF.[6,9]

Respiratory Acidosis

In this acid-base disorder, hypercarbia is the primary abnormality and is most frequently caused by pulmonary disease.[144] Abnormal neuromuscular function as a direct cause of respiratory acidosis is seldom seen in ICUs, but occasionally hypoventilation is a presenting symptom of a motor neuron disease, myopathy, prolonged blockade of the neuromuscular junction, or critical illness neuropathy or is associated with major spinal trauma. Common causes of respiratory acidosis in medical and surgical ICUs are summarized in Table 7–2.

The clinical manifestations of respiratory acidosis are reflected by hyper-

carbia and hypoxia. Few patients presumably have all the symptoms, and patients who chronically retain carbon dioxide may have none at all. Patients with profound hypercarbia (PaCO$_2$ values of 175 mm Hg) with crystal clear mentation have been reported.[26,93]

Most patients with hypercarbia are fatigued and drowsy from the increased work of breathing. As hypercarbia worsens, patients become irritable and coarse multifocal twitches and asterixis develop. Tremors may be seen but can be from beta-adrenergic agents such as albuterol. Overdose of these agents may cause a fine tremor, often only evident with outstretched hands or when magnified by placing a card on the fingers. Carroll and Rothenberg[26] made the important point that many patients fall asleep exhausted when hypoxemia is relieved at any level of PaCO$_2$.

Headaches worse at night or early in the morning are typical of chronic hypercarbia and may not be common in acute cases.[12,39] Papilledema has been

**Table 7–2 COMMON CAUSES OF
RESPIRATORY ACIDOSIS**

Narcotics, sedatives, muscle relaxants
Thoracic injury
Pleural effusion
Pneumothorax
Upper airway obstruction
Asthma, chronic obstructive pulmonary disease
Pulmonary edema
Neuromuscular disorders
   Spinal cord injury at or above C-3
   Amyotrophic lateral sclerosis
   Guillain-Barré syndrome, critical illness
     neuropathy
   Myasthenia gravis
   Polymyositis

noted in patients with acute pulmonary disorders, but the mechanism — cerebral vasodilatation or increased venous pressure — is not entirely clear. Polycythemia is not a contributory cause in most cases. Profound carbon dioxide narcosis is seldom seen, but earlier reports mentioned seizures, flaccid paralysis, and unresponsive coma.[122] Death may soon follow. Recovery cannot be expected in hypercapnic patients who become comatose, presumably also because of severe shock associated with extremely high PCO_2 levels.

Respiratory Alkalosis

Alveolar hyperventilation is often observed as a response to hypoxia or metabolic acidosis or with a specific disorder from an almost inexhaustible list of disorders (Table 7–3). Respiratory alkalosis is most frequently seen with metabolic acidosis in ICUs. Because many other factors are present, neurogenic central hyperventilation, a condition often associated with pontine lesions, is virtually impossible to diagnose in medical and surgical ICUs. Spontaneous hyperventilation may frequently occur after major surgery and is largely determined by postoperative delirium or pain.

Typical symptoms of respiratory alkalosis are lightheadedness and drowsiness, but a consistent decrease in level of consciousness is seldom produced. Tetanic cramps may occur but are rare. Respiratory alkalosis may in-

Table 7–3 COMMON CAUSES OF RESPIRATORY ALKALOSIS

Mechanical ventilation
Pulmonary disorders
  Adult respiratory distress syndrome
  Pulmonary emboli
  Chronic obstructive pulmonary disease
Anxiety, postoperative pain
Sepsis syndrome (early)
Liver failure
Central neurogenic
Salicylate, analeptic overdose
Thyroid hormone excess

Table 7–4 COMMON CAUSES OF METABOLIC ACIDOSIS

Elevated Anion Gap	Normal Anion Gap
Renal failure	Diarrhea
Ketoacidosis	Hyperalimentation
Lactic acidosis	Hypoaldosteronism

duce seizures in patients with previous stroke or epilepsy.

Metabolic Acidosis

The neurologic manifestations of metabolic acidosis with a normal anion gap (difference between unmeasured anions and cations in serum) are attributed either to cardiovascular collapse resulting in diffuse hypoxic-ischemic damage or to associated electrolyte disorders (discussed in separate sections) (Table 7–4).

Lactate acidosis, however, is frequently associated with thiamine deficiency or is a direct result of a series of tonic-clonic seizures. In ICUs, lactate acidosis is more frequently seen with sepsis, cardiogenic shock, and multiorgan failure.

Metabolic Alkalosis

Metabolic alkalosis is generally associated with volume contraction.[109] Causes are listed in Table 7–5. Paresthesias and muscle cramping may be early signs of systemic alkalemia, but metabolic alkalosis more characteristically gradually decreases the level of consciousness and, as the condition worsens, leads to tonic-clonic seizures.

Table 7–5 COMMON CAUSES OF METABOLIC ALKALOSIS

Volume chloride depletion
Diuretic therapy
Endocrine
  Cushing's disease
  Primary aldosteronism
Massive blood transfusion

Hypocalcemia has been implicated as a predisposing factor for seizures in this situation, but the relation is weak.

ELECTROLYTE DISORDERS

Electrolyte derangements are common to nearly all patients with critical illness. Many electrolyte disorders directly produce central nervous system symptoms, but symptoms can be attributed to adverse effects of treatment as well. This situation is exemplified by the potential ravages of rapid correction in patients with severe hyponatremia.

The most pertinent challenges to the brain adaptive capacity are disturbances of body fluid osmolality (Fig. 7–1). Although hyponatremia and hypernatremia are common clinical problems, the electrolyte abnormality itself is not the cause of neurologic manifestations but rather causes the hypo-osmolar or hyperosmolar state. Conditions that produce pseudohyponatremia (for example, hypoproteinemia or paraproteinemia) are not symptomatic except possibly in hyper-glycemia. These osmolality changes result in changes in the content of organic osmolytes ("idiogenic osmols"). (Idiogenic osmols complement the gap between measured change of osmolality and the total changes contributed by electrolytes.) Hypo-osmolality results in the shifting of water into the brain from an osmotic gradient. The resulting brain edema produces signs of hyponatremia and is corrected by loss of the major categories of osmolytes (glutamate, glutamine, taurine, myo-inositol, and creatine) and with them brain water. The brain adaptation to hyperosmolality is not the reverse, but in acute hyperosmolality, rapid electrolyte accumulation from CSF, plasma, and extracellular fluid results in correction of intracellular brain water.[82,83,138]

Hyponatremia

In hospital-based studies, hyponatremia is the most common electrolyte disorder. In most patients, the syndrome of inappropriate secretion of antidiuretic hormone (SIADH) is diagnosed in hypo-

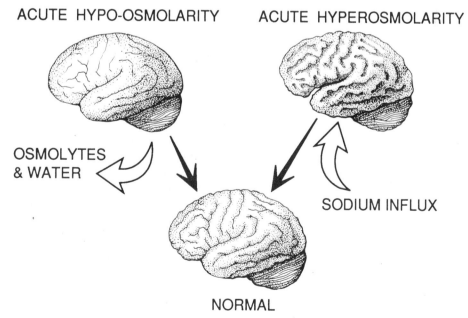

ACUTE HYPO-OSMOLARITY   ACUTE HYPEROSMOLARITY

OSMOLYTES & WATER

SODIUM INFLUX

NORMAL

Figure 7–1. Brain adaptation in acute changes of osmolarity.

natremia, but in 30% of the patients, hyponatremia can be attributed to hyperglycemia, severe renal failure, or excessive administration of free water.[4] In other series of patients with hyponatremia, depending on the medical or surgical population, a high incidence of congestive heart failure and hypovolemia associated with diuretic therapy was found. The potential causes of hyponatremia in critically ill patients are shown in Table 7–6.

The early neurologic manifestations of hyponatremia are nonspecific and can easily be overlooked. Although many patients may have headache, nausea, and vomiting, more often patients with hyponatremia have symptoms of global confusion, delirium, or profound drowsiness.[8,10] The most consistent clinical symptom in hyponatremia is progressive impaired responsiveness when serum sodium values reach 125 mEq/L. With advancing hyponatremia, the depression of consciousness progresses substantially and generalized tonic-clonic seizures are common. Nonconvulsive status or a prolonged ictal state after a cluster of generalized tonic-clonic seizures may complicate the interpretation of the level of consciousness (see Chapter 2). Patients with rapidly developing hyponatremia (to values less than 110 mEq/L) become unresponsive, and many have additional seizures. Seizures in patients with hyponatremia may signify a higher risk of poor outcome, but in many patients, the underlying condition that led

Table 7–6 COMMON CAUSES OF HYPONATREMIA

Syndrome of inappropriate antidiuretic hormone
Postoperative fluid overload (gastrointestinal and cardiovascular procedures)
Iatrogenic hypotonic fluid loading
Hypovolemic state (gastrointestinal, skin, or renal loss)
Diuretics (thiazide)
Hypothyroidism
Hypoadrenalism
Pseudohyponatremia

to hyponatremia is the main determinant of poor outcome.

Pertinent signs and symptoms of hyponatremia do not occur until plasma sodium concentration is less than 125 mmol/L, but irritability, restlessness, and confusion can occur at higher levels in patients who have a rapid decrease in sodium levels. As a rule, symptoms are more likely to occur if hyponatremia develops acutely than if it occurs over a longer period. It should be emphasized that some patients may have severe muscle cramps. Hyponatremia may result in very severe generalized cramps in limbs and abdominal muscles. Hemiparesis from hyponatremia alone has been reported in older literature in a few case reports, with complete resolution after correction, but recent reports of focal neurologic signs in hyponatremia are not available.

In the past decade, three possible neurologic syndromes associated with hyponatremia have emerged, each with specific clinical features.

CENTRAL PONTINE MYELINOLYSIS

The name *central pontine myelinolysis* (CPM), first coined by Adams and colleagues,[2] implies that demyelination is at the base of the pons, but later descriptions noted occasional extension into the tegmentum. Focal areas of myelinolysis may also be present in the thalamus, characteristically in the lateral portion.[37,61]

Central pontine myelinolysis is associated with severe debilitating disease, such as systemic advanced cancer or chronic alcoholism. It has also been described in patients with major osmolality fluctuations, such as severely burned patients,[92] patients with Reye's syndrome (after mannitol therapy), and patients who have had liver transplantation. Nevertheless, CPM has become a clinical entity that is frequently linked to rapid correction of severe hyponatremia.[13,14,19,24,30,76]

The clinical manifestations of CPM

can be diverse, but flaccid quadriplegia, pseudobulbar palsy, or facial weakness and inability to swallow or speak are prominent.[46,94,145,146] Quadriplegia may be more pronounced in the arms in some patients; in others, hemiparesis is evident. The central location in the pons precludes neuro-ophthalmologic signs except in patients with extension of demyelination beyond its central localization, in which nystagmus, abducens palsy, miosis, and limitation of conjugate eye movement in the horizontal direction are present. CPM may manifest as a locked-in syndrome with only eye blinking as a means of communication, but in contrast to occlusion of the basilar artery, recovery usually takes place within days.

Pontine lesions may not be manifested clinically by neurologic symptoms other than behavioral changes. Emotional lability, such as crying, is associated with pseudobulbar palsy in CPM, but restless behavior and irritability may be seen with only subtle neurologic signs.[113]

Central pontine myelinolysis characteristically is difficult to diagnose clinically after liver transplantation.[21,38] Many patients are drowsy, often because of increased ammonia from graft rejection and acute electrolyte derangements or acute renal failure. Pseudobulbar signs and generalized hyperreflexia may not be present initially. If magnetic resonance imaging (MRI) of the brain is not performed, the diagnosis can be missed and may become evident only at postmortem examination. The incidence of CPM in liver transplantation therefore is not known. In the Mayo Clinic series, the prevalence of CPM after orthotopic liver transplantation was 1%. All patients affected had impaired levels of consciousness alone and no typical pseudobulbar signs.[21]

Extrapontine lesions may occur simultaneously but are manifested differently. On the basis of autopsy material, it is estimated that approximately 10% of patients with CPM have extrapontine lesions,[148] usually found in the cauda,

putamen, lateral thalamus, and lateral geniculate nucleus. Delayed onset of movement disorders—3 weeks to 5 months after rapid correction of hyponatremia and subsequent clinical diagnosis of CPM—has been described, and they can be successfully treated.[90,134,135]

Acute parkinsonism responds to levodopa substitution. Generalized dystonia or predominant orolingual dystonia and athetosis may occur months after the initial event; response to trihexyphenidyl (maximum of 40 mg/d) or tiapride (maximum of 900 mg/d) is good. In 1991, a dramatic recovery to the point of independent life was reported in a patient treated with thyrotropin-releasing hormone injections,[140] but spontaneous recovery from CPM is well known.

Magnetic resonance imaging has facilitated the diagnosis of CPM ante mortem and has carefully characterized the disorder. Computed tomography (CT) scanning, however, with detailed views of the pons may also yield clearly distinctive abnormalities. Most commonly, a symmetrical oval area of prolonged T1 or T2 relaxation is found (Fig. 7–2A), but lesions in the bases of the pontes may also be trident- or bat-shaped because horizontal tracts are preferentially involved and vertical tracts are spared (Fig. 7–2B and C). It may take 2 weeks before lesions appear on sagittal MRI.

Magnetic resonance imaging may reveal extrapontine lesions, which, as mentioned previously, may be present in the lateral thalamus and subcortical white matter.[96,99] Bilateral thalamic involvement of the lateral and centromedian nucleus may be typical in extrapontine myelinolysis, differentiating it from the bilateral paramedian thalamic infarctions.

Follow-up MRI may show resolution of the T1 hypointensity, presumably as a result of diminished edema in the area of demyelination. The extrapontine manifestations resolve first.[57] No correlation exists between persistent MRI findings and subsequent potential for recovery.

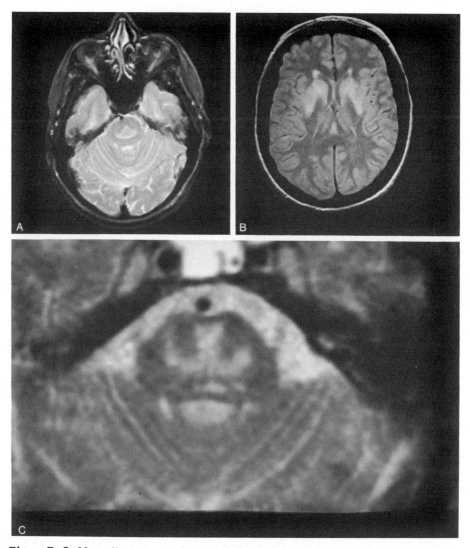

Figure 7–2. Magnetic resonance images. *A*, Central pontine location of lesion. *B*, Extra-pontine lesions in caudate nucleus and putamen bilaterally. *C*, Typical trident shape in central pontine myelinolysis.

POSTOPERATIVE HYPONATREMIA SYNDROME IN YOUNG HEALTHY WOMEN

A fulminant neurologic disorder associated with severe (and probably unrecognized) hyponatremia has been specifically linked to elective surgery.[5,15] The condition is rare, because in the first retrospective survey, 15 healthy women were seen in 15 medical centers in 10 years.[5] Two days after the operation, all patients had grand mal seizures followed within 1 hour by respiratory arrest. In many of the patients, serum sodium levels were not routinely measured postoperatively, and the nonspecific signs of early hyponatremia, such as nausea, vomiting, and headache, were not recognized as such. Excessive administration of free water led to sodium levels generally less than 110 mmol/L.

Many patients had fixed, dilated pupils after resuscitation; four patients died, and nine patients remained in a vegetative state. The remaining two patients, who survived with moderate deficits, had been treated immediately after the first seizure. CT scan in these patients may show obliteration of sulci and basal cisterns but may give negative results. Autopsy demonstrated demyelination in addition to cerebral edema. (Brain swelling may have caused the respiratory arrest from compression of the medulla through herniation.) Both CT scan and postmortem findings may be the result of hypoxic brain damage (see Chapter 6).

An intriguing feature of this syndrome is the female preponderance. Most reported patients are healthy women undergoing abdominal, gynecologic, cosmetic, or other mostly relatively minor elective procedures. This syndrome of postoperative hyponatremia in women with cerebral edema has been tentatively linked to sodium-potassium - adenosinetriphosphatase pump dysfunction, because sex differences in this pump have been found in animal studies.

Postoperative severe hyponatremia with respiratory arrest has also been documented in patients with transurethral prostatectomy, usually associated with bladder irrigation. Nevertheless, in many male patients, the outcome is good despite seizures.[15] Hyponatremia can be severe in post-transurethral prostatectomy, but serum osmolality is quite high from bladder absorption of hypertonic glycine, frequently used as an irrigant. Rapid excretion of the glycine by the kidney restores plasma osmolality. (It is important to make this distinction rather than attribute sex differences to complications of hyponatremia.)

In the first postoperative hours, many patients may also have morphine pumps for pain control, and currently the doses are often self-administered. Repeated doses of morphine may cause vomiting and, together with liberal fluid administration in the immediate postoperative course, may lead to rapidly evolving hyponatremia.

A review of all postoperative respiratory and cardiac arrests in women during 1976 to 1992 in Rochester, Minn, was negative for associated severe hyponatremia.[147] In this period, 1498 of 290,815 women (0.5%) who had surgical procedures experienced postoperative cardiac or respiratory arrest. In none of these patients was severe hyponatremia of less than 125 mmol/L found. New-onset postoperative seizures occurred in three elderly patients with hyponatremia, but all had hyponatremia associated with a severe life-threatening illness. The true prevalence of this disorder carefully outlined by Arieff[5] needs to be further determined, but our data convince us that the entity is extremely uncommon.

A variant syndrome of central diabetes mellitus and insipidus, reported in 1990, is controversial and has not gained universal acceptance or credibility.[43] Again, severe hyponatremia after elective surgery in previously healthy women resulted in seizures and respiratory arrest 15 to 56 hours after recovery from the surgical procedure. Hyponatremia (mean, 116 ± 2 mmol/L) was attributed to SIADH and excessive administration of free water, but loss of isotonic fluids associated with frequent vomiting or nasogastric suction often was present as well.

After seizures and respiratory arrest, decorticate posturing was soon followed by loss of virtually all brain stem reflexes. The clinical course is very much like that of the postoperative hyponatremic syndrome.

Some interesting features were brain edema on CT scan in all patients and concomitant diabetes insipidus and hyperglycemia. Whether this clinical syndrome represents a new entity or, much more likely, simply reflects systemic manifestations in patients who became brain dead from severe cerebral edema after prolonged resuscitation remains unclear. Transtentorial herniation and ischemic infarcts of pituitary lobes and the hypothalamus were found and tentatively linked to clinical findings of diabetes mellitus and insipidus, but both these abnormalities alone are also compatible with brain death or with brain-swelling–induced compression of the diencephalon against the clivus, resulting in hypothalmic infarcts.

OSMOTIC DEMYELINATION SYNDROME

Although directly related to the correction of hyponatremia, this well-described clinical phenomenon remains an enigma.[29,71] In their report on eight patients treated over a 5-year period at two institutions, Sterns and associates[129–131] postulated that myelinolytic lesions seen in the deep cortical cell layers and in the pons result from iatrogenic rapid correction of hyponatremia. Possible etiologic considerations are the "grid" phenomenon, suggesting strangulation of myelinated fibers by surrounding edema in the pons, and "osmotic endothelial injury," which implies that rapid osmotic changes of endothelial cells in the gray matter may release myelotoxic factors.

A 1991 experimental study, however, offered a novel hypothesis based on the finding that lost osmoles are not rapidly replaced when needed.[138] Loss of osmoles in hyponatremia treated with rapid infusion of hypertonic saline is offset not by an accumulation of osmoles but by electrolyte reaccumulation and a much slower increase in osmoles. The absence of osmole protection and increased high ionic strength may be harmful to protein interactions in oligodendrocytes, but whether this explanation is sufficient has not yet been unarguably shown.

The clinical features of this syndrome tend to be stereotypical. After correction of severe hyponatremia with hypertonic saline, patients awake without any major appreciable deficit only to have gradual deterioration 2 to 3 days later. A biphasic course occurred in half of Arieff's patients with severe postoperative hyponatremia.[5] After rapid correction of serum sodium deficiency, patients significantly improve in level of consciousness but continue to complain of throbbing headaches and nausea. New-onset vomiting and seizures mark the beginning of a lapse into an unresponsive coma, occasionally with a fatal course. Some clinical features (but not the pathologic findings) may be reminiscent of delayed anoxic-hypoxic encephalopathy, as reported by Plum and coworkers[110] (see Chapter 6).

Pathologic data for these patients are scarce, but one carefully documented case report noted multifocal demyelination without any evidence of massive brain edema.[29] This rare syndrome may be considered a variant of CPM and may occur less frequently if hyponatremia is prudently managed.

TREATMENT OF SEVERE HYPONATREMIA

Many guidelines for intervention in acute hyponatremia have been proposed,[19,102,106,128] but trials in human subjects are lacking. Readers are referred to many excellent editorials on this subject.[19,77,102]

The clinical dilemma is that acute severe hyponatremia (for example, decrease of 20 to 40 mmol/L in 24 hours) may, in predisposed patients, be associated with severe brain edema resulting in irreversible herniation, and rapid correction (more than 24 mmol/L a day) may result in CPM or osmotic demyelination syndrome. In addition, both conditions remain rare complications in patients with severe hyponatremia.

Treatment of acute severe hyponatremia should depend on whether symptoms are present. In the vast majority of patients, fluid overload causes hyponatremia, but other triggers should be identified and corrected (Table 7–6). It may be prudent to increase the serum sodium concentration to values of 125 mmol/L with 3% hypertonic saline. Additional furosemide or any other loop diuretic may be appropriate to decrease excess free water, but the initial diuretic response may be unpredictable and may lead to unexpected higher sodium values.

Treatment of symptomatic hyponatremia, usually noticed by progressive decrease in alertness and generalized seizures, is begun with 3% hypertonic saline. Hypertonic saline with 512 mEq of sodium has a concentration of 0.5 mEq/mL. With an average of 50% of body weight, 1 mL/kg of 3% hypertonic saline increases the serum sodium concentration by 1 mEq/kg. Therefore, a safe correction guideline is to administer 0.5 mL/kg per hour of 3% hypertonic saline until the plasma sodium value reaches 125 mEq/L, but the infusion rate can be doubled to 1 mL/kg per hour if seizures persist. Plasma sodium concentration should be checked every hour to prevent rapid correction and, more important, "overcorrection" to values above 140 mEq/L. Patients who do not improve and who continue to have seizures should be loaded with phenytoin rather than with further increase in the rate of sodium administration or, worse, rapid infusion of 100 to 300 mL of hypertonic saline.

Patients may benefit from a short course of dexamethasone (for example, 4 mg given four times a day) when sodium correction is unexpectedly rapid. Data in rats suggest that demyelination can be prevented with high doses of corticosteroids.[107,117] One approach is given in Figure 7–3.

Hypernatremia

Elderly critically ill patients are susceptible to hypernatremia when there is no access to water.[87,126] Hypernatremia is usually the result of water depletion in excess of sodium, but hypernatremia can occur in states of euvolemia or hypervolemia. Common examples are excess administration of hypertonic sodium bicarbonate to correct metabolic acidosis, and malfunction of the dialysate-proportioning system during hemodialysis.

It is not surprising that failure to replace insensible losses from the skin and respiratory tract is the most common cause of hypernatremia in ICUs. Another common cause is sustained infusion of large volumes of isotonic sodium chloride in patients with hypotonic fluid loss or shock.[126] The most frequently encountered causes of hypernatremia in the ICU are listed in Table 7–7.

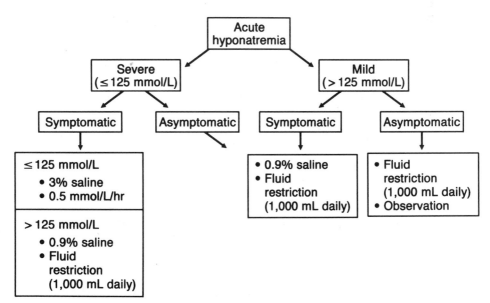

Figure 7–3. Algorithm for treatment of severe acute hyponatremia.

Table 7-7 COMMON CAUSES OF HYPERNATREMIA

Increased insensible fluid loss
  Fever
  Respiratory infection
  Burns
Osmotic diarrhea (lactulose); osmotic diuresis
Diabetes insipidus
Massive brain swelling (any cause)
Head injury
Brain death
Drugs
  Lithium
  Demeclocycline
  Amphotericin
  Methoxyflurane
  Cisplatin
Hypertonic saline administration
  Sodium bicarbonate
  Dialysis fluids

CLINICAL FEATURES

A fair degree of concordance exists between the clinical manifestations of hypernatremia and the extracellular fluid deficit. Although hypernatremia has its greatest effect on the central nervous system, other features immediately suggest a hyperosmolar state. Signs of extracellular volume depletion are dehydration, skin tenting, dry mucous membranes, and tachycardia. These signs are less obvious in elderly patients. Most patients are drowsy, but periods of diminished arousability may be interspersed with periods of restlessness and confusion. In many elderly patients, a mild degree of Alzheimer's disease or vascular dementia may be unmasked or aggravated by hypernatremia. Focal motor signs, as in hyponatremia, do not occur. Generalized seizures are unusual, even in patients with marked increase in sodium levels (greater than 160 mmol/L). Asterixis and myoclonus have been described but are generally seen in patients who also have hepatic encephalopathy. Other very infrequent clinical manifestations are rigidity, tremor, myoclonus, and chorea.[8,127] A primary neurologic disorder resulting in hypernatremia is more likely than the converse.

As dehydration and hypernatremia become severe, patients become unresponsive. The clinical course may be fulminant in postoperative patients or patients in whom hemodialysis is associated with technical problems.

Arieff and Carroll's study[7] on hyperglycemia and hypernatremia showed that most patients remained alert when plasma osmolality remained under 350 mosm/kg. Progressive drowsiness occurred beyond this critical value. Usually, however, there is a marked overlap between the degree of hypernatremia and the degree of coma.

The degree of hypernatremia may not significantly increase the probability of neurologic sequelae. Although permanent cognitive changes, attentional deficits, and faulty memory are common in patients who survive severe hypernatremia, in many patients the underlying clinical condition determines outcome and morbidity.[101] Mortality from severe hypernatremia (greater than 160 mmol/L) can be 70% in susceptible patients. The chance of recovery in patients who remain alert at peak sodium values is high irrespective of the pace of correction chosen.

TREATMENT

The ideal rate of fluid resuscitation in hypernatremic patients is not known but may in part depend on the rate at which hypernatremia develops. Fatal cerebral edema, often accompanied by grand mal seizures, occurred in patients within 24 hours after acute hypernatremia had been corrected. As in hyponatremia, overly rapid correction may be hazardous, but clinical evidence is lacking. In hypovolemic patients, intravascular volume should be replaced with isotonic saline or colloids, and a reduction of 1 to 2 mEq/L of sodium per hour may be prudent. Hypernatremia may reoccur if the underlying systemic disease is not corrected.

Hypokalemia

Most critically ill patients seem to have hypokalemia at some stage in their

Table 7-8 COMMON CAUSES OF HYPOKALEMIA

Gastrointestinal
  Vomiting
  Fistula
  Nasogastric suction
Skin losses
  Profound sweating
  Burns
Drugs
  Loop or thiazide diuretics
  Amphotericin B
  Adrenergics
  Insulin
  Penicillin derivatives
  Others
Neoplastic disorders
  Acute leukemia
  Primary hyperaldosteronism
Metabolic disorders
  Hypocalcemia
  Hypomagnesemia
  Metabolic alkalosis

clinical course, and often there is more than one reason for potassium deficiency. Common causes for hypokalemia are gastrointestinal, renal, and skin losses (Table 7-8). Any of these disturbances can lead to profound hypokalemia, but in many persons, the nasogastric suctioning puts them at risk. Nasogastric suctioning can cause extracellular fluid volume deficits that result in increased serum concentration of aldosterone, which in turn results in increased renal excretion of potassium and thus hypokalemia. The development of metabolic alkalosis from nasogastric suctioning may also cause an increase in renal potassium excretion.

MYOPATHY

Potassium depletion from any cause may lead to severe muscle weakness and, in its extreme form, to quadriplegia and respiratory failure. Many patients with potassium losses remain symptom-free, but neurologic manifestations are inevitable with plasma potassium concentrations of less than 2 mEq/L. When the serum potassium level becomes less than normal (less than 3 mEq/L), total body potassium stores are likely significantly depleted. With significant total body potassium depletion, electrocardiographic changes are often seen, including prominent U waves, ST segment changes, dampened T wave, and, more important, atrial and ventricular arrhythmias.

Muscle weakness usually progresses over several days in the ICU. Proximal leg, neck, and trunk muscle weakness is an early sign. Many patients cannot sit without help or lift their head from the pillow.[89] Aching pain in the back and fleshy muscles is common. Muscle cramps, nocturnal myoclonus, and symptoms mimicking restless leg syndrome may become extremely disruptive at night and result in additional fatigue and exhaustion. In exceptional cases, hypokalemia may be associated with rapid ascending weakness and respiratory failure suggesting Guillain-Barré syndrome, but sensory symptoms, cranial nerve deficits, and areflexia are usually absent. Distal muscles seldom become prominently involved, but if they do, they recover first after correction. Ventilatory failure, difficulty swallowing secretions, and slurred speech have been described, but as mentioned previously, usually the electrocardiographic abnormalities and progressive weakness have already prompted rapid correction.

Most patients with severe hypokalemia have a mild degree of rhabdomyolysis. Rhabdomyolysis (see Chapter 3) is not significant enough to result in its classic manifestations with compartment syndromes or acute tubular necrosis. Widespread muscle pain that may have started in the calves is present. Muscles are firmly swollen and extremely tender to touch. Many patients complain of intensifying pain with movement. Creatine kinase levels are increased, as they are in patients with moderate weakness from hypokalemia alone. The mechanism of rhabdomyolysis in severe hypokalemia is not known, but correction of hypokalemia results in marked improvement in a few weeks, as it does in patients with abnormal muscle biopsy findings.

TREATMENT

Correction in patients with severe hypokalemia is usually at a maximum rate of 10 to 20 mEq/h, but the rate may be tripled in patients with severe weakness. More than 20 mEq/h may, however, result in potentially life-threatening heart block and should in general be avoided, including in patients with severe muscle pain. Patients may have a relapse of proximal weakness after potassium correction, usually from rapid entry of potassium into depleted cells. Therefore, the potassium correction should be continued until most of the weakness has resolved. Permanent neurologic deficits have not been described after rapid or slow intravenous correction of potassium concentration.

Hyperkalemia

Increased plasma potassium levels may alter the electrical excitability of nerve and muscle membranes, usually when the concentration reaches 7 mEq/L.

Hyperkalemia is common in medical ICUs because a disproportionately large number of the patients have renal failure. Other frequent causes are pseudohyperkalemia from hemolysis during venipuncture, pseudohyperkalemia associated with severe thrombocytosis or leukocytosis, and hyperkalemia associated with succinylcholine use.

Hyperkalemia has also been anecdotally described in patients on cardiac bypass. In these patients, increased plasma potassium may be induced by washout of ischemic underperfused areas during bypass or may be caused by rewarming after hypothermia. Most commonly, hyperkalemia is encountered in patients with renal or adrenal failure. Hypoadrenalism is the most common adrenal disorder resulting in hyperkalemia, is potentially life-threatening, and probably is overlooked for

Table 7–9 COMMON CAUSES OF HYPERKALEMIA

Pseudohyperkalemia
Renal disorders
Hypoadrenalism
Pharmacologic agents
   Potassium-sparing diuretics
   Angiotensin-converting enzyme inhibitors
   Cyclosporine
   Succinylcholine
Diabetic ketoacidosis
Multiple blood transfusions

some time in the ICU. Certain drugs, often those that impair renal function, may increase potassium levels (Table 7–9).

CLINICAL FEATURES

The pathophysiologic consequences of hyperkalemia (potassium concentrations greater than 7.5 mEq/L) are predominantly cardiac. Cardiac conduction abnormalities can lead to widening of the PR interval and QRS complex, but initial changes are a peaking, narrowed T wave and a shortened QT interval. Ventricular fibrillation may occur.

The relationship between hyperkalemia and cardiac manifestations is not always clear, particularly when the rise in potassium concentration is gradual. Neurologic manifestations may precede cardiac manifestations. Neurologic manifestations may become more evident than cardiac manifestations in patients who have hypercalcemia, which may protect the heart from dysrhythmias.

Similar to hypokalemia, hyperkalemia may result in proximal leg weakness with inability to lift the legs from the bed.[23,78,111] Percussion myotonia can be demonstrated in some patients. Burning dysesthesias without objective sensory loss are very common. When hyperkalemia is not appreciated, the condition may worsen to quadriplegia and respiratory failure. Transient diplopia has been ascribed to myotonia in the internal and external ocular muscles. Facial and pharyngeal muscles may be affected, but this progression has been anecdotal; otherwise, cranial nerve deficits are uncommon. Some patients may have generalized myotonia in the forearms, hands, and calves.

TREATMENT AND OUTCOME

In life-threatening hyperkalemia, efforts should be directed at all levels, that is, stabilization of the heart with calcium carbonate, increased potassium influx with insulin and glucose or bicarbonate, and elimination of total body potassium stores with cation-exchange resins or dialysis if necessary. In less critical situations, efforts should be directed at correcting the underlying cause, eliminating potassium sources, and increasing potassium excretion (for example, by cation-exchange resins, diuretics, or dialysis). All patients recover from weakness within 1 to 4 hours after treatment, and any failure should suggest other causes.

Hypophosphatemia

The true incidence of severe phosphorus depletion in the ICU is not known, but the patient population is certainly predisposed. Critically ill patients have an increased need of phosphate. Most instances of depletion are associated with long-term antacid therapy, hemodialysis, hyperalimentation with phosphate-poor solutions, and sepsis[20,22,54,63,68,73,75,123] (Table 7–10). In 10% to 20% of patients, the cause of

Table 7–10 COMMON CAUSES OF HYPOPHOSPHATEMIA

Malabsorption syndrome (bypass surgery)
Prolonged vomiting or gastric suction
Gram-negative and gram-positive sepsis
Hepatic failure
Burns
Chronic alcoholism
Pharmacologic agents
   Catecholamines
   Thiazide diuretics
   Antacids

hypophosphatemia is unknown. In patients with severe burns, profound hypophosphatemia often occurs in the recovery phase, presumably from increased anabolism during healing. Mild asymptomatic hypophosphatemia may occur in patients with respiratory alkalosis either from mechanical ventilation with relatively large tidal volumes or from spontaneous hyperventilation. In other patients, mild hypophosphatemia may become more profound after glucose infusion, particularly in those who are starved and emaciated.

The neurologic manifestations can be realistically expected only when serum phosphate levels are below 1 mg/dL, and neuromuscular manifestations are usually present.[73] For seizures and neuromuscular manifestations to occur, a substantial decrease below 0.5 mg/dL must take place.

ACUTE FLACCID AREFLEXIC PARALYSIS

A salient feature of this generally uncommon condition is its rapid onset and progression. Usually within 1 day, perioral paresthesias are followed by virtually complete quadriplegia, ptosis, and difficulty swallowing. Sensory ataxia may occur. This dramatic progression of symptoms is seldom seen in ICUs staffed by physicians aware of the dangers of suboptimal supplementation in these patients.

A probably much more common manifestation of severe hypophosphatemia is diaphragmatic weakness associated with proximal muscle weakness.[49,53,116] Diaphragmatic failure associated with hypophosphatemia results in an inability to be weaned from the ventilator. In patients with chronic pulmonary disease and any medical or surgical critical illness, hypophosphatemia may markedly contribute to the already high propensity for weaning failure. Phosphorus depletion has been shown to improve inspiratory pressures, and supplementation therefore may optimize the clinical conditions for weaning from the ventilator.

HYPOPHOSPHATEMIC ENCEPHALOPATHY

An incompletely delineated encephalopathy associated with phosphorus depletion has been described.[75,123]

Severe hypophosphatemia may be associated with combative behavior, acute confusional state, seizures, and coma. Tremor, ataxia, nystagmus, and bilateral abducens paresis have been noted, closely mimicking Wernicke's encephalopathy. Many other clinical manifestations have been reported, including asterixis, tremors, ataxia, and pseudobulbar palsy, but many of these reported features have not been confirmed by neurologists. In addition, changes in level of consciousness are more likely to be associated with marked hypoxia from alveolar hypoventilation that is caused by diaphragmatic weakness.

TREATMENT

In the vast majority of the patients, oral phosphate supplementation is preferred and can be easily achieved by increasing milk products in the diet or by adding standard oral preparations. In severe cases, intravenous phosphate supplementation at a dose of 2 mg/kg every 6 hours is appropriate.[80,137] The neurologic findings completely resolve when the serum phosphate concentration returns to values above 1.5 mg/dL.

Hyperphosphatemia

A small rise in serum phosphate concentration is sufficient to cause a decrease in serum ionized calcium. Therefore, an increase in serum phosphate results in clinical manifestations from hypocalcemia. Hyperphosphatemia may affect many organs, but deposition of amorphous calcium phosphate usually occurs in chronic conditions. Acute hyperphosphatemia is invariably associated with acute hypocalcemia, which may be severe enough to cause tonic-clonic seizures and tetany.

Table 7–11 COMMON CAUSES OF HYPOMAGNESEMIA

Parenteral nutrition
Acute pancreatitis
Bowel surgery
Renal disorders
   Acute tubular necrosis
   Postdiuretic-phase renal
     transplantation
Endocrine disorders
   Hypoparathyroidism
   Hyperaldosteronism
Pharmacologic agents
   Antibiotic combinations
   Antineoplastic drugs

Hypomagnesemia

Magnesium depletion is common in the ICU from loss of gastrointestinal fluid, prolonged parenteral nutrition, or abdominal surgical procedures associated with depleted magnesium stores[16,27,64,66] (Table 7–11).

CLINICAL FEATURES

The frequent association of magnesium deficiency with hypocalcemia, hypokalemia, and alkalosis markedly confounds its clinical manifestations. In addition, magnesium administration alone often results in correction of other laboratory abnormalities. The biochemical significance of hypomagnesemia, therefore, remains somewhat obscure.

Magnesium deficiency readily induces muscular twitching, myoclonus, startle responses, and postural tremor.[69] Trousseau's and Chvostek's signs, carpopedal spasm, and, rarely, tetany have also been reported but are most characteristic of hypocalcemia. In many patients, periods of anxiety and fear, dilated pupils, sweating, tachycardia, hostile behavior, and hallucinations develop, in some associated with downbeat nystagmus[120] and ataxia. Unrecognized severe hypomagnesemia may predispose to tonic-clonic seizures.

TREATMENT

Hypomagnesemia, defined as a plasma level of less than 1.7 mg/dL, should be treated immediately, especially in patients with seizures, although threshold levels are generally less than 1 mEq/L. Magnesium sulfate in a dose of 2 g of a 10% solution should be administered over a 2-minute period and be followed by infusion of 12 g in 1 L of fluid over a 12-hour period. A more prudent schedule in patients with less urgent manifestations is intramuscular injection with 1 g of magnesium sulfate every 4 hours.

Hypermagnesemia

At the neuromuscular junction, magnesium competes with calcium and displaces it from its target site. As a result, release of acetylcholine and, to a large extent, the excitability of the muscle membrane decrease. Its effects on the central nervous system are less well characterized but may be related to stabilization of the synaptic membrane, which leads to decreased excitability.

Most commonly, hypermagnesemia occurs with the use of magnesium-containing antacids and laxatives in patients with renal failure or in eclamptic mothers[132] (Table 7–12).

Clinical features generally appear when serum magnesium levels exceed 4 mg/dL. Magnesium levels reaching 10 mg/dL almost certainly result in severe weakness and areflexia.

The typical neurologic manifestations of magnesium excess are usually not present in clinical conditions without exogenous intake of magnesium. Chronic renal failure, lithium therapy, hypothyroidism, hyperparathyroidism

with renal disease, and pheochromocytoma indeed may all cause a patient to be susceptible to increases of serum magnesium, but in these instances, transmission block of the neuromuscular junction is generally not clinically relevant.

CLINICAL FEATURES

Increasing plasma levels of magnesium lead to nausea, vomiting, cutaneous flushing, and dry mouth. A decrease in deep tendon reflexes is typical. In some patients, progression of limb weakness is rapid and bifacial weakness occurs. Extraocular and oropharyngeal muscles become involved, and some patients may become "locked in." Decreased level of consciousness is not a feature of hypermagnesemia.

TREATMENT

Gradual improvement over days can be expected when no further magnesium or magnesium-containing substances are administered. In severe cases with heart block, calcium gluconate (10 mL of a 10% solution) reverses hypermagnesemia. Occasionally, patients do not recover completely, and they may have underlying myasthenic syndromes.[17]

Hypocalcemia

Hypocalcemia signifies a poor prognosis in patients who are critically ill. Causes frequently encountered in the ICU are outlined in Table 7–13.[40,95] Approximately half the total serum calcium is protein-bound, primarily by albumin. Differences in serum albumin concentration and state of hydration may cause variations in serum total calcium concentration.[150] The effect of albumin can be corrected by use of the following formula: adjusted measured serum calcium equals serum calcium plus 0.8 (4 minus serum albumin). A decrease in the concentration of serum albumin by 1 g/dL produces a decrease in

Table 7–12 COMMON CAUSES OF HYPERMAGNESEMIA

Exogenous magnesium intake
  Antacids
  Eclampsia treatment
Hemodialysis with high magnesium content
Rhabdomyolysis
Endocrine disorders
Acute diabetic ketoacidosis

Table 7–13 COMMON CAUSES OF HYPOCALCEMIA

Hypoalbuminemia
Gram-negative sepsis
Acute pancreatitis
Fat embolism
Severe crush injury
Postsurgical thyroid operation
Pharmacologic agents
  Chemotherapy
  Pentamidine and foscarnet
  Anticonvulsants

total serum calcium from 0.8 to 1 mg/dL, but the ionized fraction of calcium remains unchanged. Hypocalcemia associated with hypoalbuminemia does not cause symptoms because the ionized fraction remains similar.

CLINICAL FEATURES

Signs and symptoms of hypocalcemia have been well characterized.[41,42,47,118,149] Paresthesias in the hands and feet and around the lips are early signs but almost certainly go unnoticed in critically ill patients. Muscle cramps, carpopedal spasm, and laryngeal stridor may follow as hypocalcemia progresses. Plantar flexion of the toes, arching of the feet, and contraction of calf muscles may also be cardinal signs.

Chvostek's sign is frequently found (twitching of the mouth alone should not be interpreted as diagnostic because it may occur in 25% of normal patients).[58] This typical sign in hypocalcemia is elicited by tapping three fingers over the branches of the facial nerve anterior to the external auditory meatus. A positive response is indicated by twitching of all ipsilateral facial muscles (lip at angle of mouth, ala nasi, lateral angle of eye), although there may be a graded response. Latent tetany may also be demonstrated when a blood pressure cuff on one arm is inflated above the systolic blood pressure (Trousseau's sign) for at least 5 minutes.[81] Flexion of the fingers and adduction of the thumb produce a *main d'accoucheur.*

Hypocalcemia may produce papilledema, sometimes without an overt increase in CSF pressure.[108] Tonic-clonic seizures occur when serum calcium concentration is less than 3 mEq/L. In occasional cases, focal or nonconvulsive status may develop. Seizures stop after correction of hypocalcemia, but grand mal seizures may evolve into status epilepticus. Persistent coma from hypocalcemia is seldom seen, and if present, it is usually the result of anoxia associated with laryngeal stridor or poorly controlled status epilepticus.

TREATMENT

Hypocalcemia can be promptly corrected by a 2-hour intravenous infusion with 20 to 40 mL of a 10% solution of calcium gluconate followed by oral administration of calcium, 5 g/d. Muscle spasm, however, may persist for several hours after normalization of the calcium concentration. Virtually no patient has major neurologic sequelae after treatment.

Hypercalcemia

Hypercalcemia may result from primary hyperparathyroidism and malignant disease with or without metastasis. Neurologic manifestations are nonspecific and are usually found in patients with significant dehydration. Findings include marked drowsiness and impaired concentration, which occasionally progress to unresponsive coma. Many patients recover after general measures have been taken to correct dehydration.

ENDOCRINE EMERGENCIES

Patients with primary endocrine crisis are often gravely ill and present with dramatic clinical manifestations. At the other side of the spectrum, stressors in the ICU, whether major surgical procedures, infection, or multidrug regimens, may challenge the endocrine axis. Neurologic manifestations are common in patients in endocrine crises, and early recognition is fundamental to successful management.

Nonketotic Hyperosmolar State

The physiologic changes in nonketotic hyperosmolar state (NKHS) are predominantly hyperglycemia with no or only minimal ketosis and extreme dehydration, reflected in greatly increased plasma osmolality. Type II diabetes has been undiagnosed at the time of presentation in one third of patients with NKHS.

Nonketotic hyperosmolar state can occur as a complication of any bacterial infection or septic shock, extensive burns, acute pancreatitis, hyperalimentation, use of corticosteroids, and peritoneal dialysis (Table 7–14). However, postoperative NKHS is very common, and, in fact, most patients with NKHS are seen in surgical ICUs.[36,121] NKHS can be triggered by drugs with a known hyperglycemic effect (for example, furosemide, dopamine) or by fever in the first days after major surgical procedures. Seki[121] found that, on average, NKHS occurred on the sixth day after coronary bypass (range, 3 to 10 days).

Table 7–14 PRECIPITANTS OF HYPEROSMOLAR HYPERGLYCEMIC NONKETOTIC STATE

Drugs
  Thiazide diuretics
  Phenytoin
  Beta-adrenergic blocking agents
  Steroids
Hypovolemia
  Severe burns
  Gastrointestinal hemorrhage
Infection
  Gram-negative sepsis
  Pneumonia
Stroke
  Middle cerebral artery occlusion with swelling
  Subarachnoid hemorrhage
Miscellaneous
  Myocardial infarction
  Pulmonary embolus
  Hyperalimentation

Meticulous attention to early clinical signs and frequent serum glucose determinations may prevent diabetic patients from lapsing into this potentially fatal complication.

CLINICAL FEATURES

The classic features of NKHS consist of progressive drowsiness, coma, and occasional focal signs or focal epilepsy as the presenting sign.[48,50,67,86] In its most acute form, the syndrome can be manifested by refractory status epilepticus. Focal neurologic signs that lead admitting physicians to believe that their patients have had a stroke are aphasia, hemiparesis, and visual field defects, which have been reported in one third of patients. Transient bilateral Babinski's signs, muscle twitching, and tonic eye deviation also may occur. In patients with less severe hyperglycemia, focal seizures may dominate the clinical picture. One review of 158 patients noted seizures in about one fourth of the patients with NKHS and focal motor seizures in 19%. Epilepsia partialis continua, however, generally occurs in patients with a preexisting structural lesion, mostly a result of earlier ischemic stroke.[125] Unusual types of focal epilepsy, including stereotypical movements, speech arrest, and flashing colored lights,[51] have also been described in patients with nonketotic hyperglycemia. Extremely uncommon manifestations are opsoclonus-myoclonus,[91] choreoathetosis, hemiballismus, and posture-induced seizures (clonic and brief jerking movements triggered by active or passive change in head or arm position).[115] In many other patients, tonic-clonic seizures may be seen.

Neurologic signs and the degree of decrease in the level of consciousness appear to have a better correlation with plasma osmolality (Fig. 7–4) and serum sodium level than with absolute serum glucose concentration.[7,70] Nonketotic hyperglycemic coma often occurs with a sixfold to tenfold increase in serum glucose.

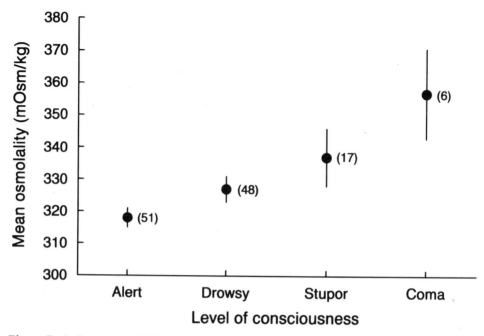

Figure 7–4. Serum osmolality and its relation to mental status in 122 patients with ketoacidosis. Numbers in parentheses indicate patients. (From Kitabchi, AE and Fisher, JN: Insulin therapy of diabetic ketoacidosis: Physiologic versus pharmacologic doses of insulin and their routes of administration. In Brownlee, M [ed]: Handbook of Diabetes Mellitus. Vol 5: Current and Future Therapies. Garland STPM Press, New York, 1981, pp 95–149, with permission of Garland Publishing.)

In patients with nonketotic hyperosmolar states, hyponatremia often occurs because increased osmotic pressure from hyperglycemia shifts fluid from cells into the extracellular fluid space. Despite hyponatremia, a hyperosmolar state exists, and efforts should be directed to correcting the hyperosmolar-hyperglycemic state and not the hyponatremia per se.

The corrected serum sodium value (calculated by increasing the serum sodium concentration by 1.3 to 1.6 mmol/L for every 5.56 mmol/L [100 mg/dL] increment in the serum glucose concentration) is a good guideline in predicting cellular dehydration and subsequent neurologic signs and symptoms.[32] Patients with hyponatremia but normal corrected serum sodium concentrations and increased plasma osmolality and hyperglycemia usually do not have neurologic signs, because dehydration is limited. On the other hand, patients with a normal, low, or high serum sodium level but a high corrected serum sodium value who are in a hyperglycemic and hyperosmolar state may have a severely depressed consciousness.

TREATMENT

Nonketotic hyperosmolar coma is associated with hypovolemia, which explains hyperglycemia (euvolemia would result in increased secretion of glucose and prevent high concentration in the blood).

A crucial element in the treatment of nonketotic hyperosmolar coma is rehydration with isotonic saline to establish adequate filling of the intravascular compartment. Insulin therapy can be withheld because of (unproven) concerns that the combination with rehydration will induce cerebral edema.

Outcome in nonketotic hyperosmolar

coma is generally determined by early recognition and proper measures. Whether aggressive correction of the hyperosmolality results in secondary insults to the brain is not supported by clinical data. Also, there are virtually no outcome data on patients who survive the insult, although the clinical impression is that many do well.[70] Nevertheless, with one third of the outcomes fatal in most medical and surgical series, mortality remains unacceptably high. The most common cause of death is the underlying disease that triggered coma.

Diabetic Ketoacidotic Coma

The hallmarks are severe hyperglycemia, ketoacidosis, and hyperosmolarity. Frequently, patients are known to have type I (juvenile-onset) diabetes, whereas nonketotic hyperosmolar coma more often occurs in type II diabetes. Ketoacidotic coma, however, may be a presenting feature.

Hyperosmolarity may be less prominent in ketoacidosis than in nonketotic states, but again degree of drowsiness may be more proportional to the severity of dehydration (Fig. 7–4). One large retrospective study of 287 episodes of diabetic ketoacidosis found only a weak correlation between H^+ concentrations and the degree of coma and confirmed the clinical impression that many diabetic patients with severe metabolic acidosis are alert.[119]

Focal signs are extremely uncommon in ketoacidotic coma and suggest an underlying structural cause. Some patients with diabetic ketoacidotic coma may be hypothermic whether or not they have a serious infection. Fulminant bacterial meningitis should be considered in any patient with diabetic coma unresponsive to fluid resuscitation (see Chapter 5).

Only general guidelines to treatment of diabetic ketoacidotic coma can be given because randomized trials are lacking. Most experts in this field favor infusion with saline, 100 to 150 mmol/L in the first 12 hours and 50 to 70 mmol/ L thereafter.[52] One small randomized study on the effect of additional bicarbonate infusion showed no advantage in patients with an initial pH of 6.9 to 7.1.[100] A study comparing different regimens of insulin therapy concluded that intravenous infusion of insulin (low doses), saline, and dextrose, with the addition of bicarbonate only if the pH was less than 7.1, was superior to other regimens.[62] Use of colloid in an attempt to restore the circulating volume is not supported by any controlled trial and is not without risk and expense.[56]

Most patients survive the metabolic derangement without any significant residual deficit. Cerebral edema during treatment of diabetic ketoacidosis is a rare but nearly uniformly fatal complication.[28,33] The occurrence of massive cerebral edema, mostly in children and adolescents, is unpredictable, and high-risk patients have not been identified.[34,44]

The clinical presentation of cerebral edema associated with treatment of diabetic acidosis is striking. After initial biochemical and clinical improvement, the patient rapidly relapses into coma with posturing, soon followed by fixed and dilated pupils. In many patients, the clinical criteria of brain death are present within 1 to 2 hours. Clinical deterioration may occur up to 24 hours after initiation of therapy. Increased muscle tone, gegenhalten, or focal seizures may herald the drowsiness. Papilledema may be present but only in patients who already have decerebrate posturing. The classic stages of transtentorial herniation are usually not present, and most patients have sudden respiratory arrest and immediate loss of brain stem reflexes. Treatment with mannitol, fluid restriction, and corticosteroids is unsuccessful in most cases, but rapid initiation of mannitol (2 g/kg of body weight) and fluid restriction (1.3 L/m^2 per 24 hours) occasionally salvages patients. Favorable outcome has been reported, but many patients may have residual severe cognitive deficits and ataxia. In 1987, an isolated growth hormone deficiency was described in a patient who recovered from cerebral edema.[65]

Computerized tomography scanning may demonstrate signs of cerebral edema, marked by decrease in size of the lateral ventricles and obliteration of the ambient cisterns. Findings on the initial CT scan do not predict later occurrence of cerebral edema. Two serial CT scan studies showed that brain swelling (defined as decreased size of ventricles or cisterns) was present before treatment, was largely unchanged after 6 to 8 hours of treatment, and resolved significantly a week after treatment.[59,74] Fatal cerebral edema, however, did not occur. Hoffman and associates,[59] therefore, raised the possibility that fatal edema during treatment may be merely a progression of an already initiated physiologic process.

Two major hypotheses have emerged over the years. Again, cerebral edema may be explained in terms of *idiogenic osmoles* that serve to protect the brain from shrinkage at the time of profound dehydration. Unfortunately, these molecules may slowly dissipate and their unwanted presence consequently may lead to brain edema when fluid infusion rapidly results in a hypo-osmotic state. However, this hypothesis lacks good support, because no correlation could be found with any of the following treatment modes or biochemical factors: excessive hypotonic fluid replacement, serum sodium values, osmolality, and insulin protocols. Others suggested that a Na^+/H^+ exchanger may be involved.[136] This hypothesis would indeed support the pretreatment subclinical presence of cerebral edema and temporal relation with insulin and fluid treatment.

This Na^+/H^+ exchanger can be activated by insulin, as convincingly demonstrated in other tissues (for example, muscle).[72] This activation results in sodium influx into the cells and brain swelling. There may be a rationale for Na^+/H^+ exchanger inhibitors such as amiloride (which, on the basis of molecular properties, should be able to cross the blood-brain barrier),[136] but clinical and experimental studies have not yet been performed.

Hypoglycemia

In most patients in the ICU, a hypoglycemic episode is a consequence of treatment with insulin. In others, inadequate management of parenteral nutrition can be held responsible for symptomatic episodes of hypoglycemia.[88]

Use of beta-blockers may generate hypoglycemia in insulin-treated diabetic patients but, more importantly, may also mask typical symptoms of hypoglycemia, such as tachycardia, sweating, and tremor.[55] These symptoms of hyperepinephrinemia may theoretically also go unnoticed in heavily sedated patients in the ICU. Other triggering events for significant hypoglycemia are fulminant hepatic failure, sepsis, and drugs with stimulating effects on insulin (Table 7–15).

The symptoms of hypoglycemia are produced by an adrenergic reaction and include pallor, sweating, tachycardia, sensation of hunger, anxiety, and palpitations (at times interpreted as critical care psychosis).

Neurologic symptoms cannot be predicted from blood glucose levels, but the depth of coma may have some correlation with the degree of hypoglycemia. Surprisingly, some patients with severe biochemical hypoglycemia are fully awake or only mildly disoriented. When

Table 7–15 CAUSES OF HYPOGLYCEMIA IN THE INTENSIVE CARE UNIT

Drugs
  Insulin
  Ouabain
  Beta-adrenergic blocking agents
  Pentamidine
Sepsis
Hepatic failure
Alimentary
  Postprandial after gastrectomy
  Discontinuing total parenteral alimentation

hypoglycemia develops slowly, blurred vision, slurred speech, and transient focal motor deficits are prominent.[97] Patients who become comatose quickly awaken after intravenous administration of glucose but may remain unconscious after prolonged hypoglycemic coma or after a concomitant tonic-clonic seizure. Seizures in hypoglycemia may occur in diabetic patients with previous strokes and rapid shifts in blood glucose concentration. In probably the largest series of patients with symptomatic hypoglycemia admitted to an emergency room, 9 of 125 visits were associated with seizures, usually tonic-clonic, but most patients were known epileptics or alcoholics. The neurologic manifestations of hypoglycemia are summarized in Table 7–16.

The principal signs and symptoms of hypoglycemia are behavior changes marked by confusion, vacant stare, or, in the extreme situation, unresponsiveness to pain stimuli. Marked chorioathetosis with facial grimacing at the time of hypoglycemia has been reported.[105] Transient hemiplegia has been associated with severe hypoglycemia.[143] Normalization of blood glucose concentration results in resolution of hemiplegia within minutes.

Episodes of hypoglycemia are treated with glucose in the range of 25 to 50 mL of 50% solution, and further deterioration should be prevented, often with simple measures. Severe hypoglycemic reactions may also be treated with glucagon. As alluded to earlier, most patients recover completely. The delay in recognition and the duration of coma probably determine neurologic sequelae. Patients with hypoglycemic coma of long duration (estimated to be approximately 4 to 6 hours) have a great chance of persistent vegetative state or severe disabling cerebellar signs.[3]

Many patients in whom autopsy was completed after prolonged hypoglycemic coma had selective neuronal vulnerability consisting of damage in the hippocampus, the striatum, and, in particular, the cerebellum.[11,124] Associated hypotension or marked hypoxia from gastric aspiration or hypoventilation in patients with prolonged hypoglycemia may be a confounding factor. Damage in the hippocampus may now be recognized on MRI (Fig. 7–5).

Thyroid Storm

An endocrine disorder of major importance is sudden thyrotoxicosis. Thyroid storm frequently occurs in patients with incomplete control but may be the first presentation of thyroid imbalance.[18]

The key clinical features (Table 7–17) are hyperthermia, tachycardia, and delirium.[45,139,142] Early in the course, patients may be anxious, nervous, and overreactive.

Marked psychiatric symptoms with vivid visual and acoustic hallucinations are occasionally present.[79,85] Untreated patients lapse into coma and may have decorticate posturing, prominent pyramidal signs with profound spasticity, pathologic brain stem reflexes, bilateral clonus, and Babinski's signs.[104]

Elderly patients may display a distinctive clinical syndrome of apathetic thyrotoxicosis (patients who "quietly and peacefully sink into coma and die an absolutely relaxed death without activation"[133]). Other distinctive features of apathetic thyrotoxicosis are absence of eye signs except for profound blepharoptosis and proximal myopathy. Patients with severe thyrotoxicosis more

Table 7–16 NEUROLOGIC MANIFESTATIONS OF HYPOGLYCEMIA

Presenting Symptom	Patient Visits, n*
Coma or stupor	55
Behavioral changes	38
Drowsiness	10
Dizziness, tremor	10
Seizures	9
Sudden hemiparesis	3

From Malouf and Brust,[88] with permission from Annals of Neurology.
*$n = 125$.

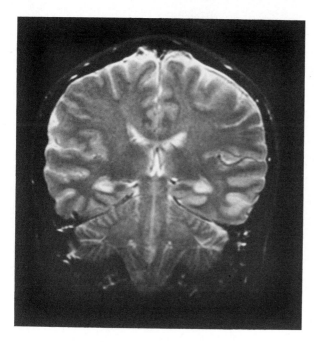

Figure 7–5. Magnetic resonance image, T2-weighted, of severe hippocampal damage after severe hypoglycemic insult. (Courtesy of Dr. B. F. Boeve, Department of Neurology, Mayo Clinic, Rochester, MN.)

often have periorbital puffiness and proptosis, which may be more prominent unilaterally (Fig. 7–6). Hyperthermia (often greater than 104°F) with excessive sweating and moist skin is a rather specific symptom. Multinodular thyromegaly is another frequent finding but may be absent in 10% of the patients.

Hyperthyroidism may be accompanied by acute thyrotoxic myopathy.[141] This entity is characterized by rapid muscular weakness associated with diaphragmatic failure, but unfortunately accurate documentation is scarce. To complicate matters further, thyrotoxicosis may be associated with myasthenia gravis and familial periodic paralysis.

Prompt treatment with propylthiouracil, propranolol, and corticosteroids results in a favorable outcome. Excess of circulating thyroid hormone may also be removed by plasma exchange or peritoneal dialysis. Emergency thyroid surgery may be indicated in patients with thyroid storm not controlled by these measures. Fatal outcome may be a consequence of irreversible congestive heart failure, extreme dehydration, and hypoglycemia, but many patients survive.

Myxedema Coma

The encephalopathy of hypothyroidism can be expected in patients with previously treated thyroid disease but may also develop from new-onset autoimmune thyroiditis. Other important triggers are bacterial infections, trauma, and recent thyroid surgery. Anesthesia, barbiturates, phenothiazines, and, in particular, imipramine may result in exacerbation of myxedema.[84] Exposure to cold is a well-recognized trig-

---

Table 7–17 CLINICAL FEATURES OF THYROID STORM

Hyperthermia
New-onset tachyarrhythmias
Jaundice
Delirium, stupor, coma
Proptosis, ophthalmoplegia
Pyramidal signs
Tremor, myoclonic jerks
Brisk tendon reflexes

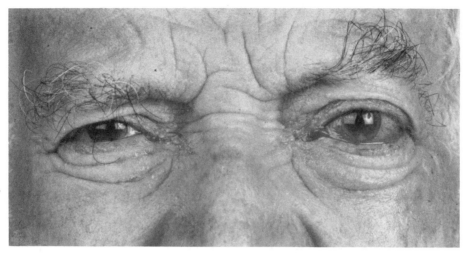

Figure 7–6. Proptosis in patient with hyperthyroidism.

ger, and one should be alert for a thyroid disorder in comatose patients during the cold season.

In patients with myxedema coma, the clinical characteristics are those of metabolic encephalopathy, with seizures and multifocal myoclonus. Tapping of muscles frequently leaves a transient local swelling that resembles myotonia. Tendon reflexes are diminished and may have a prolonged recovery phase. The typical features of hypothyroidism in patients with myxedema coma are usually present: dry, rough skin with yellow discoloration, puffy face and eyelids, and loss of outer eyebrows. Most patients hypoventilate and are cyanotic.[114] Hypothermia and bradycardia may also be the predominant findings.

It is important to recognize that associated metabolic factors, such as hypoglycemia, hyponatremia, and hypercalcemia, may cause coma.

Aggressive treatment of myxedema includes mechanical ventilation, fluid resuscitation in patients with hypotension, and parenteral administration of T_4 (500 μg, intravenous push).[31] Addison's disease may coexist; therefore, many patients need additional hydrocortisone (100 mg, intravenously). Conversely, hypothyroidism is not uncommon in Addison's disease, and after corticosteroid therapy, abnormal results of the thyroid-stimulating hormone test may normalize.

Hypothermia usually responds rapidly to correction of T_4 and triiodothyronine (T_3) levels. Except in patients with severe hypothermia (less than 90°F), additional support other than blankets is not necessary. Heating blankets, however, may worsen shock.

Outcome of myxedema coma is good if the patient survives the initial phase. Hylander and Rosenqvist[60] analyzed factors associated with fatal outcome and concluded that old age, initial hypothermia, shock, and excessive hormone doses of T_3 to correct hypothyroid state predicted poor outcome.

Adrenal Crisis

Acute adrenal insufficiency (Addison's disease) is a potential problem in any ICU. Adrenal crisis typically occurs in patients previously treated with steroids in whom the dose was not increased during intervals of stress.

Sepsis, recent major surgery, or use of drugs that interfere with hepatic biosynthesis or with the peripheral action of steroids (for example, ketoconazole, barbiturates, phenytoin, spironolactone) may predispose patients to Addison's disease.

Addison's disease is manifested by rapidly evolving shock and dehydration. Laboratory diagnosis reveals a plasma cortisol value of less than 15 μg/L, but the triad of hyponatremia, hyperglycemia, and hyperkalemia is also supportive. Many patients complain of migratory myalgias and weakness, and flexion pseudocontractures of the knees and hips are often present.[35] Pain may occur in any weak muscle, but the thigh muscles are particularly tender. Creatine kinase concentration may reach extremely high values and decrease after substitution. Electromyographic examination of affected muscles may show myopathic features with short duration and low-amplitude potentials.

Alternatively, weakness in an addisonian crisis may be associated with hyperkalemic myopathy[111] with flaccid tetraplegia or, in exceptional cases, with a Guillain-Barré–like syndrome.[1,25,98] The clinical features of Addison's disease are listed in Table 7–18.[103] Hyperpigmentation in scars, in mucous membranes, and along the gingival margin is a leading sign but may not be present.

The encephalopathy of adrenal insufficiency may have features of profound perceptual impairment, with lethargy progressing to coma. Bilateral papilledema has been described but only in association with pathologically demonstrated cerebral edema. In patients with severe electrolyte abnormalities and profound hypotension, "encephalopathie addisonienne," a term introduced by Klippel in 1899, may be difficult to diagnose.

Substitution of cortisol by corticosteroids (for example, hydrocortisone, 300 mg/day intravenously) and replacement of sodium and water deficit and electrolytes are the mainstays of treating the addisonian crisis. Outcome in most patients is good if the underlying cause is recognized and appropriately treated.

CONCLUSIONS

The correlation between neurologic features and acid-base derangements or severe electrolyte disorders is based on the first, rapid sign of recovery when the abnormality is being corrected. Electrolyte abnormalities are prevalent in critical illness. In principle, to produce neurologic symptoms, electrolyte abnormalities have to be severe, with substantial deviation from normal values but often also with a shift in a very short time span. However, patients can be asymptomatic.

The most common hospital- and ICU-associated electrolyte abnormality is hyponatremia. Causes in the postoperative period, in which hyponatremia is frequent, are morphine use that leads to vomiting in susceptible patients, water retention, and liberal use of fluids often given to overcome postoperative oliguria. Severe, unrecognized hyponatremia may cause seizures, respiratory arrest, and vegetative state or progression to brain death, particularly in young women. The condition is fortunately extremely rare. In many other patients, a single seizure or decrease in level of consciousness is seen. Although considerable debate has centered on the speed of correction, and some investigators insist that the issue is currently unresolved, many believe that correction of

Table 7–18 MAJOR SYMPTOMS AND SIGNS OF ADDISON'S DISEASE IN 100 PATIENTS

Findings	Patients, %
Weakness and fatigability	100
Weight loss	100
Hyperpigmentation	92
Hypotension	88
Hyponatremia	88
Hyperkalemia	64
Gastrointestinal symptoms	56
Postural dizziness	12
Muscle and joint pains	6
Hypercalcemia	6
Vitiligo	4

From Nerup,[103] with permission of Acta Endochronologica.

severe hyponatremia should be gradual to prevent demyelination in the pons. An important practical consideration is that overcorrection to values above 140 mEq/L may be a contributory cause of central pontine myelinolysis. One guideline is to correct the plasma sodium concentration to a value above 125 mmol/L with 3% hypertonic saline administered at 0.5 mL/kg per hour.

Other electrolyte abnormalities (potassium, phosphate, calcium, and magnesium) produce limb weakness, diaphragm weakness (hypophosphatemia alone), tetanic cramps, or occasional tonic-clonic seizures.

Endocrine crises are often perplexing not only in the initial presentation but also in the neurologic sequelae of biochemical correction. If recognition is delayed, hyperglycemic or hypoglycemic coma may cause severe cognitive defects. Cerebral edema after treatment of diabetic ketoacidosis, most often in children and young adults, is a fatal complication. Aggressive management of cerebral edema with conventional therapy may save an occasional patient but often at the expense of persistent disability. Hypothyroid coma or thyroid storm can be suspected by changes in skin color and heart rate and, in patients with hyperthyroidism, by proptosis and conjunctional injection. Addison's disease may cause weakness, but the laboratory features of hyponatremia, hyperglycemia, and hyperkalemia are usually detected and corrected in the ICU before progression to marked encephalopathy and coma.

REFERENCES

1. Abbas, DH, Schlagenhauff, RE, and Strong, HE: Polyradiculopathy in Addison's disease: Case report and review of literature. Neurology 27:494–495, 1977.

2. Adams, RD, Victor, M, and Mancall, EL: Central pontine myelinolysis: A hitherto undescribed disease occurring in alcoholic and malnourished patients. Arch Neurol Psychiatry 81:154–172, 1959.

3. Agardh, C-D, Rosén, I, and Ryding, E: Persistent vegetative state with high cerebral blood flow following profound hypoglycemia. Ann Neurol 14:482–486, 1983.

4. Anderson, RJ, Chung, H-M, Kluge, R, and Schrier, RW: Hyponatremia: A prospective analysis of its epidemiology and the pathogenetic role of vasopressin. Ann Intern Med 102:164, 1985.

5. Arieff, AI: Hyponatremia, convulsions, respiratory arrest, and permanent brain damage after elective surgery in healthy women. N Engl J Med 314:1529–1535, 1986.

6. Arieff, AI: Acid-base balance in specialized tissues: Central nervous system. In Seldin, DW and Giebisch, G (eds): The Regulation of Acid-Base Balance. Raven Press, New York, 1989, pp 107–121.

7. Arieff, AI and Carroll, HJ: Nonketotic hyperosmolar coma with hyperglycemia: Clinical features, pathophysiology, renal function, acid-base balance, plasma-cerebrospinal fluid equilibria and the effects of therapy in 37 cases. Medicine (Baltimore) 51:73–94, 1972.

8. Arieff, AI and Guisado, R: Effects on the central nervous system of hypernatremic and hyponatremic states. Kidney Int 10:104–116, 1976.

9. Arieff, AI, Kerian, A, Massry, SG, and DeLima, J: Intracellular pH of brain: Alterations in acute respiratory acidosis and alkalosis. Am J Physiol 230:804–812, 1976.

10. Arieff, AI, Llach, F, and Massry, SG: Neurological manifestations and morbidity of hyponatremia: Correlation with brain water and electrolytes. Medicine (Baltimore) 55:121–129, 1976.

11. Auer, RN: Progress review: Hypoglycemic brain damage. Stroke 17:699–708, 1986.

12. Austen, FK, Carmichael, MW, and Adams, RD: Neurologic manifestations of chronic pulmonary insufficiency. N Engl J Med 257:579–590, 1957.

13. Ayus, JC, Krothapalli, RK, and Arieff, AI: Changing concepts in treatment of severe symptomatic hyponatremia: Rapid correction and possible relation to central pontine myelinolysis. Am J Med 78:897–902, 1985.

14. Ayus, JC, Olivero, JJ, and Frommer, JP: Rapid correction of severe hyponatremia with intravenous hypertonic saline solution. Am J Med 72:43–48, 1982.

15. Ayus, JC, Wheeler, JM, and Arieff, AI: Postoperative hyponatremic encephalopathy in menstruant women. Ann Intern Med 117:891–897, 1992.

16. Barton, CH, Vaziri, ND, Martin, DC, et al: Hypomagnesemia and renal magnesium wasting in renal transplant recipients receiving cyclosporine. Am J Med 83:693–699, 1987.

17. Bashuk, RG and Krendel, DA: Myasthenia gravis presenting as weakness after magnesium administration. Muscle Nerve 13:708–712, 1990.

18. Bennett, MH and Wainwright, AP: Acute thyroid crisis on induction of anaesthesia. Anaesthesia 44:28–30, 1989.

19. Berl, T: Treating hyponatremia: Damned if we do and damned if we don't. Kidney Int 37:1006–1018, 1990.

20. Betro, MG and Pain, RW: Hypophosphataemia and hyperphosphataemia in a hospital population. Br Med J 1:273–276, 1972.

21. Blue, PR, Wijdicks, EFM, Steers, JL, et al: Central pontine myelinolysis in liver transplantation (abstract). Ann Neurol.

22. Boston Veterans Administration Medical Center: Postoperative hypophosphatemia: A multifactorial problem. Nutr Rev 47:111–116, 1989.

23. Brady, HR, Goldberg, H, Lunski, C, and Uldall, PR: Dialysis-induced hyperkalaemia presenting as profound muscle weakness. Int J Artif Organs 11:43–44, 1988.

24. Brunner, JE, Redmond, JM, Haggar, AM, et al: Central pontine myelinolysis and pontine lesions after rapid correction of hyponatremia: A prospective magnetic resonance imaging study. Ann Neurol 27:61–66, 1990.

25. Calbarese, LH and White, CS: Musculoskeletal manifestations of Addison's disease. Arthritis Rheum 22:558, 1979.

26. Carroll, GC and Rothenberg, DM: Carbon dioxide narcosis: Pathological or "pathillogical" (editorial). Chest 102:986–988, 1992.

27. Chernow, B, Bamberger, S, Stoiko, M, et al: Hypomagnesemia in patients in postoperative intensive care. Chest 95:391–397, 1989.

28. Clements, RS Jr, Blumenthal, SA, Morrison, AD, and Winegrad, AI: Increased cerebrospinal-fluid pressure during treatment of diabetic ketosis. Lancet ii:671–675, 1971.

29. Clifford, DB, Gado, MH, and Levy, BK: Osmotic demyelination syndrome: Lack of pathologic and radiologic imaging correlation. Arch Neurol 46:343–347, 1989.

30. Cluitmans, FHM and Meinders, AE: Management of severe hyponatremia: Rapid or slow correction? Am J Med 88:161–166, 1990.

31. Cook, DM and Boyle, PJ: Rapid reversal of myxedema madness with triiodothyronine (letter). Ann Intern Med 104:893–894, 1986.

32. Daugirdas, JT, Kronfol, NO, Tzamaloukas, AH, and Ing, TS: Hyperosmolar coma: Cellular dehydration and the serum sodium concentration. Ann Intern Med 110:855–857, 1989.

33. Duck, SC, Weldon, VV, Pagliara, AS, and Haymond, MW: Cerebral edema complicating therapy for diabetic ketoacidosis. Diabetes 25:111–115, 1976.

34. Duck, SC and Wyatt, DT: Factors associated with brain herniation in the treatment of diabetic ketoacidosis. J Pediatr 113:10–14, 1988.

35. Ebinger, G, Six, R, Bruyland, M, and Somers, G: Flexion contractures: A forgotten symptom in Addison's disease and hypopituitarism (letter). Lancet ii:858, 1986.

36. Ellison, DA and Forman, DT: Transient hyperglycemia during abdominal

aortic surgery. Clin Chem 36:815–817, 1990.

37. Endo, Y, Oda, M, and Hara, M: Central pontine myelinolysis: A study of 37 cases in 1,000 consecutive autopsies. Acta Neuropathol (Berl) 53:145–153, 1981.

38. Estol, C J, Faris, AA, Martinez, AJ, and Ahdab-Barmada, M: Central pontine myelinolysis after liver transplantation. Neurology 39:493–498, 1989.

39. Faden, A: Encephalopathy following treatment of chronic pulmonary failure. Neurology 26:337–339, 1976.

40. Falk, SA, Birken, EA, and Baran, DT: Temporary postthyroidectomy hypocalcemia. Arch Otolaryngol Head Neck Surg 11 4:168–174, 1988.

41. Fonseca, OA and Calverley, JR: Neurological manifestations of hypoparathyroidism. Arch Intern Med 120:202–206, 1967.

42. Frame, B: Neuromuscular manifestations of parathyroid disease. In Vinken, PJ and Bruyn, GW (eds): Handbook of Clinical Neurology, Vol 27. North-Holland Publishing Company, Amsterdam, 1976, pp 283–320.

43. Fraser, CL and Arieff, AI: Fatal central diabetes mellitus and insipidus resulting from untreated hyponatremia: A new syndrome. Ann Intern Med 112:11 3–119, 1990.

44. Garre, M, Boles, JM, Garo, B, and Mabin, D: Cerebral oedema in diabetic ketoacidosis: Do we use too much insulin? (letter) Lancet i:220, 1986.

45. Gavin, LA: Thyroid crises. Med Clin North Am 75:179–193, 1991.

46. Goebel, HH and Herman-Ben Zur, H: Central pontine myelinolysis: A clinical and pathological study of 10 cases. Brain 95:495–504, 1972.

47. Gotta, H: Tetany and epilepsy. Arch Neurol Psychiatry 66:714–721, 1951.

48. Grant, C and Warlow, C: Focal epilepsy in diabetic non-ketotic hyperglycaemia. Br Med J 290:1204–1205, 1985.

49. Gravelyn, TR, Brophy, N, Siegert, C, and Peters-Golden, M: Hypophosphatemia–associated respiratory muscle weakness in a general inpatient population. Am J Med 84:870–876, 1988.

50. Guisado, R and Arieff, AI: Neurologic manifestations of diabetic comas: Correlation with biochemical alterations in the brain. Metabolism 24:665–679, 1975.

51. Harden, CL, Rosenbaum, DH, and Daras, M: Hyperglycemia presenting with occipital seizures. Epilepsia 32:215–220, 1991.

52. Harris, GD, Fiordalisi, I, and Finberg, L: Safe management of diabetic ketoacidemia. J Pediatr 113:65–68, 1988.

53. Hasselstrom, L, Wimberley, PD, and Nielsen, VG: Hypophosphatemia and acute respiratory failure in a diabetic patient. Intensive Care Med 12:429–431, 1986.

54. Hayek, ME and Eisenberg, PG: Severe hypophosphatemia following the institution of enteral feedings. Arch Surg 124:1325–1328, 1989.

55. Heller, SR, MacDonald, IA, Herbert, M, and Tattersall, RB: Influence of sympathetic nervous system on hypoglycaemic warning symptoms. Lancet ii:359–363, 1987.

56. Hillman, K: Fluid resuscitation in diabetic emergencies: A reappraisal. Intensive Care Med 13:4–8, 1987.

57. Ho, VB, Fitz, CR, Yoder, CC, and Geyer, CA: Resolving MR features in osmotic myelinolysis (central pontine and extrapontine myelinolysis). AJNR Am J Neuroradiol 14:163–167, 1993.

58. Hoffman, E: The Chvostek sign: A clinical study. Am J Surg 96:33–37, 1958.

59. Hoffman, WH, Steinhart, CM, El Gammal, T, et al: Cranial CT in children and adolescents with diabetic ketoacidosis. AJNR Am J Neuroradiol 9:733–739, 1988.

60. Hylander, B and Rosenqvist, U: Treatment of myxoedema coma: Factors associated with fatal outcome. Acta Endocrinol 108:65–71, 1985.

61. Illowsky, BP and Laureno, R: Encephalopathy and myelinolysis after rapid correction of hyponatraemia. Brain 110:855–867, 1987.

62. Jos, J, Oberkampf, B, Couprie, C, et al: Comparaison de deux modes de traitement de l'acidocétose diabétique de

Moses, H III: Nonketotic hyperglycemia appearing as choreoathetosis or ballism. Arch Intern Med 142:154–155, 1982.

116. Rie, MA: Hypophosphatemia and diaphragmatic contractility (letter). N Engl J Med 314:519, 1986.

117. Rojiani, AM, Prineas, JW, and Cho, E-S: Alteration in myelin degradation in electrolyte induced demyelination (EID) by steroid/colchicine (abstract). J Neuropathol Exp Neurol 47:307, 1988.

118. Rose, GA and Vas, CJ: Neurological complications and electroencephalographic changes in hypoparathyroidism. Acta Neurol Scand 42:537–550, 1966.

119. Rosival, V: The influence of blood hydrogen ion concentration on the level of consciousness in diabetic ketoacidosis. Ann Clin Res 19:23–25, 1987.

120. Saul, RF and Selhorst, JB: Downbeat nystagmus with magnesium depletion. Arch Neurol 38:650–652, 1981.

121. Seki, S: Clinical features of hyperosmolar hyperglycemic nonketotic diabetic coma associated with cardiac operations. J Thorac Cardiovasc Surg 91:867–873, 1986.

122. Sieker, HO and Hickam, JB: Carbon dioxide intoxication: The clinical syndrome, its etiology and management with particular reference to the use of mechanical respirators. Medicine (Baltimore) 35:389–423, 1956.

123. Silvis, SE, DiBartolomeo, AG, and Aaker, HM: Hypophosphatemia and neurological changes secondary to oral caloric intake: A variant of hyperalimentation syndrome. Am J Gastroenterol 73:215–222, 1980.

124. Simon, RP, Meldrum, BS, Schmidley, JW, et al: Mechanisms of selective vulnerability: Hypoglycemia. In Powers, W J and Raichle, ME (eds): Cerebrovascular Diseases. Raven Press, New York, 1987, pp 13–25.

125. Singh, BM and Strobos, RJ: Epilepsia partialis continua associated with nonketotic hyperglycemia: Clinical and biochemical profile of 21 patients. Ann Neurol 8:155–160, 1980.

126. Snyder, NA, Feigal, DW, and Arieff, AI: Hypernatremia in elderly patients: A heterogenous, morbid, and iatrogenic entity. Ann Intern Med 107:309–319, 1987.

127. Sparacio, RR, Anziska, B, and Schutta, HS: Hypernatremia and chorea: A report of two cases. Neurology 26:46, 1976.

128. Sterns, RH: Severe symptomatic hyponatremia: Treatment and outcome: A study of 64 cases. Ann Intern Med 107:656–664, 1987.

129. Sterns, RH: Neurological deterioration following treatment for hyponatremia. Am J Kidney Dis 13:434–437, 1989.

130. Sterns, RH, Riggs, JE, and Schochet, SS Jr: Osmotic demyelination syndrome following correction of hyponatremia. N Engl J Med 314:1535–1542, 1986.

131. Sterns, RH, Thomas, DJ, and Herndon, RM: Brain dehydration and neurologic deterioration after rapid correction of hyponatremia. Kidney Int 35: 69–75, 1989.

132. Swift, TR: Weakness from magnesium-containing cathartics: Electrophysiologic studies. Muscle Nerve 2:295–298, 1979.

133. Thomas, FB, Mazzaferri, EL, and Skillman, TG: Apathetic thyrotoxicosis: A distinctive clinical and laboratory entity. Ann Intern Med 72:679–685, 1970.

134. Tinker, R, Anderson, MG, Anand, P, et al: Pontine myelinolysis presenting with acute parkinsonism as a sequel of corrected hyponatraemia (letter). J Neurol Neurosurg Psychiatry 53:87–88, 1990.

135. Tison, FX, Ferrer, X, and Julien, J: Delayed onset movement disorders as a complication of central pontine myelinolysis. Mov Disord 6:171–173, 1991.

136. Van der Muelen, JA, Klip, A, and Grinstein, S: Possible mechanism for cerebral oedema in diabetic ketoacidosis. Lancet ii:306–308, 1987.

137. Vannatta, JB, Whang, R, and Papper, S: Efficacy of intravenous phosphorus therapy in the severely hypophosphatemic patient. Arch Intern Med 141: 885–887, 1981.

138. Verbalis, JG and Gullans, SR: Hyponatremia causes large sustained reductions in brain content of multiple organic osmolytes in rats. Brain Res 567:274–282, 1991.

139. Verhagen, WIM and Schimsheimer, RJ: Neurologic disease and thyrotoxic storm: A clinical and electrophysiological study. Electromyogr Clin Neurophysiol 26:27–32, 1986.

140. Wakui, H, Nishimura, S, Watahiki, Y, et al: Dramatic recovery from neurological deficits in a patient with central pontine myelinolysis following severe hyponatremia. Jpn J Med 30:281–284, 1991.

141. Waldenström, J: Acute thyrotoxic encephalo- or myopathy: Its cause and treatment. Acta Med Scand 121:251–294, 1945.

142. Waldstein, SS, Slodki, SJ, Kaganiec, GI, and Bronsky, D: A clinical study of thyroid storm. Ann Intern Med 52:626–642, 1960.

143. Wallis, WE, Donaldson, I, Scott, RS, and Wilson, J: Hypoglycemia masquerading as cerebrovascular disease (hypoglycemic hemiplegia). Ann Neurol 18:510–512, 1985.

144. Weinberger, SE, Schwartzstein, RM, and Weiss, JW: Hypercapnia. N Engl J Med 321:1223–1231, 1989.

145. Weissman, JD and Weissman, BM: Pontine myelinolysis and delayed encephalopathy following the rapid correction of acute hyponatremia. Arch Neurol 46:926–927, 1989.

146. Wiederholt, WC, Kobayashi, RM, Stockard, JJ, and Rossiter, VS: Central pontine myelinolysis: A clinical reappraisal. Arch Neurol 34:220–223, 1977.

147. Wijdicks, EFM and Larson, TS: Absence of postoperative hyponatremia syndrome in young, healthy females. Ann Neurol 35:626–628, 1994.

148. Wright, DG, Laureno, R, and Victor, M: Pontine and extrapontine myelinolysis. Brain 102:361–385, 1979.

149. Yang, S, Wang, C, and Feng, Y: Neurologic and psychiatric manifestations in hypoparathyroidism: Clinical analysis of 71 cases. Chin Med J (Engl) 97:267–277, 1984.

150. Zaloga, GP, Chernow, B, Cook, D, et al: Assessment of calcium homeostasis in the critically ill surgical patient: The diagnostic pitfalls of the McLean-Hastings nomogram. Ann Surg 202:587–594, 1985.

Chapter 8

NEUROLOGIC COMPLICATIONS OF ACUTE RENAL DISEASE

UREMIC ENCEPHALOPATHY
DISEQUILIBRIUM SYNDROME
HYPERTENSIVE ENCEPHALOPATHY
NEUROMUSCULAR DISORDERS

Acute renal failure often defines critical illness in patients admitted to intensive care units (ICUs). The risk for renal involvement in any critical illness is extraordinarily high, often ending in hemodialysis.

The clinical features of uremic, or disequilibrium encephalopathy range from drowsiness to manifestations typical of any metabolic encephalopathy, such as asterixis. Its clinical features may be few or many, subtle or overwhelming. The recognition of uremic encephalopathy is not trivial, because in many ICUs, its signs and symptoms are usually an indication to initiate hemodialysis. Most patients have a favorable response to dialysis therapy. The neurologic manifestations of chronic renal failure have been tailored to the most common clinical problems seen in critically ill patients and those that may pose difficulty in assessment during consultation in ICUs. Hypertensive encephalopathy is included in this chapter because of its interrelation with acute renal failure.

UREMIC ENCEPHALOPATHY

Many causes are possible in patients with signs of encephalopathy associated with acute renal failure, and more than one cause may be operative (Table 8–1). Nonetheless, it is possible to set apart the clinical presentation of uremic encephalopathy.

Clinical Features

Gradually progressive confusion, drowsiness, multifocal myoclonus, and asterixis are collectively recognized as signs and symptoms of uremic encephalopathy, but none is pathognomonic for the disorder.[13,62,63,66]

If rapidly progressive renal failure is associated with severe uremia, it will undoubtedly produce clinical signs of a metabolic encephalopathy. However, many reports of uremic encephalopathy show a poor correlation between the degree of uremia and the degree of altered consciousness.

Each patient reacts differently to the consequences of severe and abrupt reduction of renal function. Uremic encephalopathy usually is signaled by sudden onset of drowsiness or obtundation. However, patients often appear alert but are easily distracted and lack sustained attention. Many patients

Table 8-1 SYSTEMIC ABNORMALITIES IN ACUTE RENAL FAILURE THAT MAY CONFOUND SIGNS OF UREMIC ENCEPHALOPATHY

Prolonged hypotension
Hyponatremia
Hypocalcemia
Metabolic alkalosis
Congestive heart failure and anemia
Drug toxicity (penicillin, digoxin)[37,53,80]

with acute uremia act blasé about their often critical condition. Perseveration and motor impersistence are early signs of uremic encephalopathy, but in other patients, early manifestations predominantly are intermittent explosive panic spells, aggressive behavior, restlessness, disorganized and rambling speech, and hallucinatory symptoms. The natural history of uremic encephalopathy is progression into unresponsive coma with frontal release signs. Nuchal rigidity may be seen in one third of the patients. Cranial nerve deficits were noted in studies before the computed tomography (CT) scan era, but the value of these findings is uncertain. Of interest are mild facial asymmetries in 11 of 13 patients with uremia that were reported in earlier work by Locke and associates.[61]

Focal signs are uncommon but may be only transiently present in about one fourth of the patients. Dense hemiplegia, however, generally points to structural central nervous system damage. In exceptional patients, slurred speech with irregular pitch and loudness is evident and initially may suggest drug intoxication from sudden reduction of the glomerular filtration rate. Asterixis of the tongue may also impair speech.

Abnormal limb movements are common in patients with metabolic encephalopathy associated with acute renal failure. Tetany may occur in patients with associated hypocalcemia, but carpopedal spasm is seldom seen (see Chapter 7). Trousseau's sign may be found, but again trismus and spasms of the facial muscles are generally not present.

Multifocal myoclonus is frequent in uremic encephalopathy,[91] and its incidence is probably higher in uremic encephalopathy than in other encephalopathies. Myoclonus can be identified by repetitive jerks or shocklike involuntary movements—focal, segmental, or generalized—and involves many muscles.[24]

Asterixis is often seen in uremic encephalopathy and is a well-appreciated clinical sign in ICUs and in chronic dialysis units. It appears predominantly in drowsy patients and can be elicited by asking the patient to hold out the arms or by hip flexion-abduction.[88] When tongue asterixis and limb asterixis occur together, puckering of the lips, sustained baring of the teeth, and protrusion of the tongue demonstrate bursts of arrhythmic movements (1/s) in the face and tongue muscles[1] (Fig. 8-1). Asterixis has been fully characterized by electromyography, although its origin remains unknown. Shahani and Young[88] showed in a study of 70 patients with asterixis of various types that lapses of posture appeared as silent periods of 50 to 200 milliseconds in tonically active muscles. Although common in dialysis units, asterixis is not characteristic of uremic encephalopathy and may also be seen in hepatic encephalopathy and severe hypercarbia. Unilateral asterixis typically occurs in structural brain lesions.

In most patients with uremic encephalopathy, CT scan is negative, but occasionally subacute or chronic subdural hematoma is unexpectedly seen. In a well-documented case report, severe white matter hypodensities on CT scan not associated with hypertension appeared to be reversible after dialysis.[54]

Results of electroencephalography (EEG) are nonspecific and may demonstrate shift of spectral power into the delta frequencies. If the objective of EEG recording is to exclude seizures or nonconvulsive status in obtunded patients, it should be emphasized that bilateral spike and wave abnormalities can be expected in 14% of patients with

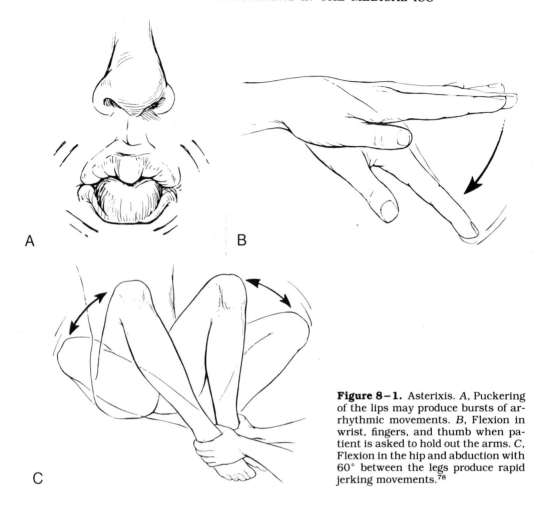

Figure 8-1. Asterixis. *A*, Puckering of the lips may produce bursts of arrhythmic movements. *B*, Flexion in wrist, fingers, and thumb when patient is asked to hold out the arms. *C*, Flexion in the hip and abduction with 60° between the legs produce rapid jerking movements.[78]

chronic renal failure.[49] The accuracy and precision of EEG recording in the ICU are obviously confounded by suboptimal conditions and other metabolic or pharmacologic factors; therefore, its clinical usefulness is very limited and it may not help in predicting outcome.

Studies of cerebrospinal fluid findings in uremia have not been reported recently, but studies in the 1950s showed that most patients with uremic encephalopathy may have increased protein values between 80 and 100 mg. Pleocytosis (from 7 to 600 leukocytes/mm^3) may be found in half of patients with uremic encephalopathy.[65] Neurologists evaluating patients with uremic encephalopathy for possible meningitis need to be aware of the relatively frequent occurrence of nonspecific neck stiffness and pleocytosis, and the risk of bleeding from uremic platelet dysfunction. (In immunosuppressed patients, the threshold for examination of the cerebrospinal fluid is obviously lower.) Administration of large doses of cryoprecipitate or desmopressin acetate (DDAVP) shortens bleeding time in preparation for lumbar puncture.

Treatment

Hemodialysis has reduced the mortality from acute renal failure, and resolution of clinical signs of uremic encephalopathy should be expected if no major (even brief) hypoxic or hypotensive event has led to additional insults. Failure to improve should certainly be anticipated if acute renal failure has resulted from an episode of hypotension, a common clinical occurrence in ICUs. Overall mortality from acute renal failure, however, remains between 20% and 72% and is determined by the number of associated systemic complications.[21] Outcome of encephalopathy of renal failure is further discussed in Chapter 17.

DISEQUILIBRIUM SYNDROME

The disequilibrium syndrome of hemodialysis is fortunately rare and, therefore, its diagnosis requires exclusion of conditions that may simulate this entity. Moreover, the disequilibrium syndrome seldom appears with all its clinical features. A presentation with only a few pertinent clinical signs is more common. Predisposing factors have not been consistently identified, but the risk may be proportionally increased if blood urea nitrogen values are initially high, dialysis is rapid, and large surface membranes are used (Table 8–2).

The pathophysiologic process of disequilibrium syndrome is obscure, but several hypotheses have been suggested.[43] A unifying hypothesis may be the "reverse urea shift," which implies a less rapid decrease in the concentration of urea and osmolality in the cerebrospinal fluid than in the blood. This phenomenon is associated with a paradoxical acidosis in the cerebrospinal fluid despite an increase in plasma pH after rapid hemodialysis. Cerebrospinal

fluid acidosis probably is a result of more rapid diffusion of carbon dioxide than of bicarbonate across the blood-brain barrier. Intracellular acidosis of brain cells can result in an increase of brain intracellular osmolality, which contributes to cerebral edema.

Clinical Features

The typical clinical picture of disequilibrium syndrome, usually appearing at the end of a dialysis procedure and almost invariably associated with the first treatment,[59] begins with restlessness, agitation, and combative behavior. Headache may be prominent and is bifrontal, throbbing, and more severe in a reclining position. Myoclonic jerks in proximal muscles and cramps are occasionally reported as early signs. The time course of clinical presentation is often rapid. Sudden cortical blindness may become apparent during dialysis, developing within minutes. Complete recovery can be expected within 2 weeks.[71] Monocular blindness from an anterior ischemic optic neuropathy has been described but is more often associated with an episode of marked hypotension.[87] Many patients lapse into coma with extensor posturing, frequently preceded by one or two generalized tonic-clonic seizures. Therapeutic measures are unsuccessful when patients become comatose, and many may die within a few hours after onset. A CT scan may demonstrate slitlike ventricles, effacement of sulci, and obliteration of ambient cisterns, and autopsy studies have indeed demonstrated massive swelling of white matter without evidence of border-zone infarction or intracranial hemorrhage. Fortunately, this course is extremely rare. Variants of the disequilibrium syndrome that can appear deceptively benign, however, are well known in dialysis units.

Most hemodialyzed patients have clinical signs indicative but not characteristic of disequilibrium syndrome. These mild clinical signs of headache,[7] restlessness, and tremor in extremities

---

Table 8–2 ASSOCIATED FACTORS AND POTENTIAL CAUSES OF DISEQUILIBRIUM SYNDROME

Hyponatremia
Hypo-osmolality
Hyperphosphatemia
Rapid dialysis (450–500 mL/min)
Large dialysis membrane
Surface area > 1 m² and initially high blood
  urea nitrogen value

subside after the procedure but may again occur when hemodialysis is repeated. Usually, these symptoms disappear after a few sessions and very frequently after adjustment of the rate and fluid composition of dialysis.

Another rare condition is hard water syndrome. The predominant causes are hypercalcemia and hypermagnesemia from failure of a water treatment process in locations with high content of calcium and magnesium in water. Characterized by lethargy, headache, dysarthria, seizures, hallucinations, and burning sensations of the skin, the syndrome has some similarities with the classic disequilibrium syndrome, but most patients are extremely confused and have vivid hallucinations and considerable muscle weakness. Acute intoxication with aluminum or other trace materials (copper, zinc) from tubing lines also may occur, but only a few well-documented cases have been reported.[5,23] As alluded to previously, various other disorders (largely anecdotal) may superficially resemble disequilibrium syndrome and are decidedly rare (Table 8–3).

Biochemical changes may mimic disequilibrium syndrome and are usually a result of technical errors. Hyponatremia is noted when plasma is allowed to equilibrate with hypotonic dialysis fluid. Several other potential causes of hyponatremia have been described, but the most frequent is failure to connect the concentrate container or failure to test the dialysate before the start of the procedure. The resulting hypo-osmolar hypervolemia may cause marked hemolysis that is associated with shock. Seizures are frequent.

Table 8–3 DIFFERENTIAL DIAGNOSIS OF DISEQUILIBRIUM SYNDROME

Hypoxic-ischemic encephalopathy (associated with severe hypotension)[44]
Air embolism
Subdural hematoma[10,55,58]
Hypernatremia
Hyponatremia
Wernicke's encephalopathy[30,35]
Hypoglycemia associated with beta-blockade

Treatment

To prevent recurrence of disequilibrium syndrome, the addition of hyperosmotic or hyperoncotic solute, such as glycerol or mannitol, or the substitution of sodium bicarbonate for sodium lactate in the dialysate has been suggested.[3]

Whether postdialysis cerebral edema occurs subclinically is unclear, but one CT and EEG study showed no appreciable changes in brain density and ventricular size or background in EEG findings.[8] Therefore, increase of slow wave activity with delta wave burst and early loss of posterior alpha rhythm may indicate the potential for disequilibrium in selected patients.[42,79] It is probably worthwhile to monitor EEG recordings if disequilibrium syndrome is suspected, and abnormalities should lead to preventive measures such as shortened and more frequent hemodialyses.

Prophylactic administration of anticonvulsant drugs is generally not indicated, usually because many seizures are often related to concomitant hyponatremia and will not recur after sodium correction. Phenytoin loading may be indicated in patients with recurrent seizures. One session of hemodialysis or 24 hours of continuous ambulatory peritoneal dialysis[92] should not influence the therapeutic window of phenytoin.

HYPERTENSIVE ENCEPHALOPATHY

There is conclusive evidence that the incidence of hypertensive encephalopathy has declined considerably over the years. Certainly, improved surveillance and aggressive drug treatment have resulted in a much lower incidence, but improved definition of the clinical entity in the era of the CT scan and magnetic resonance imaging (MRI) should be considered an important factor as well.

For many reasons, many critically ill patients have a sudden significant rise in systolic blood pressure, but hyper-

Table 8–4 CAUSES OF HYPERTENSIVE ENCEPHALOPATHY IN THE INTENSIVE CARE UNIT

Antihypertensive withdrawal syndrome
Acute parenchymal renal disease
Pharmaceutical agents
Major thermal burns
Eclampsia
Aortic dissection
Systemic vasculitis
Surgery for pheochromocytoma or renin-producing tumor
Multitrauma (head injury, spinal cord injury with dysautonomia)

tensive encephalopathy develops in only a small proportion of patients.

Frequent causes of hypertensive encephalopathy are listed in Table 8–4. Sudden withdrawal of antihypertensive treatment in patients with long-standing hypertension is probably the most frequent, and acute parenchymal renal disease is the next most frequent. Drug-induced causes of hypertensive encephalopathy have been reported in single cases and are often without any warning.[47] The most recent reported cases are associated with erythropoietin treatment.[20,33] Postoperative causes of hypertension, such as cross-clamping of the aorta in coronary bypass surgery, renal vascularization, heart transplantation, and carotid endarterectomy, have been well recognized, but many anesthesiologists anticipate these surges in blood pressure and correct them promptly. Occasionally, pregnant women with preeclampsia are admitted to a medical ICU for blood pressure control.

The pathology of hypertensive encephalopathy has infrequently been studied. The study by Chester and associates[27] in the late 1970s, which consisted of a systematic pathologic examination, is probably the most informative to date.

The most common vascular change in hypertensive encephalopathy is fibrinoid necrosis of arterioles in virtually any target organ besides the brain. Patients with long-lasting hypertension may have additional hyalinization and medial hypertrophy. Many arterioles may show obliteration caused by fibrin thrombi, with recanalization in some. Microscopic examination often reveals miliary infarction in the brain and occasionally petechial hemorrhages.[48]

Cerebral edema was absent in most autopsy cases, including patients with increased cerebrospinal fluid pressure and papilledema. Generally, the vascular and intravascular changes in any patient with hypertensive encephalopathy probably should be regarded as a direct result of endothelial damage, platelet aggregation, release of platelet factors and thromboxane, increased blood viscosity, and, finally, microangiopathic hemolytic anemia and intravascular coagulation.

Earlier explanations of hypertensive encephalopathy are probably too simple.[46,47] They include the breakthrough concept (forced dilation of cerebral blood vessels, causing disruption of the blood-brain barrier, increase in cerebral blood flow, leakage of plasma proteins, and resultant focal or generalized edema). A second but less likely theory is the overregulation concept, which assumes exaggerated vasoconstriction of arterioles resulting in cerebral ischemia.[93,94] Recent studies with single photon emission CT indicated regional hyperperfusion, supporting the existence of a vasodilatory mechanism.[85]

In most patients with clinical signs of hypertensive encephalopathy, diastolic blood pressure is significantly increased (greater than 120 mm Hg). Equally important in the definition of hypertensive crisis is whether there is end organ damage. Outcome in patients with hypertensive encephalopathy is generally not determined by the degree of brain edema but depends on acute congestive heart failure, pulmonary edema, acute anuria requiring emergency dialysis, and microangiopathic hemolytic anemia.

The pathophysiologic trigger of target organ involvement other than the brain is not clarified, but arteries are alternately constricted and dilated (sausage string), often with endothelial damage and overlying platelet thrombi. Platelet-derived growth factors eventually lead to vascular proliferation of smooth muscle cells and further narrowing of vessels.

Patients with a sudden increase in blood pressure have signs of left ventricular failure manifested by paroxysmal dyspnea at night, wheezing, or sustained orthopnea. In extreme conditions, the patient may look pale, slightly cyanotic, cold, and sweaty. In the most advanced cases, severe pulmonary edema may occur.

Coincident with left ventricular failure is the potential for renal failure. Renal failure associated with hypertensive encephalopathy is typically defined as a twofold or greater increase in blood urea nitrogen or creatinine concentration. Proteinuria, microscopic hematuria, and red cell casts can be expected with urinalysis. Peripheral blood smears may show target cells and schistocytes. These indicators of microangiographic hemolytic anemia are common in patients with renal failure.

Clinical Features

The clinical picture of hypertensive encephalopathy is typified by severe, throbbing, generalized headache associated with vomiting and nausea, decreased level of consciousness, transient neurologic signs, and seizures.[102] Early hypertensive encephalopathy may be difficult to appreciate in patients who also have significant congestive heart failure and hypoxia. The severity of the headache in hypertensive encephalopathy is not related to the systolic or diastolic blood pressure level. Headaches in hypertensive encephalopathy are seldom continuous over the day but more often brief with sudden brief surges of throbbing generalized occipital or unilateral face pain. Very frequently, coughing or straining triggers a brief attack of pulsating headache, which is relieved when the patient assumes the sitting position. Headache in patients with malignant hypertension may be extremely intense but usually develops gradually. A temporal profile with a split-second onset should raise the clinical suspicion of a subarachnoid or cerebellar hemorrhage that resulted in hypertension rather than the converse.

The mechanism of headaches in malignant hypertension is obscure. Sudden increases in blood pressure may result in dilatation of intracranial arteries or displacement of pain-sensitive intracranial structures at the base of the skull.

Another characteristic clinical feature is clouding of consciousness. In the accelerated phase of hypertension, an acute confusional state is common.

Common in patients with hypertensive encephalopathy are visual disturbances. Blurred vision (reported in 20% to 50% of patients) is the most frequent complaint. Some patients may have cortical blindness accompanied by vivid visual hallucinations.[50,60] Loss of color vision at the ictus or as a permanent sequela of malignant hypertensive crisis has been reported in exceptional cases. Some patients may have visual perseveration.[31]

Papilledema is a frequent presenting feature of hypertensive encephalopathy, varying from early disc hyperemia to impressively engorged retinal veins with multiple splinter hemorrhages and obliterated optic cups. The diagnosis of hypertensive encephalopathy becomes problematic in the absence of this finding. Malignant hypertensive crisis frequently occurs in patients with long-standing hypertension; therefore, papilledema may be part of a widespread retinopathy with soft exudates, gray discoloration of the retina, epithelial necrosis with serous detachment of the retina, and dilated and tortuous arterioles. Obscurations may be prominent and are usually bilateral but may alternate. This short-lasting (seconds rather than minutes) blindness usually occurs in patients with rapidly progressive papilledema. Obscurations may appear several times a day and are common immediately after a change in posture. Some of these transient episodes may last minutes, but again with complete resolution of symptoms. Outcome is favorable after control of blood pressure. Effective control of hypertension results in resolution of papilledema in 6 to 8 weeks. However, blurred disc margins and abnormalities of the peripapillary retinal nerve fiber layer may remain for months.[70]

Hemiparesis and aphasia are uncommon manifestations and should point to an underlying vascular event. Two prospective series reported conflicting results.[46,56] In a study from Harlem Hospital center, 10 of 34 patients with an initial admission diagnosis of malignant hypertension had lateralizing signs, but they were associated with cerebral infarction.[46] In contrast, a Scandinavian study reported focal signs in 23% of 64 patients with admission diastolic blood pressures of 135 mm Hg or more.[56] Most patients had permanent limb weakness after treatment of blood pressure, but clinical details and imaging studies were not given.

Generalized tonic-clonic seizures may accompany hypertensive encephalopathy. Myoclonus and asterixis are not features of hypertensive encephalopathy except in patients who have marked uremia and need dialysis. Peripheral facial palsy is a well-documented early presentation of malignant hypertension. The condition, tentatively linked to hemorrhage within the facial canal, is more frequent in children and young adults and resolves completely.[90]

Both CT scan and MRI can be very helpful in the evaluation of hypertensive encephalopathy. A fairly consistent abnormal finding is diffuse or focal areas of lucency with diminished attenuation values, most frequently in the parietal and occipital white matter.[52,54,81,99] Some patients may have generalized diffuse hypodensity of the white matter, which most likely reflects cerebral edema. Cortical effacement may also be present in the acute stage.[36]

Most reports with serial MRI studies demonstrate reversal of white matter

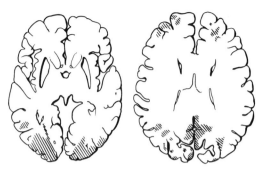

Figure 8–2. Magnetic resonance imaging patterns of hypertensive encephalopathy.

edema,[38,45] but residual hypodensity in the centrum semiovale may remain. Although the degree of encephalopathy is not related to the degree of white matter disease on CT scan, many patients with marked papilledema, seizures, and acute confusional state have white matter abnormalities on CT scan. Usually, MRI images are consistent with the CT scan patterns, but T2-weighted images may also preferentially show abnormalities in the pons, the cerebellum, and the basal ganglia. In some patients, compression of the fourth ventricle may cause obstructive hydrocephalus, which resolves after blood pressure control.[38,99]

In many patients, MRI demonstrates increased T2 signals in the bilateral occipital lobes or at the parieto-occipital junction and superior frontal lobes (Fig. 8–2).

Treatment

Irrespective of what triggered the event, early aggressive treatment of hypertensive encephalopathy limits the progression of the cascade of events and increases the chances of satisfactory outcome.[56] Current recommendations are summarized in Table 8–5.[22,39,83] The experience with esmolol is growing, and it may become a first-line drug in patients without bronchospastic disease. The goal is to reduce the mean arterial blood pressure by 20% within a few hours. This target value is crucial,

Table 8–5 EMERGENCY TREATMENT OF HYPERTENSIVE ENCEPHALOPATHY

Drug	Dosage
Sodium nitroprusside	0.3–10 μg/kg/min IV; maximal dose in 10 min
Diazoxide	50–150 mg by IV bolus repeated or 15–30 mg/min by IV infusion
Labetalol hydrochloride	20–80 mg by IV bolus every 10 min or 2 mg/min by IV infusion

Data from Gifford[39] and Calhoun and Oparil.[22]

because blood flow autoregulatory limits are altered in long-standing hypertension, producing a shift of both lower and upper limits toward higher pressures. Decreasing blood pressure more than 25% of the baseline value may result in failure of the brain to maintain unchanged metabolism through extraction of more oxygen from the blood. Single seizures are usually not treated with antiepileptic drugs, but phenytoin should be given intravenously if episodes recur. A loading dose of phenytoin may be used to cover the first days during recovery from the clinical manifestations of hypertensive encephalopathy. In patients with eclampsia, magnesium sulfate (therapeutic level of magnesium, 2 to 3 mmol/L) is preferred and is more successful in seizure management than phenytoin or diazepam.[28]

Treatment of brain edema, if present at all, is extremely controversial, and therapeutic options are limited. Mannitol may be given to patients who remain stuporous and have CT scan evidence of white matter hypodensity with effacement of the ambient cisterns despite normalization of blood pressure. Mannitol may be contraindicated in patients with renal failure. The value of intracra-

nial pressure monitoring has not been systematically studied, and monitoring is probably not indicated in early treatment, although others have an opposing view.[41]

NEUROMUSCULAR DISORDERS

Neuromuscular involvement is inevitable in patients with long-standing renal failure but may take weeks to months to become prevalent. In the ICU, generalized weakness associated with acute renal failure is very often due to muscle weakness. Weakness from polyneuropathy is found in chronic renal disease but also appears in patients who require admission to an ICU for management of decompensated renal function. Considerable information has accumulated about polyneuropathies and mononeuropathies in renal failure, and a comprehensive account can be found in Bolton and Young's monograph.[18]

Myopathy

The catabolic state in acute renal failure may produce muscle weakness, particularly when nutritional needs are not met (see Chapter 3). Muscle mass vanishes if patients with acute renal failure do not receive adequate caloric intake (up to 50 kcal/kg per day). Loss of muscle mass alone may be a sufficient explanation for "weakness." Nevertheless, in patients with chronic renal failure, maintenance hemodialysis, and osteomalacia, proximal weakness from myopathy is well recognized and often documented on electromyography by motor unit potentials with reduced duration and amplitude together with large numbers of polyphasic potentials. Muscle fiber degeneration in myopathy associated with chronic renal failure is at times evident only by electron microscopic examination.[57] Abnormalities in vitamin D metabolism or aluminum may contribute, but the pathways to muscle necrosis have not been elucidated. Electrolyte abnormalities from acute renal failure are virtually never severe enough to produce muscle weakness but may certainly contribute when neuromuscular blocking agents have been used. A recent prospective study identified hypermagnesemia and renal failure as important factors in the otherwise poorly understood post-vecuronium paralysis syndrome (see Chapter 3).[86]

Muscle cramps also may occur during hemodialysis, often late during dialysis. Rapid fluid removal or hypo-osmolality may be implicated, and significant relief can be achieved with a hypertonic (50%) dextrose intravenous injection or hypertonic saline infusion.[74,75,89]

Polyneuropathy of Renal Disease

Polyneuropathy is seen in approximately 60% of patients with renal disease, but this number is largely derived from series with patients receiving hemodialysis regularly.[4,9,18,32,51,76] A fully developed motor and sensory polyneuropathy is not seen in patients with mild renal failure that does not (yet) necessitate hemodialysis. A relation with plasma creatinine level has been reported, and moderate-to-severe mixed polyneuropathy indeed can be expected in patients with creatinine levels above 6 mg/dL. Below this level, the incidence of severe polyneuropathy is low, although many patients have loss of vibration sense and absent ankle jerks. Polyneuropathy is not seen in patients with new-onset acute renal failure, but when it is present, systemic vasculitis must be strongly considered as an underlying mechanism (see Chapter 11).

The pathologic basis of uremic polyneuropathy is axonal degeneration with secondary demyelination from accumulation of toxins such as molecules of medium molecular weight. (For an extensive discussion of the so-called middle molecule hypothesis, see the review by Bolton and Young.[18]) Other researchers continue to question primary axonal

damage and favor the hypothesis that both axons and Schwann cells are targets.[84]

Most patients at presentation have predominantly sensory symptoms with stocking hypoesthesia to light touch and loss of ankle jerks.[9,18] Vibratory thresholds increase later, and distal motor weakness worsens to the point of inability to stand and walk unsupported. An acute, fulminant, severe motor polyneuropathy has been repeatedly reported, and the rapid clinical course, sometimes a month after first dialysis,[64,68,69,82] results in a bed-bound state. The condition closely mimics Guillain-Barré syndrome but is never associated with ophthalmoplegia, severe dysautonomia, or need for mechanical ventilation. In many reported patients, renal failure is stable and no association with rapid worsening of kidney function is found. In many, underlying sepsis is implicated as a trigger; therefore, the differentiation from the recently described critical illness neuropathy (see Chapters 3 and 5) becomes virtually impossible. A fulminant motor neuropathy has also been found in patients without clinical evidence of sepsis. This unusual clinical course of uremic polyneuropathy has been estimated to occur in 0.6% of dialyzed patients.[84]

Outcome from fulminant uremic neuropathy is unpredictable, but a satisfactory outcome with independent mobility after dialysis has been reported.[9] In a 1993 series of patients, improvement was seen after more frequent use of dialysis.[82] In others, however, severe muscle wasting and severe footdrop remained, despite hemodialysis and renal transplantation, after years of follow-up.[68,84]

In most patients with renal failure, the course is more indolent. Tingling in the legs is frequently the first complaint. Burning pain is rare, and recent studies of thermal thresholds found little evidence for involvement of small fibers.[2] Restless legs and nocturnal cramps are common and disrupt sleep. Nocturnal cramps in the calf muscles are painful and often occur in the first few hours of sleep. Restless legs are equally common in patients with early uremic polyneuropathy, and these prickling and crawling sensations are only transiently relieved by movements. These symptoms can be relieved with clonazepam, 2 mg at night; carbamazepine, 300 to 1000 mg daily; bromocriptine, 7.5 mg; carbidopa-levodopa, 25 to 100 mg; or verapamil, 120 mg.[6,19,95,97,98]

Whether clinically significant autonomic neuropathy is present is controversial.[96] The causes of hypotension after dialysis may include excessive ultrafiltration or acute hypovolemia from hemorrhage. Nevertheless, reduced baroreceptor sensitivity was found in one study that used Valsalva's maneuver and the amyl nitrite test. Other studies have shown normal adrenergic responses[34,74] and normal responses to physiologic testing with Valsalva's maneuver, head-up tilt, cold pressor test, and sustained hand grip.[29,72]

Uremic polyneuropathy may progress to different degrees of severity, but most patients, whether receiving long-term hemodialysis or peritoneal dialysis, will have signs of mild polyneuropathy. Renal transplantation results in improvement both clinically and electrophysiologically, often striking in severe cases and often within weeks of transplantation.[16,77]

Electrodiagnostic studies in patients with uremic polyneuropathy largely show reduction of the amplitudes of muscle and sensory compound action potential, reflecting axonal damage. Conduction in sural nerves is invariably lost. Nielsen[77] found a statistically significant relation between creatinine clearance and motor nerve conduction of the peroneal nerve. The course of uremic neuropathy as measured by motor conduction velocity is variable, and most patients have relatively constant values over years or gradual improvement after dialysis or renal transplantation. In Bolton's series,[15] occasional transient worsening in nerve conduction velocity was seen in patients with intercurrent illness.

Mononeuropathies

Acute mononeuropathies in patients with renal failure are rare. Most mononeuropathies are associated with placement of temporary catheters or long-term use of arteriovenous shunts.[17] A potential complication from temporary access procedures in patients requiring hemodialysis is a retroperitoneal hematoma. Perforation of the iliac vein during insertion of a catheter through the femoral vein results in acute flank or abdominal pain and femoral neuropathy.[12] (Diagnosis and management of psoas hematoma are discussed in Chapter 10.)

The most common neuropathy in patients receiving long-term dialysis is carpal tunnel syndrome.[11,14,25] It occurs in both sexes with equal incidences and appears at any time, but only after several years of dialysis. The incidence of carpal tunnel syndrome is virtually the same in patients with peritoneal dialysis. Carpal tunnel syndrome is most commonly caused by amyloid deposition from increased serum levels of β_2-microglobulin.[26,67] Regular electrodiagnostic studies are necessary in dialyzed patients, because the results of sectioning of the flexor retinaculum in these patients are disappointing once both motor and sensory symptoms have been present for more than 2 years.[40,73,101] This outcome undoubtedly reflects concomitant uremic neuropathy. Therefore, early surgery in patients with sensory symptoms is recommended; only then may it prevent loss of hand function.[73,101]

Upper arm (brachial artery, antecubital vein) shunts may cause multiple brachial mononeuropathies, particularly in patients with diabetes. Shunt ligation leads to improvement.[100]

CONCLUSIONS

Neurologists do not routinely see patients with uremic encephalopathy or hypertensive encephalopathy. Rapid favorable response to dialysis or antihypertensive treatment does not strongly impel internists to call in a neurologist. Both encephalopathies are characterized clinically by confusion and clouding of consciousness. In uremic encephalopathy, asterixis and tremor (although nonspecific) are frequent; in hypertensive encephalopathy, papilledema, cortical blindness, or seizures predominate. Both disorders have marked renal failure in common. Hemodialyzed patients may have problems that occur during hemodialysis, such as headache, restlessness, and tremor, that become progressively less frequent with following sessions. These symptoms are much more common than those of a typical disequilibrium syndrome. Dialyzed patients have a low proclivity for this entity, which is linked to rapid dialysis and large dialysis membranes.

Neuromuscular manifestations of renal failure are usually long-term effects, but when acute, they should point to a possible systemic vasculitis (see Chapter 11). Restless legs with discomfort that is difficult to manage is a common manifestation of uremic polyneuropathy. Remarkable improvement in polyneuropathy has been noted after renal transplantation, noticeable within weeks in some patients.

REFERENCES

1. Adams, RD and Foley, JM: The neurological disorder associated with liver disease. Res Publ Assoc Nerv Ment Dis 32:198–237, 1953.

2. Angus-Leppan, H and Burke, D: The function of large and small nerve fibers in renal failure. Muscle Nerve 15:288–294, 1992.

3. Arieff, AI: More on the dialysis disequilibrium syndrome (editorial). West J Med 151:74–76, 1989.

4. Asbury, AK, Victor, M, and Adams, RD: Uremic polyneuropathy. Arch Neurol 8:413–428, 1963.

5. Bakir, AA, Hryhorczuk, DO, Berman, E, and Dunea, G: Acute fatal hyperaluminemic encephalopathy in undialyzed and recently dialyzed uremic patients. ASAIO Trans 32:171–176, 1986.

6. Baltodano, N, Gallo, BV, and Weidler, DJ: Verapamil vs quinine in recumbent nocturnal leg cramps in the elderly. Arch Intern Med 148:1969–1970, 1988.

7. Bana, DS, Yap, AU, and Graham, JR: Headache during hemodialysis. Headache 12:1–14, 1972.

8. Basile, C, Miller, JDR, Koles, ZJ, et al: The effects of dialysis on brain water and EEG in stable chronic uremia. Am J Kidney Dis 9:462–469, 1987.

9. Bazzi, C, Pagani, C, Sorgato, G, et al: Uremic polyneuropathy: A clinical and electrophysiological study in 135 short- and long-term hemodialyzed patients. Clin Nephrol 35:176–181, 1991.

10. Bechar, M, Lakke, JPWF, van der Hem, GK, et al: Subdural hematoma during long-term hemodialysis. Arch Neurol 26:513–516, 1972.

11. Benz, RL, Siegfried, JW, and Teehan, BP: Carpal tunnel syndrome in dialysis patients: Comparison between continuous ambulatory peritoneal dialysis and hemodialysis populations. Am J Kidney Dis 11:473–476, 1988.

12. Bhasin, HK and Dana, CL: Spontaneous retroperitoneal hemorrhage in chronically hemodialyzed patients. Nephron 22:322–327, 1978.

13. Biasioli, S, D'Andrea, G, Feriani, M, et al: Uremic encephalopathy: An updating. Clin Nephrol 25:57–63, 1986.

14. Bicknell, JM, Lim, AC, Raroque, HG Jr, and Tzamaloukas, AH: Carpal tunnel syndrome, subclinical median mononeuropathy, and peripheral polyneuropathy: Common early complications of chronic peritoneal dialysis and hemodialysis. Arch Phys Med Rehabil 72:378–381, 1991.

15. Bolton, CF: Peripheral neuropathy associated with chronic renal failure. Can J Neurol Sci 7:89–96, 1980.

16. Bolton, CF, Baltzan, MA, and Baltzan, RB: Effects of renal transplantation on uremic neuropathy: A clinical and electrophysiologic study. N Engl J Med 284:1170–1175, 1971.

17. Bolton, CF, Driedger, AA, and Lindsay, RM: Ischaemic neuropathy in uraemic patients caused by bovine arteriove-

nous shunt. J Neurol Neurosurg Psychiatry 42:810–814, 1979.

18. Bolton, CF and Young, GB: Neurological Complications of Renal Disease. Butterworths, Boston, 1990, pp 1–256.

19. Brodeur, C, Montplaisir, J, Godbout, R, and Marinier, R: Treatment of restless legs syndrome and periodic movements during sleep with L-dopa: A double-blind, controlled study. Neurology 38:1845–1848, 1988.

20. Buckner, FS, Eschbach, JW, Haley, NR, et al: Hypertension following erythropoietin therapy in anemic hemodialysis patients. Am J Hypertens 3:947–955, 1990.

21. Bullock, ML, Umen, AJ, Finkelstein, M, and Keane, WF: The assessment of risk factors in 462 patients with acute renal failure. Am J Kidney Dis 5:97–103, 1985.

22. Calhoun, DA and Oparil, S: Treatment of hypertensive crises. N Engl J Med 323:1177–1183, 1990.

23. Campistol, JM, Cases, A, Botey, A, and Revert, A: Acute aluminum encephalopathy in an uremic patient. Nephron 51:103–106, 1989.

24. Chadwick, D and French, AT: Uraemic myoclonus: An example of reticular reflex myoclonus? J Neurol Neurosurg Psychiatry 42:52–55, 1979.

25. Chanard, J, Lavaud, S, Toupance, O, et al: Carpal tunnel syndrome and type of dialysis membrane used in patients undergoing long-term hemodialysis (letter). Arthritis Rheum 29:1170–1171, 1986.

26. Charra, B, Calemard, E, Uzan, M, et al: Carpal tunnel syndrome, shoulder pain and amyloid deposits in long-term hemodialysis patients (abstract). Kidney Int 26:549, 1984.

27. Chester, EM, Agamanolis, DP, Banker, BQ, and Victor, M: Hypertensive encephalopathy: A clinicopathologic study of 20 cases. Neurology 28:928–939, 1978.

28. Cunningham, FG and Lindheimer, MD: Hypertension in pregnancy. N Engl J Med 326:927–932, 1992.

29. Davies, IB, Mathias, CJ, Sudera, D, and Sever, PS: Agonist regulation of α-adrenergic receptor responses in man. J Cardiovasc Pharmacol 4 (Suppl): S139–S143, 1982.

30. Descombes, E, Dessibourg, C-A, and Fellay, G: Acute encephalopathy due to thiamine deficiency (Wernicke's encephalopathy) in a chronic hemodialyzed patient: A case report. Clin Nephrol 35:171–175, 1991.

31. Dinsdale, HB: Hypertensive encephalopathy. Neurol Clin 1:3–16, 1983.

32. Dyck, PJ, Johnson, WJ, Lambert, EH, and O'Brien, PC: Segmental demyelination secondary to axonal degeneration in uremic neuropathy. Mayo Clin Proc 46:400–431, 1971.

33. Edmunds, ME, Walls, J, Tucker, B, et al: Seizures in haemodialysis patients treated with recombinant human erythropoietin. Nephrol Dial Transplant 4:1065–1069, 1989.

34. Faber, MD, Dumler, F, Zasuwa, GA, and Levin, NW: Relationship between sympathetic dysfunction and hemodialysis instability. ASAIO Trans 33:280–285, 1987.

35. Faris, AA: Wernicke's encephalopathy in uremia. Neurology 22:1293–1297, 1972.

36. Fisher, M, Maister, B, and Jacobs, R: Hypertensive encephalopathy: Diffuse reversible white matter CT abnormalities. Ann Neurol 18:268–270, 1985.

37. Geyer, J, Höffler, D, Demers, HG, and Niemeyer, R: Cephalosporin-induced encephalopathy in uremic patients (letter). Nephron 48:237, 1988.

38. Gibby, WA, Stecker, MM, Goldberg, HI, et al: Reversal of white matter edema in hypertensive encephalopathy (letter). AJNR Am J Neuroradiol 10 (Suppl):S78, 1989.

39. Gifford, RW Jr: Management of hypertensive crises. JAMA 266:829–835, 1991.

40. Gilbert, MS, Robinson, A, Baez, A, et al: Carpal tunnel syndrome in patients who are receiving long-term renal hemodialysis. J Bone Joint Surg [Am] 70:1145–1153, 1988.

41. Griswold, WR, Viney, J, Mendoza, SA, and James, HE: Intracranial pressure monitoring in severe hypertensive en-

cephalopathy. Crit Care Med 9:573–576, 1981.

42. Hampl, H, Klopp, HW, Michels, N, et al: Electroencephalogram investigations of the disequilibrium syndrome during bicarbonate and acetate dialysis. Proc Eur Dial Transplant Assoc 19:351–359, 1983.

43. Harris, CP and Townsend, JJ: Dialysis disequilibrium syndrome. West J Med 151:52–55, 1989.

44. Harris, RD, Campbell, JK, Howard, FM, et al: Neurovascular complications of dialysis and transplantation. Stroke 5:725–729, 1974.

45. Hauser, RA, Lacey, M, and Knight, MR: Hypertensive encephalopathy. Magnetic resonance imaging demonstration of reversible cortical and white matter lesions. Arch Neurol 45:1078–1083, 1988.

46. Healton, EB, Brust, JC, Feinfeld, DA, and Thomson, GE: Hypertensive encephalopathy and the neurologic manifestations of malignant hypertension. Neurology 32:127–132, 1982.

47. Houston, MC: Pathophysiology, clinical aspects, and treatment of hypertensive crises. Prog Cardiovasc Dis 32:99–148, 1989.

48. Hudson, AJ and Hyland, HH: Hypertensive cerebrovascular disease: A clinical and pathologic review of 100 cases. Ann Intern Med 49:1049–1072, 1958.

49. Hughes, JR: Correlations between EEG and chemical changes in uremia. Electroencephalogr Clin Neurophysiol 48:583–594, 1980.

50. Jellinek, EH, Painter, M, Prineas, J, and Russell, RR: Hypertensive encephalopathy with cortical disorders of vision. Q J Med 33:239–256, 1964.

51. Jennekens, FGI, Dorhout Mees, EJ, and van der Most van Spijk, D: Clinical aspects of uraemic polyneuropathy. Nephron 8:414–426, 1971.

52. Jesperson, CM, Rasmussen, D, and Hennild, V: Focal intracerebral oedema in hypertensive encephalopathy visualized by computerized tomographic scan. J Intern Med 225:349–350, 1989.

53. Josse, S, Godin, M, and Fillastre, JP:

54. Cefazolin-induced encephalopathy in a uraemic patient (letter). Nephron 45:72, 1987.

54. Komatsu, Y, Shinohara, A, Kukita, C, et al: Reversible CT changes in uremic encephalopathy (letter). AJNR Am J Neuroradiol 9:215–216, 1988.

55. Kopitnik, TA Jr, deAndrade, R Jr, Gold, MA, and Nugent, GR: Pressure changes within a chronic subdural hematoma during hemodialysis. Surg Neurol 32:289–293, 1989.

56. Krogsgaard, AR, McNair, A, Hilden, T, and Nielsen, PE: Reversibility of cerebral symptoms in severe hypertension in relation to acute antihypertensive therapy: Danish Multicenter Study. Acta Med Scand 220:25–31, 1986.

57. Layzer, RB: Neuromuscular Manifestations of Systemic Disease. Contemporary Neurology Series, Vol 25. F. A. Davis Company, Philadelphia, 1985.

58. Leonard, A and Shapiro, FL: Subdural hematoma in regularly hemodialyzed patients. Ann Intern Med 82:650–658, 1975.

59. Levin R: Dialysis disequilibrium syndrome (letter). West J Med 152:77, 1990.

60. Liebowitz, HA and Hall, PE: Cortical blindness as a complication of eclampsia. Ann Emerg Med 13:365–367, 1984.

61. Locke, S, Merrill, JP, and Tyler, HR: Neurologic complications of acute uremia. Arch Intern Med 108:519–530, 1961.

62. Lockwood, AH: Metabolic encephalopathies: Opportunities and challenges. J Cereb Blood Flow Metab 7:523–526, 1987.

63. Lockwood, AH: Neurologic complications of renal disease. Neurol Clin 7:617–627, 1989.

64. Lynch, PG, Yuill, GM, and Nicholson, JAH: Acute polyneuropathy complicating chronic renal failure. Nephron 8:278–288, 1971.

65. Madonick, MJ, Berke, K, and Schiffer, I: Pleocytosis and meningeal signs in uremia: Report on sixty-two cases. Arch Neurol Psychiatry 64:431–436, 1950.

66. Mahoney, CA and Arieff, AI: Uremic encephalopathies: Clinical, biochemical,

and experimental features. Am J Kidney Dis 2:324–336, 1982.

67. McClure, J, Bartley, CJ, and Ackrill, P: Carpal tunnel syndrome caused by amyloid containing β_2 microglobulin: A new amyloid and a complication of long term haemodialysis. Ann Rheum Dis 45:1007–1011, 1986.

68. McGonigle, RJS, Bewick, M, Weston, MJ, and Parsons, V: Progressive, predominantly motor, uraemic neuropathy. Acta Neurol Scand 71:379–384, 1985.

69. Meyrier, A, Fardeau, M, and Richet, G: Acute asymmetrical neuritis associated with rapid ultrafiltration dialysis. Br Med J 2:252–254, 1972.

70. Miller, NR: Walsh and Hoyt's Clinical Neuro-Ophthalmology, ed 4, Vol 1. Williams & Wilkins, Baltimore, 1982, pp 175–211.

71. Moel, DI and Kwun, YA: Cortical blindness as a complication of hemodialysis. J Pediatr 93:890–891, 1978.

72. Naik, RB, Mathias, CJ, Wilson, CA, et al: Cardiovascular and autonomic reflexes in haemodialysis patients. Clin Sci 60:165–170, 1981.

73. Naito, M, Ogata, K, and Goya, T: Carpal tunnel syndrome in chronic renal dialysis patients: Clinical evaluation of 62 hands and results of operative treatment. J Hand Surg [Br] 12:366–374, 1987.

74. Nakashima, Y, Fouad, FM, Nakamoto, S, et al: Localization of autonomic nervous system dysfunction in dialysis patients. Am J Nephrol 7:375–381, 1987.

75. Neal, CR, Resnikoff, E, and Unger, AM: Treatment of dialysis-related muscle cramps with hypertonic dextrose. Arch Intern Med 141:171–173, 1981.

76. Nielsen, VK: The peripheral nerve function in chronic renal failure. I. Clinical symptoms and signs. Acta Med Scand 190:105–111, 1971.

77. Nielsen, VK: The peripheral nerve function in chronic renal failure: VIII. Recovery after renal transplantation. Clinical aspects. Acta Med Scand 195:163–170, 1974.

78. Noda, S, Ito, H, Umezaki, H, and Minato, S: Hip flexion: Abduction to elicit asterixis in responsive patients. Ann Neurol 18:96–97, 1985.

79. Noriega-Sanchez, A, Martinez-Maldonado, M, and Haiffe, RM: Clinical and electroencephalographic changes in progressive uremic encephalopathy. Neurology 28:667–669, 1978.

80. Pascual, J, Liaño, F, and Ortuño, J: Cefotaxime-induced encephalopathy in an uremic patient (letter). Nephron 54:92, 1990.

81. Rail, DL and Perkin, GD: Computerized tomographic appearance of hypertensive encephalopathy. Arch Neurol 37:310–311, 1980.

82. Ropper, AH: Accelerated neuropathy of renal failure. Arch Neurol 50:536–539, 1993.

83. Rubenstein, EB and Escalante, C: Hypertensive crisis. Crit Care Clin 5:477–495, 1989.

84. Said, G, Boudier, L, Selva, J, et al: Different patterns of uremic polyneuropathy: Clinicopathologic study. Neurology 33:567–574, 1983.

85. Schwartz, RB, Jones, KM, Kalina, P, et al: Hypertensive encephalopathy: Findings on CT, MR imaging, and SPECT imaging in 14 cases. AJR Am J Roentgenol 159:379–383, 1992.

86. Segredo, V, Caldwell, JE, Matthay, MA, et al: Persistent paralysis in critically ill patients after long-term administration of vecuronium. N Engl J Med 327:524–528, 1992.

87. Servilla, KS and Groggel, GC: Anterior ischemic optic neuropathy as a complication of hemodialysis. Am J Kidney Dis 8:61–63, 1986.

88. Shahani, BT and Young, RR: Asterixis — A disorder of the neural mechanisms underlying sustained muscle contraction. In Shahani, M (ed): The Motor System — Neurophysiology and Muscle Mechanisms. Elsevier, Amsterdam, 1976, pp 301–316.

89. Sherman, RA, Goodling, KA, and Eisinger, RP: Acute therapy of hemodialysis-related muscle cramps. Am J Kidney Dis 2:287–288, 1982.

90. Siegler, RL, Brewer, ED, Corneli, HM, and Thompson, JA: Hypertension first seen as facial paralysis: Case reports

and review of the literature. Pediatrics 87:387–389, 1991.

91. Stark, RJ: Reversible myoclonus with uraemia. Br Med J 282:1119–1120, 1981.

92. Steele, WH, Lawrence, JR, Elliott, HL, and Whiting, B: Alterations of phenytoin protein binding with in vivo haemodialysis in dialysis encephalopathy. Eur J Clin Pharmacol 15:69–71, 1979.

93. Strandgaard, S and Paulson, OB: Cerebral blood flow and its pathophysiology in hypertension. Am J Hypertens 2:486–492, 1989.

94. Tamaki, K, Sadoshima, S, Baumbach, GL, et al: Evidence that disruption of the blood-brain barrier precedes reduction in cerebral blood flow in hypertensive encephalopathy. Hypertension 6 Suppl I:I-75–I-81, 1984.

95. Telstad, W, Sørensen, Ø, Larsen, S, et al: Treatment of the restless legs syndrome with carbamazepine: A double blind study. Br Med J [Clin Res] 288:444–446, 1984.

96. Vita, G, Messina, C, Savica, V, and Bellinghieri, G: Uraemic autonomic neuropathy. J Auton Nerv Syst 30 (Suppl):S179–S184, 1990.

97. von Scheele, C: Levodopa in restless legs. Lancet ii:426–427, 1986.

98. Walters, AS, Hening, WA, and Chokroverty, S: Review and videotape recognition of idiopathic restless legs syndrome. Mov Disord 6:105–110, 1991.

99. Weingarten, L, Barbut, D, Filippi, C, and Zimmerman, RD: Acute hypertensive encephalopathy: Findings on spin-echo and gradient-echo MR imaging. AJR Am J Roentgenol 162:665–670, 1994.

100. Wytrzes, L, Markley, HG, Fisher, M, and Alfred, HJ: Brachial neuropathy after brachial artery-antecubital vein shunts for chronic hemodialysis. Neurology 37:1398–1400, 1987.

101. Zamora, JL, Rose, JE, Rosario, V, and Noon, GP: Hemodialysis-associated carpal tunnel syndrome: A clinical review. Nephron 41:70–74, 1985.

102. Ziegler, DK, Zosa, A, and Zileli, T: Hypertensive encephalopathy. Arch Neurol 12:472–478, 1965.

Chapter 9

NEUROLOGIC MANIFESTATIONS OF ACUTE HEPATIC FAILURE

GENERAL CONSIDERATIONS
HEPATIC ENCEPHALOPATHY

Hepatic failure in critically ill patients commonly occurs as part of multiorgan failure. Too often, patients with long-standing cirrhosis are admitted with sudden onset of hepatic encephalopathy from acute gastrointestinal hemorrhage that causes rapid nitrogenous overload. Acute hepatic failure, however, may be an isolated emergency.

A particularly challenging management problem is sudden massive hepatic necrosis.[48] The most important cause of fulminant hepatic failure is viral hepatitis, but it is also associated with acetaminophen, halothane, carbon tetrachloride, hepatic vein occlusion (Budd-Chiari syndrome), Wilson's disease, Reye's syndrome,[38] and acute fatty liver of pregnancy. The management of acute liver diseases has evolved in surprising ways during recent years as a result of successful liver transplantation.

This chapter illustrates the clinical characteristics of acute hepatic encephalopathy. In addition, critical care management of fulminant hepatic failure and treatment of cerebral edema in this condition are emphasized.

GENERAL CONSIDERATIONS

Patients with acute liver failure need intensive care management for many reasons. Mortality is extraordinarily high (up to 90%) in patients with fulminant hepatic failure but can be reduced to 60% when liver transplantation is appropriately timed.[1,9,19] The results of this emergency procedure depend on the degree of the encephalopathy.

One series reported survival of 12 of 17 patients with fulminant hepatic failure, but half the patients had hepatic encephalopathy of stage I or II.[6] The likelihood of patients with stage IV encephalopathy surviving liver transplantation is low, but reports of small series during the late 1980s have claimed survival with a good level of performance.[1,19] Differences in outcome in the category of patients with stage IV encephalopathy probably reflect different degrees of coma and whether secondary brain stem damage has occurred. In the present classification of hepatic encephalopathy, stage IV indicates a sharp cutoff from stage III and has been linked to coma without further specification other than absence or presence of motor response to painful stimuli. Glasgow coma scores, which represent several stages of supratentorial or brain stem involvement, have not been systematically used in these patients. Whether further subdivision in motor responses adds to the present classification in terms of prognosis is not known, but change in the motor scale may more reliably guide treatment decisions than changes in the commonly used, rather broad categories of hepatic encephalopathy.

Progression to acute renal failure complicates the clinical picture of liver failure. In patients with fulminant hepatic failure, oliguric renal failure coexists in approximately 75% of those who become comatose from liver failure, and deteriorating renal function may require hemodialysis.[40,44]

Another important complication in acute hepatic failure is a coagulopathy that is often severe enough to warrant plasmapheresis or plasma infusions. Platelet infusions are usually indicated in patients with severe hemorrhage and in those about to undergo invasive procedures. Fresh frozen plasma is often used to replace coagulation factors, but the effect is short-lived.

Metabolic derangements can affect the level of consciousness. These include dilutional hyponatremia, hypoglycemia, and metabolic alkalosis. The impact of these acute metabolic changes on staging of hepatic encephalopathy is small when they are transient. Progression into higher stages of hepatic encephalopathy in fulminant hepatic failure should not be readily attributed to multifactorial systemic factors but is often associated with the emergence of brain edema. Persistent hypotension may occur in patients with hepatic failure that is associated with high cardiac output and low peripheral vascular resistance. Infusion of norepinephrine and vasopressin is required not only to overcome the systemic effects but also to minimize the risk for additional hypoxic-ischemic encephalopathy. The prognosis in patients who eventually need vasopressin for pressure control is poor.

HEPATIC ENCEPHALOPATHY

Traditionally, the degree of hepatic encephalopathy has been described in terms of clinical stages. There is some variation in the description of each stage in the literature, but the differences between adjacent stages are clear enough for the stages to be helpful in day-to-day clinical practice (Table 9–1). Until now, clinical studies have used these staging scales without much difficulty, probably because the steps between the stages are large. A formal interobserver and intraobserver variation study has not been performed, but there is no compelling reason to believe that this method of staging of hepatic encephalopathy is invalid or poorly reproducible. Additional use of the motor component of the Glasgow coma scale score is useful.

Clinical Features

Psychiatric changes are frequently noted, and the earliest abnormality

Table 9–1 SIGNS AND SYMPTOMS OF HEPATIC ENCEPHALOPATHY

Stage	Psychiatric	Neurologic
I	Apathy, anxiety, restlessness, short attention span, inverted sleep patterns, impaired calculations	Impaired handwriting, tremor, slowed coordination
II	Personality change, disorientation (time), poor recall, disobedience	Asterixis, ataxia, dysarthria, paratonia
III	Bizarre behavior, disorientation (place), delirium, paranoia, drowsy but arousable	Seizures, marked hyperreflexia, hyperpnea, myoclonus
IV	Coma	Coma (abnormal flexion or extension responses), brisk oculocephalic responses, sluggish pupillary reactions to light

is apathy or euphoria.[62] Personality changes, usually querulousness and impaired judgment, may also be noted.[51] Hypersomnia can be an early feature, with prolongation of nocturnal sleep as well as extreme daytime sleepiness, but in others sleep inversion with agitated delirium at night may be more prominent.[51]

Progression into the next stages of hepatic encephalopathy is characterized by changes in the level of consciousness. Fluctuations in attention and slow responses to requests are typically present. Patients are not capable of registration, retention, or recall. The immediate memory span for digits is severely reduced. Overactivity, disorientation for place, delusions, and repetitive picking movements become evident in stage III hepatic encephalopathy. The paranoid content of delusions often results in panic reactions with tachycardia, facial flushing, and tremor. Outbursts of anger and hostility are fairly typical in this stage of encephalopathy.[23]

Patients with fulminant hepatic failure experience a very condensed process of development of hepatic encephalopathy.[50] They quickly become jaundiced, and fever and marked dehydration develop. The disorder may begin with excitement and delirium, at times interrupted by focal or generalized tonic-clonic seizures. Multifocal myoclonus and startle responses can easily be produced by hand clap. Fragmentary speech and paraphasic errors are very frequently seen. Within 24 to 48 hours after the first manifestations, patients may lapse into coma with spontaneous extensor responses, but some patients have sudden deterioration into stage IV encephalopathy.

Any of the four major acid-base abnormalities may be encountered in patients with hepatic encephalopathy, but respiratory or metabolic alkalosis is most frequent.[49] Most patients with fulminant hepatic failure hyperventilate, and the result is low $PaCO_2$ with alkalemia. Respiratory alkalosis most likely results from increased respiratory drive triggered by accumulating toxins (such as ammonia) in the blood. One study found that short-chain fatty acids, which are increased in hepatic encephalopathy, produced central hyperventilation in the rabbit.[56] The significance of alkalosis in hepatic encephalopathy was bolstered by Plum and Posner,[45] who strongly implied that encephalopathy without respiratory or metabolic alkalosis was not likely hepatic in origin.

Papilledema is absent in severe hepatic encephalopathy. Very infrequently, papilledema appears early in patients with rapidly progressing brain edema, but it should point to a structural rather than a metabolic cause. Only patients with Reye's syndrome may have early papilledema from cerebral edema. The same stipulation may apply for patients with fulminant hepatic failure, but published data are not available. The cause of papilledema is not clear, as exemplified by a case report that demonstrated pathologic evidence of central retinal vein occlusion in Reye's syndrome.[55]

The pupils of patients with early hepatic encephalopathy are normal and in middle position, and light reflexes are preserved. In end-stage encephalopathy and later stages of Reye's syndrome, the pupil reaction becomes sluggish and eventually disappears. Oculocephalic responses, although brisk, usually remain normal but may transiently disappear.[26] Brisk oculocephalic responses are frequently found in patients with hepatic encephalopathy and are probably characteristic. In occasional patients with higher stages of encephalopathy, very brisk oculocephalic responses may give the impression that both globes are floating.

Eye movement abnormalities are rare. Transient ocular bobbing and dysconjugate gaze have been reported to occur after treatment of hepatic encephalopathy, with disappearance after improvement of serum ammonia levels.[12] Plum and Posner[45] noted transient downward gaze in their series of patients with hepatic coma, a phenomenon also reported in anoxic coma.[32]

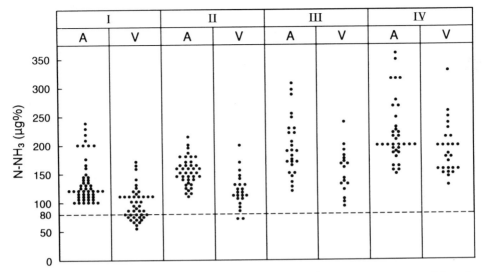

Figure 9–1. Arterial (A) and venous (V) ammonia levels in various stages of hepatic encephalopathy.

Motor responses may fluctuate over time and are usually closely correlated with the depth of coma. The extensor posturing characteristically seen in stage IV encephalopathy may be completely reversible after correction of plasma ammonia.[14] The correlation between arterial ammonia concentration and degree of hepatic encephalopathy is weak, but not when broad categories are compared with one another (Fig. 9–1). The muscle tone in patients with hepatic encephalopathy is usually impressively increased, and gegenhalten is common, with exaggerated tendon reflexes and Babinski's reflexes. When extensor posturing occurs in the course of fulminant hepatic failure, brain death can be expected within a few hours. At this point, aggressive treatment of cerebral edema is indicated and may completely reverse the clinical manifestations.

Asterixis (see Chapter 8) is infrequent in acute hepatic encephalopathy from fulminant hepatic necrosis, but focal muscle twitching and generalized myoclonus may occur. Seizures have occasionally been noted in severe stages of Reye's syndrome, just before complete flaccidity and loss of pupillary reflexes.

In general, the clinical presentation of hepatic encephalopathy can be impressively colorful, but the disorder may resolve without any residual findings on examination after liver transplantation or successful medical treatment.

Pathogenesis

The neuropathologic features of hepatic encephalopathy may, like those of any other metabolic encephalopathy, vary between complete absence of any light microscopic features and gross cerebral edema. Some glial changes, however, are distinctive in hepatic encephalopathy. Alzheimer type II astrocytes may occur in clusters and are identified by enlarged nuclei with inclusion bodies positive to periodic acid–Schiff testing. These changes are often found in the gray matter of the cerebrum and cerebellum and in the putamen and globus pallidus. In Reye's syndrome that is marked by a selective mitochondrial injury, cerebral edema is the only characteristic feature at autopsy.[13]

A unifying hypothesis of the biochemical changes and causes of hepatic encephalopathy has not yet emerged. (A potential mechanism is summarized in

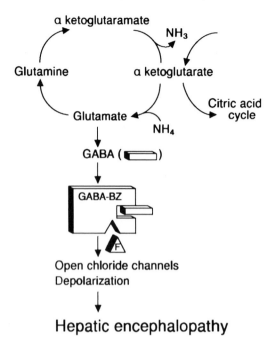

Figure 9–2. The gamma-aminobutyric acid–benzodiazepine (GABA-BZ) receptor complex and its relation to hepatic encephalopathy. F = Flumazenil. (Modified from Morris, JC and Ferrendelli, JA: Metabolic encephalopathy. In Pearlman, AL and Collins, RC [eds]: Neurobiology of Disease. Oxford University Press, New York, 1990, pp 356–379.)

Figure 9–2.) The correlation between degree of encephalopathy and concentration of ammonia in the blood is imprecise, but ammonia continues to be pivotal in the mechanism of hepatic encephalopathy and perhaps causes an imbalance of excitatory and inhibitory neurotransmitters. Ammonia is generated in the gastrointestinal tract from the degradation of amines, amino acids, and purines. Failure of liver function results in impaired conversion of ammonia to urea and glutamine and consequently a buildup of glutamate. As a result of the linkage of ammonia with glutamate, gamma-aminobutyric acid (GABA) is formed. GABA produces an inhibitory action after depolarization through the opening of chloride channels. The degree of hepatic encephalopathy is more closely correlated with cerebrospinal fluid levels of GABA.

The GABA-benzodiazepine receptor complex,[31] present in synaptic neural membranes, can be manipulated[10] and may provide a new rationale for treatment of hepatic encephalopathy. Patients treated with drugs that antagonize the GABA-benzodiazepine receptor (for example, flumazenil) may have both clinical and electroencephalographic improvement.[5,24,29,57] Further support for this hypothesis of the effect of benzodiazepines on GABA receptor neurotransmission has been the recent discovery of an increase in endogenous benzodiazepines in body fluids in patients with hepatic encephalopathy,[39] in animal models,[4] and in uptake of benzodiazepine measured by positron emission tomography scanning.[53] The evidence that flumazenil, a benzodiazepine receptor antagonist, controls hepatic encephalopathy is at present weak, but successful treatment with flumazenil has been reported in some uncontrolled series. Dramatic awakening from hepatic coma as soon as 30 seconds after the injection of flumazenil and sustained remission after repeated injections have been reported.[3]

In a preliminary series of nine patients with fulminant hepatic failure, 6 of 11 episodes of hepatic encephalopathy were successfully reversed with flumazenil.[24] Unsuccessful treatment in stage IV encephalopathy has been tentatively explained by the existence of secondary factors, such as hypoxic brain damage, cerebral edema, and hypoglycemia. Controlled studies are under way on flumazenil in fulminant hepatic failure complicated by severe encephalopathy. Undoubtedly, flumazenil has an important role in patients with fulminant hepatic failure who have repeated injections of benzodiazepines and may help in correctly assessing the stage of hepatic encephalopathy when emergency transplantation is considered.

Other possible explanations of the mechanism of hepatic encephalopathy are controversial. Mercaptans (responsible for fetor hepaticus), short-chain fatty acids, and depletion of neurotransmitters, such as norepinephrine and dopamine, have been implicated.[63] The significance of these factors alone or in combination remains unknown, although in Reye's syndrome, abnormalities in short- and medium-chain fatty acids have a prominent role. An extensive survey of the possible toxins can be found in several excellent reviews on this subject.[23,30]

Laboratory Tests

Before the introduction of evoked responses in patients with hepatic encephalopathy, electroencephalography was the only objective method to measure the degree of hepatic encephalopathy. Spectral analysis of the electroencephalogram allows one to see small differences and shifts in patterns. A retrospective study noted a significant inverse correlation between the occurrence of delta waves and survival.[57] Triphasic wave patterns are defined as generalized, bilaterally synchronous, bifrontal periodic waves in patients with decreased level of consciousness.[2,21] They can be used as prognostic indicators, because triphasic wave patterns have been associated with a 50% mortality in patients with metabolic encephalopathies, including hepatic encephalopathy.[2]

The predictive value of evoked potentials for outcome in hepatic encephalopathy is unresolved.[61] Many investigators in this field claim that hepatic encephalopathy can be recognized early with abnormal visual evoked potentials, but in other studies of flash visual evoked responses, no sufficiently sensitive differences between patients with and those without encephalopathy could be demonstrated.[16,28,54]

Brain stem evoked potentials may be more promising for subclinical detection of hepatic encephalopathy. A 1990 study comparing auditory, somatosensory, and visual evoked potentials in 22 patients found that the brain stem evoked potentials were the most sensitive for detection of subclinical hepatic encephalopathy.[37]

Magnetic resonance imaging has been found to be helpful in assessing severity of liver disease. In approximately two thirds of patients with advanced liver disease, hyperintensity in the globus pallidus is found on T1-weighted images and disappears after liver transplantation. The nature of this change in paramagnetic properties in the globus pallidus, also seen in patients after prolonged parenteral feeding, is unknown. Lipid deposits or any toxic substance allowed to enter the brain from portal systemic shunting may amplify the signal intensity of the globus pallidus. Biochemical-pathologic correlation, not yet performed, may provide an understanding of its clinical significance.[47]

Medical Management

Management of hepatic encephalopathy focuses on reduction of ammonia absorption from the intestinal lumen (Table 9–2). Enemas with 20% lactose or 1% neomycin solutions adjusted to a pH of 4 usually thoroughly clean the gut. Dietary proteins are completely avoided to minimize the production of ammonia. Radical approaches in treatment-resistant patients with progressive he-

---

Table 9–2 BASIC MANAGEMENT OF HEPATIC ENCEPHALOPATHY

- Correction of hypokalemia, metabolic alkalosis, hyponatremia, hypovolemia
- Identification of possible bleeding site (e.g., varices, gastrointestinal tract)
- Protein-free diet (1500–2000 cal/d)
- Cathartics to clean protein from gut (oral magnesium citrate, 200 mL; sorbitol, 50 g/200 mL of water)
- Vitamin supplementation: folate, 1 mg/d; vitamin K, 10 mg/d; thiamine and multivitamins
- Decrease in absorption of gastrointestinal ammonia
  Neomycin, 1 g p.o. q.i.d
  Lactulose, 10–30 mg p.o. t.i.d.
  Metronidazole, 250 mg t.i.d.

Data from Rothstein and McKhann.[52]

patic encephalopathy include surgical exclusion of the colon and charcoal hemoperfusion, but success is only anecdotal.

A 1989 meta-analysis of parenteral nutrition with branched-chain amino acids concluded that this regimen resulted in significant improvement in patients with hepatic coma, but further well-designed studies are needed to settle this matter.[43] The basic management of hepatic encephalopathy therefore should include measures to minimize production of ammonia and perhaps a trial of flumazenil.

The management of fulminant hepatic failure stands out because brain edema is a direct cause of mortality.[18,58] Brain edema is significant in most patients with stage III hepatic encephalopathy caused by hepatic necrosis, not just the most critically ill, In 1991, Blei[7] summarized the potential mechanisms of brain edema in fulminant hepatic failure, which appear to involve both vasogenic and cytotoxic injuries. Animal studies have shown sodium accumulation within cells and swelling through inhibition of endothelial $Na+$, $K+$-ATPase after administration of sera from patients with stages III and IV encephalopathy. Glutamine accumulation may have an osmotic effect and may significantly enhance the generation of brain water. Another, but uncertain, possibility is primary injury to astrocytes by ammonia or other toxins, causing cytotoxic edema.[36]

Diagnosis of brain edema is facilitated by measurements of intracranial pressure (ICP). Patients with increased ICP, decreased cerebral perfusion pressure, and fulminant hepatic failure may not have ominous signs such as sudden, transient dilated pupils and spontaneous extensor responses. Computed tomography (CT) scan, however, may demonstrate effacement of cortical sulci and obliteration of basal cisterns. Two reports in 1991 and 1992[35,42] dismissed the value of CT scanning in detecting brain edema. In a recent study, however, systematic review of serial CT scanning and classification of the degree of edema showed a significant correlation between the degree of cerebral edema and the degree of hepatic encephalopathy.[59] Patients whose condition worsened to stage III often had complete disappearance of the sylvian fissures and cortical sulci. In many patients with stage III hepatic encephalopathy, the clinical and radiologic signs of cerebral edema could be reversed with conventional treatment of increased ICP (Fig. 9–3). In others, cerebral edema progressed to brain death (Fig. 9–4).

Recently, a miniaturized device composed of a small fiberoptic bundle was developed to monitor ICP after insertion

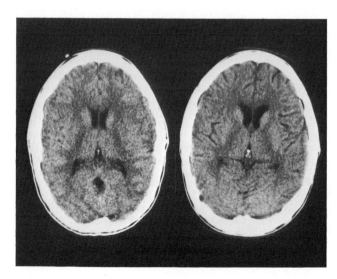

Figure 9–3. Computed tomography scans in a patient with fulminant hepatic failure. *Left,* Hepatic encephalopathy with evidence of cerebral edema (largely absent sulci and sylvian fissures). *Right,* After treatment of increased intracranial pressure and return to stage I encephalopathy. Sulci and sylvian fissures have reappeared.

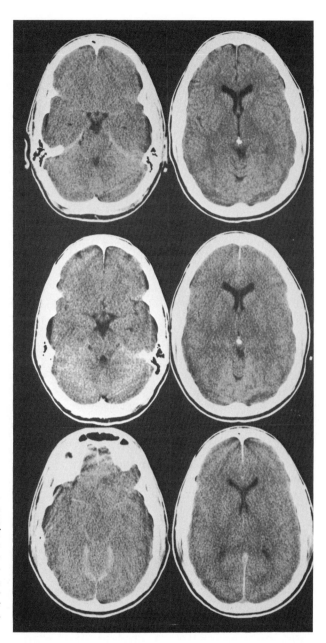

Figure 9–4. Serial computed tomography scan in a patient with rapid progression of cerebral edema. *Top row*, Normal findings. *Middle row*, Disappearance of cortical sulci and white matter discrimination of internal capsule; the third ventricle is barely visible. *Bottom row*, Complete compression of basal cisterns, compression of lateral ventricles, and attenuation of middle cerebral artery caused by clot (patient fulfilled the clinical criteria for brain death).

through a 2-mm burr hole (see Chapter 15). Insertion of the pressure monitor in the epidural space is preferable. Attempts to overcome the coagulopathy by transfusion of fresh frozen plasma or plasmapheresis result in only a very temporary correction of coagulopathy. (Plasma exchange has the additional advantage of less volume loading when a hepatorenal syndrome exists.) Blei and associates[8] surveyed all centers in the United States that performed liver transplantation and found that 1.3% of patients with epidurally placed ICP monitoring devices experienced fatal intracerebral hemorrhages; another 1.7% had nonfatal hemorrhages. Of patients with subdurally placed devices, on the other hand, 5% had fatal hemorrhages and 13%, nonfatal. When devices were placed in the parenchyma, 4% had fatal hemorrhages and 9%, nonfatal. These risks, although with considerable morbidity, remain small and are probably outweighed by the benefits of monitoring ICP and, more important, cerebral perfusion pressure. Cerebral edema on CT scanning may further guide placement of the ICP monitor, but prospective studies with serial CT scans are not yet available.

Large and sudden increases in ICP may precede the development of cerebral edema, and increases to more than 60 torr are associated with poor outcome.[25] Jenkins and colleagues[27] reported that cerebral perfusion pressure (difference between mean arterial pressure and ICP) was more closely linked to outcome in Reye's syndrome. ICP values on insertion of the device were less predictive for outcome than the calculated cerebral perfusion pressures. Cerebral perfusion pressures of 40 torr or less resulted in severe disability and death.

Monitoring ICP in patients with fulminant hepatic failure remains controversial, and many neurosurgeons are discouraged by the poor management results in some series and by the coexisting coagulopathy. Moreover, aggressive treatment of ICP may not always lead to improvement in the degree of encephalopathy because prolonged hypoglycemia and significant episodes of shock may cause additional ischemic-anoxic damage.

Several patterns of ICP may be observed during the clinical course of hepatic encephalopathy. A gradual increase in ICP is common and has been experimentally produced in pigs. Occasionally, brief increases and plateau waves may occur. These transient increases in ICP most likely indicate decreasing cerebral compliance but may also follow straining, coughing, or bucking of the ventilator. Surges of ICP occur in patients after reperfusion of the transplanted liver and during the first day after orthotopic liver transplanta-

tion as well.[33,34,46] ICP monitoring should continue at least until the second postoperative day. Improvement in hepatic function usually coincides with resolution of intracranial hypertension and, if present, with resolution of brain swelling on CT scan. In our institution, an epidural catheter is placed when a CT scan indicates edema or when stage III hepatic encephalopathy is present.

When patients with fulminant hepatic failure are admitted to the liver transplantation unit at a Mayo Clinic–affiliated hospital, the decision to place an epidural catheter is based on the Glasgow coma sum score and CT scan findings. A Glasgow coma score of 8 or CT scan evidence of brain edema determines placement, often at the same time that a patient needs to be intubated for airway protection. As alluded to earlier, correction of a coagulopathy with fresh frozen plasma is preferable at the time of placement (platelet counts less than 30,000, prothrombin ratio greater than 1.3).

Treatment of increased ICP should be initiated immediately. The first line of treatment is elevation of the head to 30°,[15,20] controlled hyperventilation, and osmotic therapy. Cerebral perfusion pressure should be maintained at more than 60 torr. A difficult management problem in patients with fulminant hepatic failure is the potential for hepatorenal syndrome. Hyperosmolarity may exacerbate renal failure, and patients with severe renal failure may temporarily require ultrafiltration to remove mannitol and excess free water. In this situation, mannitol administration can be coupled with removal of about three times the given volume by ultrafiltration performed after 15 to 30 minutes.[60] Other difficulties with mannitol administration are hypokalemia and nonketotic hyperosmolar hyperglycemia. Short-term hyperventilation with an initial range for arterial PCO_2 between 28 and 35 torr is preferable. As in many other circumstances, long-term hyperventilation is useless. In a clinical trial, prolonged hyperventilation in fulminant hepatic failure failed to decrease the number of episodes of increased ICP.[17] The core therapy for ICP reduction remains restriction of free water intake and osmotic therapy. Mannitol in low doses (0.5 g/kg) may effectively reduce ICP and increase cerebral perfusion pressure within 10 to 20 minutes of infusion, and its effect may last 4 to 6 hours. The dose of mannitol should be titrated by plasma osmolality (ideal plasma osmolality: 310 to 320 mOsm/L).[11] In patients with renal failure and in situations requiring prolonged treatment of ICP, use of tromethamine (THAM) should be strongly considered.

Usually, these measures result in lower ICP values and prevent sudden increases in ICP. Some patients, however, may need additional muscle relaxants, sedation, and barbiturates. A 1993 retrospective analysis of possible factors that preceded large increases in ICP found that fever, agitation, and arterial hypertension were significantly more common, but whether control of these factors halts progression to brain death is unclear.[41] Barbiturates can be of value in controlling ICP, although experience is limited in hepatic coma. (Barbituates are potent cerebral vasoconstrictors; thiopental in a loading dose of 4 mg/kg and a maintenance dose of 1 mg/kg per hour can reduce blood flow by 50%.) Forbes and associates[22] claimed a remarkable effect of thiopental infusion and complete recovery from stage IV encephalopathy in one third of the patients, far better than the dismal figure of 5% reported earlier in patients with stage IV disease. The risk of systemic hypotension with thiopental administration can be overcome by a decrease in the rate of infusion or temporary use of vasopressors. Sudden surges in ICP should be treated with an intravenously delivered bolus of lidocaine or thiopental. Steroids are of no use in the management of brain edema in patients with fulminant hepatic failure. In many of our patients with fulminant hepatic failure, we had to resort to barbiturates for ICP control.

CONCLUSIONS

Neurologists involved in the critical care of fulminant hepatic failure have had to rethink their laissez-faire attitude toward management of hepatic encephalopathy. Actually, hepatologists have been at the forefront, trying to convince neurologists (and neurosurgeons) that cerebral edema in fulminant hepatic failure is significant and not an epiphenomenon seen in only the most extreme cases. Although CT scanning can demonstrate flattening of sulci, disappearance of white and gray matter differentiation, and obliteration of basal cisterns as evidence of cerebral edema, results can be normal in the early stages of encephalopathy. Aggressive treatment of increased ICP may prevent progression to brain death, an obviously very unfortunate outcome after successful liver transplantation.

The timing of placement of an intracranial monitoring device is controversial. In clinical practice, a device is placed when a Glasgow coma sum score of 8 is reached, often at the same time that endotracheal intubation becomes necessary. Confounding factors (such as benzodiazepine toxicity, hypoglycemia, and hyponatremia) should be excluded first. An ICP monitor may be placed earlier in patients with early CT scan features of edema, but normal findings on CT scan should not postpone the decision to place a monitoring device. Every patient with fulminant hepatic failure has considerable coagulopathy, and intraparenchymal placement is not advised. Intracerebral hematomas, although surprisingly uncommon, have been reported with fatal outcome. These risks are low with epidural placement of an ICP monitor. Attempts to overcome the coagulopathy are only temporary and futile in many cases, and neurosurgeons have been understandably reluctant to indiscriminately place these devices. The often rapid and clinically unexpected progression of signs of brain herniation in this situation also justifies placement of a monitor.

After correction of ICP and maintenance of cerebral perfusion pressure at more than 60 torr, monitoring should continue through the transplantation procedure, because marked surges in ICP during reperfusion and during the first 24 hours after return of the patient to the intensive care unit do occur. Treatment of ICP is at times complicated by coexisting renal failure, which precludes mannitol administration. Tromethamine (THAM) is preferred in this situation. In many patients, barbiturates are needed to control ICP. Aggressive management of cerebral edema in fulminant hepatic failure and emergency liver transplantation have improved survival and reduced morbidity.

REFERENCES

1. Adams, DH, Kirby, RM, Clements, D, et al: Fulminant hepatic failure treated by hepatic transplantation (letter). Lancet ii:1037, 1986.
2. Bahamon-Dussan, JE, Celesia, GG, and Grigg-Damberger, MM: Prognostic significance of EEG triphasic waves in patients with altered state of consciousness. J Clin Neurophysiol 6:313–319, 1989.
3. Bansky, G, Meier, PJ, Ziegler, WH, et al: Reversal of hepatic coma by benzodiazepine antagonist (Ro 15-1788) (letter). Lancet i:1324–1325, 1985.
4. Basile, AS, Pannell, L, Jaouni, T, et al: Brain concentrations of benzodiazepines are elevated in an animal model of hepatic encephalopathy. Proc Natl Acad Sci USA 87:5263–5267, 1990.
5. Bassett, ML, Mullen, KD, Skolnick, P, and Jones, EA: Amelioration of hepatic encephalopathy by pharmacologic antagonism of the GABA$_A$-benzodiazepine receptor complex in a rabbit model of fulminant hepatic failure. Gastroenterology 93:1069–1077, 1987.
6. Bismuth, H, Samuel, D, Gugenheim, J, et al: Emergency liver transplantation for fulminant hepatitis. Ann Intern Med 107:337–341, 1987.
7. Blei, AT: Cerebral edema and intracranial hypertension in acute liver failure: Distinct aspects of the same problem. Hepatology 13:376–379, 1991.
8. Blei, AT, Olafsson, S, Webster, S, and Levy, R: Complications of intracranial pressure monitoring in fulminant hepatic failure. Lancet 341:157–158, 1993.
9. Brems, JJ, Hiatt, JR, Ramming, KP, et al: Fulminant hepatic failure: The role of liver transplantation as primary therapy. Am J Surg 154:137–140, 1987.
10. Butterworth, RF and Layrargues, GP: Benzodiazepine receptors and hepatic encephalopathy (editorial). Hepatology 11:499–501, 1990.
11. Canalese, J, Gimson, AES, Davis, C, et al: Controlled trial of dexamethasone and mannitol for the cerebral oedema of fulminant hepatic failure. Gut 23:625–629, 1982.
12. Caplan, LR and Scheiner, D: Dysconjugate gaze in hepatic coma. Ann Neurol 8:328–329, 1980.
13. Chang, LW, Gilbert, EF, Tanner, W, and Moffat, HL: Reye syndrome: Light and electron microscopic studies. Arch Pathol 96:127–132, 1973.
14. Conomy, JP and Swash, M: Reversible decerebrate and decorticate postures in hepatic coma. N Engl J Med 278:876–879, 1968.
15. Davenport, A, Will, EJ, and Davison, AM: Effect of posture on intracranial pressure and cerebral perfusion pressure in patients with fulminant hepatic and renal failure after acetaminophen self-poisoning. Crit Care Med 18:286–289, 1990.
16. Davies, MG, Rowan, MJ, and Feely, J: Flash visual evoked responses in the early encephalopathy of chronic liver disease. Scand J Gastroenterol 25:1205–1214, 1990.
17. Ede, RJ, Gimson, AES, Bihari, D, and Williams, R: Controlled hyperventilation in the prevention of cerebral oedema in fulminant hepatic failure. J Hepatol 2:43–51, 1986.
18. Ede, RJ and Williams, R: Hepatic encephalopathy and cerebral edema. Semin Liver Dis 6:107–118, 1986.
19. Emond, JC, Aran, PP, Whitington, PF, et al: Liver transplantation in the management of fulminant hepatic fail-

ure. Gastroenterology 96:1583–1588, 1989.

20. Feldman, Z, Kanter, MJ, Robertson, CS, et al: Effect of head elevation on intracranial pressure, cerebral perfusion pressure, and cerebral blood flow in head-injured patients. J Neurosurg 76:207–211, 1992.

21. Fisch, BJ and Klass, DW: The diagnostic specificity of triphasic wave patterns. Electroencephalogr Clin Neurophysiol 70:1–8, 1988.

22. Forbes, A, Alexander, GJM, O'Grady, JG, et al: Thiopental infusion in the treatment of intracranial hypertension complicating fulminant hepatic failure. Hepatology 10:306–310, 1989.

23. Fraser, CL and Arieff, AI: Hepatic encephalopathy. N Engl J Med 313:865–873, 1985.

24. Grimm, G, Katzenschlager, R, Schneeweiss, B, et al: Improvement of hepatic encephalopathy treated with flumazenil. Lancet ii:1392–1394, 1988.

25. Hanid, MA, Davies, M, Mellon, PJ, et al: Clinical monitoring of intracranial pressure in fulminant hepatic failure. Gut 21:866–869, 1980.

26. Heubi, JE, Daugherty, CC, Partin, JS, et al: Grade I Reye's syndrome—outcome and predictors of progression to deeper coma grades. N Engl J Med 311:1539–1542, 1984.

27. Jenkins, JG, Glasgow, JFT, Black, GW, et al: Reye's syndrome: Assessment of intracranial monitoring. Br Med J 294:337–338, 1987.

28. Johansson, U, Andersson, T, Persson, A, and Eriksson, LS: Visual evoked potential—a tool in the diagnosis of hepatic encephalopathy? J Hepatol 9:227–233, 1989.

29. Jones, EA, Basile, AS, Mullen, KD, and Gammal, SH: Flumazenil: Potential implications for hepatic encephalopathy. Pharmacol Ther 45:331–343, 1990.

30. Jones, EA and Gammal, SH: Hepatic encephalopathy. In Arias, IM, Jakoby, WB, Popper, H, et al (eds): The Liver: Biology and Pathobiology, ed 2. Raven Press, New York, 1988, pp 985–1005.

31. Jones, EA, Skolnick, P, Gammal, SH, et al: The γ-aminobutyric acid A (GABA$_A$) receptor complex and hepatic encephalopathy: Some recent advances. Ann Intern Med 110:532–546, 1989.

32. Keane, JR, Rawlinson, DG, and Lu, AT: Sustained downgaze deviation: Two cases without structural pretectal lesions. Neurology 26:594–595, 1976.

33. Keays, R, Potter, D, O'Grady, J, et al: Intracranial and cerebral perfusion pressure changes before, during and immediately after orthotopic liver transplantation for fulminant hepatic failure. Q J Med 79(n.s.):425–433, 1991.

34. LeRoux, PD, Elliott, JP, Perkins, JD, and Winn, HR: Intracranial pressure monitoring in fulminant hepatic failure and liver transplantation (letter). Lancet 335:1291, 1990.

35. Lidofsky, SD, Bass, NM, Prager, MC, et al: Intracranial pressure monitoring and liver transplantation for fulminant hepatic failure. Hepatology 16:1–7, 1992.

36. Livingstone, AS, Potvin, M, Goresky, CA, et al: Changes in the blood-brain barrier in hepatic coma after hepatectomy in the rat. Gastroenterology 73:697–704, 1977.

37. Mehndiratta, MM, Sood, GK, Sarin, SK, and Gupta, M: Comparative evaluation of visual, somatosensory, and auditory evoked potentials in the detection of subclinical hepatic encephalopathy in patients with nonalcoholic cirrhosis. Am J Gastroenterol 85:799–803, 1990.

38. Meythaler, JM and Varma, RR: Reye's syndrome in adults: Diagnostic considerations. Arch Intern Med 147:61–64, 1987.

39. Mullen, KD, Szauter, KM, and Kaminsky-Russ, K: "Endogenous" benzodiazepine activity in body fluids of patients with hepatic encephalopathy. Lancet 336:81–83, 1990.

40. Muñoz, SJ, Ballas, SK, Moritz, MJ, et al: Perioperative management of fulminant and subfulminant hepatic failure with therapeutic plasmapheresis. Transplant Proc 21:3535–3536, 1989.

41. Muñoz, SJ, Moritz, MJ, Bell, R, et al: Factors associated with severe intracranial hypertension in candidates for emergency liver transplantation. Transplantation 55:1071–1074, 1993.

42. Muñoz, SJ, Robinson, M, Northrup, B, et al: Elevated intracranial pressure and computed tomography of the brain in fulminant hepatocellular failure. Hepatology 13:209–212, 1991.

43. Naylor, CD, O'Rourke, K, Detsky, AS, and Baker, JP: Parenteral nutrition with branched-chain amino acids in hepatic encephalopathy: A meta-analysis. Gastroenterology 97:1033–1042, 1989.

44. O'Grady, JG, Gimson, AES, O'Brien, CJ, et al: Controlled trials of charcoal hemoperfusion and prognostic factors in fulminant hepatic failure. Gastroenterology 94:1186–1192, 1988.

45. Plum, F and Posner, JB: The Diagnosis of Stupor and Coma, ed 3. F. A. Davis, Philadelphia, 1980.

46. Potter, D, Peachey, T, Eason, J, et al: Intracranial pressure monitoring during orthotopic liver transplantation for acute liver failure. Transplant Proc 21:3528, 1989.

47. Pujol, A, Pujol, J, Graus, F, et al: Hyperintense globus pallidus on T_1-weighted MRI in cirrhotic patients is associated with severity of liver failure. Neurology 43:65–69, 1993.

48. Rakela, J, Lange, SM, Ludwig, J, and Baldus, WP: Fulminant hepatitis: Mayo Clinic experience with 34 cases. Mayo Clin Proc 60:289–292, 1985.

49. Record, CO, Iles, RA, Cohen, RD, and Williams, R: Acid-base and metabolic disturbances in fulminant hepatic failure. Gut 16:144–149, 1975.

50. Ritt, DJ, Whelan, G, Werner, DJ, et al: Acute hepatic necrosis with stupor or coma: An analysis of thirty-one patients. Medicine (Baltimore) 48:151–172, 1969.

51. Rothstein, JD and Herlong, HF: Neurologic manifestations of hepatic disease. Neurol Clin 7:563–578, 1989.

52. Rothstein, JD and McKhann, GM: Hepatic encephalopathy. Curr Ther Neurol Dis 3:352–356, 1990.

53. Samson, Y, Bernuau, J, Pappata, S, et al: Cerebral uptake of benzodiazepine measured by positron emission tomography in hepatic encephalopathy (letter). N Engl J Med 316:414–415, 1987.

54. Sandford, NL and Saul, RE: Assessment of hepatic encephalopathy with visual evoked potentials compared with conventional methods. Hepatology 8:1094–1098, 1988.

55. Smith, P, Green, R, Miller, NR, and Terry, JM: Central retinal vein occlusion in Reye's syndrome. Arch Ophthalmol 98:1256–1260, 1980.

56. Trauner, DA and Huttenlocher, PR: Short chain fatty acid-induced central hyperventilation in rabbits. Neurology 28:940–944, 1978.

57. van der Rijt, C and Schalm, SW: Quantitative EEG analysis and survival in liver disease. Electroencephalogr Clin Neurophysiol 61:502–504, 1985.

58. Ware, AJ, D'Agostino, AN, and Combes, B: Cerebral edema: A major complication of massive hepatic necrosis. Gastroenterology 61:877–884, 1971.

59. Wijdicks, EFM, Plevak, D, Rakela, J, and Wiesner, R: Clinical and CT scan features of brain edema in fulminant hepatic failure. Liver Transplantation and Surgery, in press.

60. Williams, R and Gimson, AES: Intensive liver care and management of acute hepatic failure. Dig Dis Sci 36:820–826, 1991.

61. Yang, S-S, Chu, N-S, and Liaw, Y-F: Somatosensory evoked potentials in hepatic encephalopathy. Gastroenterology 89:625–630, 1985.

62. Zacharski, LR, Litin, EM, Mulder, DW, and Cain, JC: Acute, fatal hepatic failure presenting with psychiatric symptoms. Am J Psychiatry 127:382–386, 1970.

63. Zieve, L and Olsen, RL: Can hepatic coma be caused by a reduction of brain noradrenaline or dopamine? Gut 18:688–691, 1977.

Chapter 10

NEUROLOGIC COMPLICATIONS ASSOCIATED WITH DISORDERS OF THROMBOSIS AND HEMOSTASIS

DISSEMINATED INTRAVASCULAR
  COAGULATION
THROMBOLYSIS AND
  ANTICOAGULATION
THROMBOTIC THROMBOCYTOPENIC
  PURPURA

Thrombocytopenias or thrombocytopathies are likely to be the prime causes of bleeding disorders in the intensive care unit (ICU). Triggers for thrombocytopenia are drugs (e.g., heparin, antibiotics), massive transfusion, and intravascular consumption. Thrombocytopathies, however, are often induced by uremia and cardiopulmonary bypass. Isolated factor deficiencies should be excluded in any event but are of limited relevance in this setting. Relatively frequent multiorgan failure in critically ill patients is an important cause of increased bleeding time, and in some patients the point may be reached at which neurologic complications emerge.

Another obvious potential for bleeding in ICUs is the use of anticoagulant and thrombolytic drugs. Both may result in neurologic complications that are often ominous. There has been surprisingly little clinical research in the prevalence of neurologic complications of coagulopathies in the critical care unit. In one retrospective series, 2 of 118 patients with disseminated intravascular coagulation had neurologic complications,[97] but prospective data are not available. Given the grim prognosis in patients with multiorgan failure and severe coagulopathy, neurologic complications may not have triggered a neurologic consultation and therefore are not detected or are detected only when autopsy is allowed. This chapter provides an overview of the most commonly seen complications.

DISSEMINATED INTRAVASCULAR COAGULATION

Not unexpectedly, much morbidity in medical and surgical ICUs is related to acute disseminated intravascular coagulation (DIC). The conditions associated with DIC are summarized in Table 10–1. In many of these conditions, primarily the thrombotic coagulopathy is responsible for significant end-organ damage, and failure to recognize these triggers results in self-perpetuation of the common pathways of clotting activation.

Patients with DIC have clinical symptoms that pertain to both hemorrhage and thrombosis. Activation of the coag-

Table 10-1 CAUSES OF DISSEMINATED INTRAVASCULAR COAGULATION IN THE INTENSIVE CARE UNIT

Sepsis or septic shock syndrome[98]
Massive blood transfusions
Burns
Aortic balloon pump or cardiopulmonary bypass
Infection after splenectomy
Toxic shock syndrome
Viremias (cytomegalovirus)[100]
Cancer (including acute leukemias)[19]
Massive tissue trauma
Aortic aneurysm*[18,30,106]
Head injury*[18,55,56,77,86,107]
Subarachnoid hemorrhage[102]
Neuroleptic malignant syndrome[27]
Cardiac arrest*[70]

*Many patients do not have clinical signs.

Table 10-2 LABORATORY SUPPORT OF DISSEMINATED INTRAVASCULAR COAGULATION

Indicator	Patients With This Finding (%)
Prolonged prothrombin time	65-75
Prolonged partial thromboplastin time	50-60
Thrombocytopenia (<60,000)	80-90
Increase in fibrin degradation products	85-100
Red cell fragments	40-50

Data from references 5, 9, and 97.

ulation system is complex and partly unresolved, but systemic circulating thrombin and plasmin both have pivotal roles. Thrombin is a product of activation of the clotting cascade and, in turn, catalyzes the breakdown of fibrinogen into fibrin monomers. These monomers polymerize into fibrin, which leads to obstructive clots in the microvasculature. Trapping of platelets into these fibrin clots results in considerable thrombocytopenia (fewer than 50,000). The laboratory diagnosis of DIC becomes likely when a decreased platelet count, decreased fibrinogen level, and prolonged prothrombin time are found. At the other end of the spectrum are the manifestations of proteolysis of fibrin by plasmin. Small fragments resulting from degradation of fibrinogen coat platelet membrane surfaces and contribute to defective platelet function in addition to the already existing thrombocytopenia. Demonstration of the fibrin degradation products by latex particle agglutination or hemagglutination test (often greater than 40 μg/mL) is a strong indicator of DIC. The laboratory indicators of DIC are summarized in Table 10-2. Recently developed sophisticated laboratory tests detect antithrombin III, increase in platelet factor 4, and increase in fibrinopeptide A. Probably the most promising test is the D-dimer assay (D-dimers are formed after plasmin digestion of cross-linked fibrin) with monoclonal antibodies, which has a high sensitivity and specificity.

The diagnosis of DIC is made most frequently by the continuing oozing of surgical wounds and arterial or venous puncture sites. In addition to these subtle clinical signs, petechiae, purpura, and, at times, large subcutaneous hematomas may develop. Intravascular fibrin and platelet deposition probably accounts for most of the clinical symptoms and determines outcome. Microthrombi compromise many organs, particularly in the pulmonary and renal circulation. Acute renal failure and acute respiratory distress syndrome are major life-threatening complications that require urgent intervention. Signs of microvascular thrombosis may also involve the skin and result in superficial gangrene.

Neurologic complications of DIC consist of intracerebral hemorrhage,[57] cerebral artery branch occlusions,[44,92,93] and, probably more common, sinus thrombosis.[15,35]

Cerebral Venous Occlusion

Patients in a hypercoagulable state are likely to have venous thrombi as well. Sinovenous occlusion with involvement of large cerebral veins, such as the superior sagittal sinus and superficial middle cerebral vein, may account for sudden focal signs and stupor.[15] Pathologic studies have thoroughly documented venous cerebral thrombosis in patients with rapid development of DIC. Little, however, is known of the risk in patients without a rapid cascade of thrombotic events.

In some patients, clinical features of cerebral venous occlusion are characterized by a sudden rapidly progressive decrease in consciousness without any warning localizing signs. Most patients (74%), however, present with severe headache, and approximately 50% present with papilledema as well. Most patients are drowsy or confused, and a considerable number have recurrent tonic-clonic seizures. To a lesser extent, focal signs are seen and are invariably associated with the development of hemorrhagic infarction that may evolve into a massive intracerebral hematoma.

Cerebral venous sinus occlusion can be adequately assessed by computed tomography (CT) scanning with infusion of contrast medium. The empty triangle, or delta, sign is pathognomonic of superior sinus thrombosis but may also appear as a false sign in patients scanned after angiographic studies for other reasons. In 1991, Ulmer and Elster found that the empty delta sign was unreliable beyond 30 to 45 minutes of contrast agent infusion.[114] Other CT scan findings are unilateral or bilateral hypodensities or mixed densities suggesting hemorrhagic infarction and increased tentorial or gyral enhancement in contrast CT scans. Occlusion of the internal cerebral veins may result in bilateral thalamic hypodensities or hemorrhages[29,39] (Fig. 10–1). Magnetic resonance imaging (MRI), however, is the method of choice in noninvasive assessment of dural sinus thrombosis.[29,73,117]

Ischemic and Hemorrhagic Strokes

Ischemic strokes are less commonly seen, although microthrombi in small-or medium-sized vessels are frequent histopathologic findings. Occlusion of major arterial branches, primarily the middle cerebral artery, may occur.[119] Anecdotal reports have mentioned subdural hematoma and subarachnoid hemorrhage. Subarachnoid hemorrhage usually is limited to the convexity. Subcortical petechial hemorrhages have recently been reported on CT scans[125] in patients with DIC and are identical to the pathologic descriptions (Fig. 10–1B and 10–1C). Often, the critical condition in these patients hampers the neurologist's ability to make the diagnosis by CT scan.

Thrombi also may lodge in the choriocapillaris, causing visual loss and metamorphopsia, but fortunately, the condition is rare and, if present, transient.[67]

Treatment

The treatment of patients with DIC depends on the underlying cause, but many neurologists favor an aggressive approach with subcutaneous administration of a low dose of heparin (80 U/kg every 4 to 6 hours).[25,40] Intravenous administration may be reasonable in patients who have associated cerebral venous thrombosis. A recently completed randomized trial (using 300 IU and 25,000 to 65,000 IU/d, with target partial thromboplastin time between 80 and 100 seconds) demonstrated striking differences in morbidity and mortality and included patients who had already had hemorrhagic infarctions.[25] Most patients in the heparin group had complete clinical recovery, whereas in the control group, most patients remained severely disabled or died. The role of heparin is unclear, however, in patients in whom an intracerebral hematoma with horizontal shift has already developed. Medical intervention with osmotic therapy is indicated, and surgical evacuation should be regarded as a last resort in these patients with continuing coagulopathy.

Alternative treatment may be perfusion of the sinus with urokinase or tis-

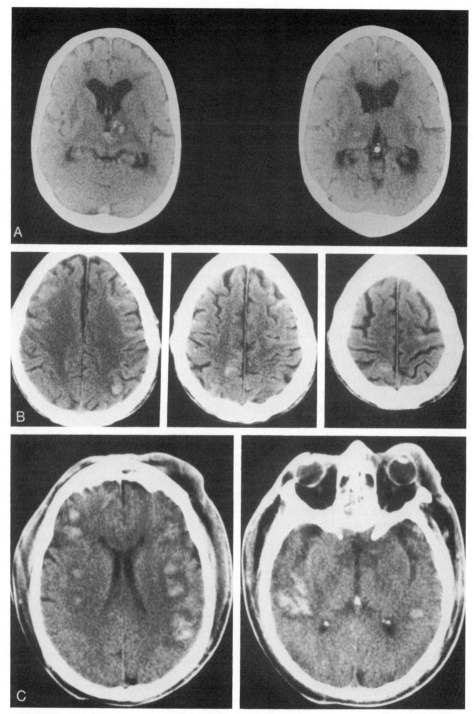

Figure 10–1. Computed tomography scan patterns in disseminated intravascular coagulation. *A*, Bilateral hemorrhagic thalamic infarction associated with deep vein thrombosis. *B*, Petechial hemorrhages in the white matter, at times following the cortex. *C*, Multiple small intracerebral hemorrhages. (Panels *B* and *C* from Wijdicks, et al,[124] with permission of the American Society of Neuroradiology.)

sue plasminogen activator (TPA),[7] and although this is promising, clinical experience is very limited.

THROMBOLYSIS AND ANTICOAGULATION

Thrombolytic therapy and anticoagulation are widely used in medical and cardiac ICUs. Streptokinase, urokinase, and, more recently, TPA are established agents for thrombolysis in selected patients with acute myocardial infarction.[1,36,37,47,48,108,121] The efficacy of thrombolytic therapy is being tested and is promising in other critical illnesses, such as pulmonary embolism, occlusion of vascular access shunts, thrombi from vascular grafts, and peripheral arterial thromboembolic disease.

The current generation of thrombolytic agents (TPA, prourokinase, streptokinase-plasminogen complex) has the potential to be more fibrin-specific and is less likely to cause an overwhelming systemic response, but bleeding into the gastrointestinal tract and retroperitoneal hematomas do occur. Allergic responses with anaphylactic shock have been reported in association with streptokinase alone.

In thrombolytic therapy, most complications have been reported in association with acute myocardial infarction. Infarcted myocardium may generate thrombi and cause ischemic stroke, but the risk is low: 1% to 2% of the patient population admitted with acute myocardial infarction.[60,65,66,105]

The Duke Databank for Cardiovascular Disease determined that in 67% of patients with strokes after acute myocardial infarction, stroke occurred within the first week (median, 4.5 days) after infarction. Transthoracic echocardiography has shown that left ventricular thrombus forms in the first week.[4] Cerebral infarction was usually confined to the carotid territory, but posterior circulation strokes occurred in approximately 25% of the patients.

Risk factors for ischemic stroke after acute myocardial infarction may include arrhythmias (particularly atrial arrhythmias), history of previous stroke, forward failure, and echocardiographic demonstration of left ventricular thrombus.

Demonstration of left ventricular thrombus or even the presence of multiple peripheral emboli does not necessarily imply a high risk of stroke.[43] The risk of ischemic stroke in patients with echocardiographically demonstrated thrombus remains low but continues to be present in the first months.

A 1987 prospective study[104] of patients with acute myocardial infarction found that within the group of patients with transthoracic echocardiographically documented left ventricular thrombi, cerebral and systemic emboli occurred significantly more often in those with protruding rather than flat thrombi and in those with portions of thrombi that moved independently from the underlying myocardium. Left ventricular aneurysm, atrial fibrillation, or the magnitude of diminished ejection fraction did not increase the risk of embolization.

Whether anticoagulation decreases the incidence of stroke associated with myocardial infarction is not resolved, but one randomized trial showed that heparin, 12,500 U administered subcutaneously every 12 hours, reduced the incidence of left ventricular thrombus, with a significant trend toward reduction of ischemic stroke (0.9% compared with 37%).[112] A 1992 meta-analysis (less reliable because of different end points) confirmed a reduction of stroke with anticoagulation therapy.[116]

Patients with in-hospital ischemic stroke associated with acute myocardial infarction may potentially benefit from intravenous or intra-arterial thrombolytic treatment. Fresh thrombus may be lysed by immediate treatment with intravenously administered TPA. In at least one study, this treatment resulted in partial or complete recanalization in 34% of the patients.[127] Intra-arterial delivery of urokinase with placement of the catheter inside the clot may be an option if the logistics are favorable, but experience is limited.

The evidence now available indicates that patients with acute myocardial infarction can substantially benefit from thrombolytic treatment. (The margin of benefit, however, may be smaller if coronary perfusion is not restored within 4 hours after occlusion.) Thrombolytic therapy (streptokinase, anistreplase, TPA) is usually combined with full doses of intravenously administered heparin for several days to prevent reocclusion, a combination that may in some cases account for the increased incidence of hemorrhagic complications. Kase and associates[53] found that activated partial thromboplastin time was excessively prolonged in two thirds of their patient population.

Thrombolytic Treatment

The cerebrovascular complications of intravenously delivered thrombolytic agents are relatively rare. Studies of thrombolysis-induced intracerebral hemorrhage have reported rates of 0.4% to 0.7%.[3,34,47,49,50] Cerebral infarcts, however, are equally frequent, and hemorrhagic transformation of a large cerebral infarct or hemorrhage in a previous or silent infarct may also occur and cannot always be reliably differentiated from a spontaneous lobar hematoma. Subdural hematomas are extremely rare (0.2% in the Thrombolysis in Myocardial Infarction, phase II [TIMI II] trial). In most large clinical trials on thrombolysis, prevalence of intracerebral complications is biased by exclusion of patients with previous strokes and patients with moderate hypertension. Moreover, in most thrombolysis trials, one third of the patients were not properly investigated and had strokes of undetermined origin.[101]

Intracerebral hemorrhage after administration of thrombolytic agents occurs within a few hours but has been reported up to 2 days after bolus injection, which weakens the associa-

tion with these short-acting agents.* In the TIMI II trial, 65% of intracranial hematomas occurred within 12 hours and 83% within 24 hours after infusion and continuous heparin treatment.

Most hematomas are localized in the subcortical white matter. In some patients, additional hematomas develop in previously infarcted areas. Unusual sites are the vermis, cerebellar hemispheres, and pons.[80] Hemorrhages in the putamen are rare but may reflect exclusion of patients with hypertension from treatment trials. The CT scan characteristics of thrombolysis-associated hemorrhage have recently been reviewed in comparison with other types of lobar hemorrhages (Fig. 10–2). More prevalent in fibrinolysis-associated hemorrhages are fluid levels inside the hematoma (indicating continuing anticoagulation), multiple parenchymal hemorrhages, and hemorrhages in multiple intracranial compartments, including the intraventricular, subdural, and subarachnoid spaces. In 75% of the patients with fibrinolysis-associated hemorrhages, hemorrhages were found in three or more compartments.[123] These characteristics are not unique to TPA or the combination with heparin, because recently the same pattern of multiple compartment involvement and fluid levels was seen in warfarin-associated intracerebral hematomas.[124] Hemorrhage in only intraventricular or subarachnoid compartments without intraparenchymal hemorrhage is rare but has been described. In Ugliette and associates' series,[113] one patient had subdural hematoma in the posterior fossa and between hemispheres, both extremely uncommon locations.

The clinical course in many patients is devastating, often progressing to brain death, so that emergency neurosurgical intervention probably will be unsuccessful. Early aggressive medical

---

*References 23, 52, 53, 72, 81, 87, 113, 123.

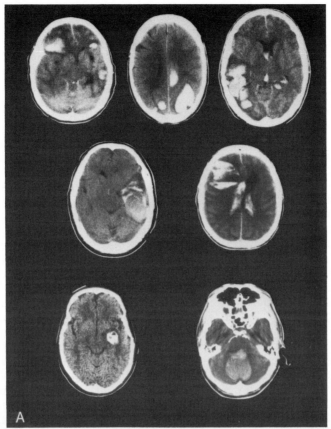

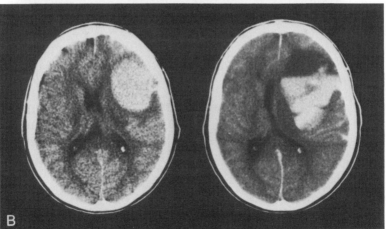

Figure 10-2. *A*, Patterns of intracerebral hematoma associated with tissue plasminogen activator. Multiple compartment hemorrhages are shown in the top row, lobar hemorrhages with prominent fluid levels in the middle row, and putamen and vermis hemorrhage in the bottom row. *B*, Sequential computed tomography scans (1 hour apart) in patient with intracerebral hematoma associated with tissue plasminogen activator. Note dramatic enlargement, fluid level, and shift. (From Wijdicks and Jack,[123] with permission of the American Heart Association.)

treatment probably does not prevent deterioration, because rapidly enlarging hematomas are common[123] (Fig. 10–2B). Outcome is poor because many patients have large-sized hematomas within hours after onset.[123]

Risk factors for intracerebral hematomas have been identified, and age of 70 years or more appears to be a major risk factor.[2] In a recent retrospective analysis, transient increased blood pressure (150/90 mm Hg or greater) tended to be more frequent in patients with intracerebral hemorrhage.[2] Only systolic blood pressure was statistically significant, a finding that suggested a systemic response rather than a direct cause of intracerebral hemorrhage.

The site of the hemorrhages in thrombolysis-associated intracerebral hematomas argues against hypertension as a major contributing factor. Patients with hypertension alone usually have bleeding in the distribution of perforating vessels, so that bleeding occurs into sites such as the basal ganglia, posterior lateral thalamus, pons, and cerebellar hemispheres. No associations have been found with specific thrombolytic agents, concomitant anticoagulant therapy, or partial thromboplastin time.

The pathophysiologic mechanism of TPA-associated intracerebral hematoma is unresolved. However, the increased incidence in the elderly and multiplicity and superficial location of hematomas may support a role for severe cerebral amyloid angiopathy in this subset of patients. Amyloid angiopathy is much more prevalent in the octogenarian, but only a few patients have severe involvement with leaky arteries.

In a few patients with TPA-associated intracerebral hematoma, severe amyloid angiopathy has been found at autopsy when specifically looked for with Congo red stain under polarized light.[123] Severe amyloid angiopathy, pathologically characterized by continuous blood leakage and fibroid necrosis, may cause only a lobar hemorrhage when the balance between clotting and hemorrhage is acutely disturbed by TPA and heparin.

Guidelines for management are summarized in Table 10–3. Probably important in the management of intracerebral hemorrhage is treatment of hypertension in a patient with continuing bleeding. Hypertension is associated with catecholamine surges and can, therefore, probably be best managed with single doses of beta-blockers such as labetalol or esmolol. The principal agents for bleeding management are cryoprecipitate, fresh-frozen plasma, and, in exceptional cases, antifibrinolytic drugs. (Antifibrinolytic drugs, however, carry the risk of coronary reocclusion and may cause extensive insoluble clots in the renal collecting system.) Rapid progression of the hematoma may warrant neurosurgical evacuation, but this procedure is likely to be unsuccessful and may not prevent progression to brain death. Mortality remains very high, and survivors are often markedly disabled. Good recovery has been reported, but only in patients with intracerebral hemorrhages small in volume. In a 1994 report of successful needle aspiration of a TPA-associated hematoma with a fluid level, outcome was good.[63]

Table 10–3 GUIDELINES FOR THE TREATMENT OF THROMBOLYSIS-ASSOCIATED INTRACEREBRAL HEMATOMAS

Step 1	Cryoprecipitate	10 units
	Fresh-frozen plasma	2 units
	Protamine	1 mg/100 U of heparin
Step 2	Bleeding time > 9 min	Platelets, 10 units
Step 3	Repeat computed tomography scan 1 to 3 h later; progression with shift	Consider neurosurgical evacuation or needle aspiration

Data from references 26 and 64.

Anticoagulant Therapy

Full anticoagulation with heparin or warfarin is frequently used in critically ill patients. Documented embolic events are common indications, but heparin is also frequently used postoperatively in patients who had major cardiac or vascular procedures. Life-threatening bleeding complications from anticoagulation are relatively rare. Cumulative risk in one study was 1% at 6 months and 5% at 1 year.[83] (These risks will probably be redefined with use of international normalized ratio measures.)

Intracerebral hemorrhage may occur during anticoagulation without any warning signs. Kase and coworkers,[54] in a review of 24 patients with anticoagulation-associated intracerebral hemorrhage, found a predilection for vermis hemorrhage, but any location is possible. Patients with anticoagulant-associated intracerebral hemorrhage generally have higher incidences of mortality and morbidity that remain unexplained. Advanced age did not increase the risk of any hemorrhagic complication of warfarin therapy, and in most studies, larger volume of hematomas could not account for this finding.[83] Serial CT scanning, however, has not been performed systematically; therefore, continued bleeding may have gone unnoticed.

Subdural hematomas, including those in the posterior fossa,[17,126,131] generally are more frequent in anticoagulated patients, often after trivial head trauma. Subarachnoid hemorrhage has been frequently mentioned in many review papers on neurologic complications of anticoagulation, but these isolated reports predate the routine use of CT scan.

Intramedullary spinal cord hemorrhages have been described in only two isolated case reports.[79,85] Intraspinal hemorrhages may occur suddenly with maximal deficit at the onset. Fortunately, a protracted course has been described that allows for immediate hemostasis. Severe sudden back pain reminiscent of coup de poignard (dagger's thrust) in epidural spinal hemorrhage may precede the spinal cord injury, but pain can be absent.[95] Aggressive medical and surgical intervention may certainly result in good ambulation and bladder control.

Spinal epidural, subarachnoid, and subdural hematomas, often in association with lumbar puncture, have been described in many isolated reports.* MRI is a superior study to myelography and CT scanning but may not be the most practical imaging study in mechanically ventilated critically ill patients. Urgent surgical decompression is warranted, but reversal of anticoagulation and conservative management have been tried in patients with extensive hematomas unsuitable for surgery. Conservative management in two patients who had extensive spinal intradural hematomas with clinically almost complete transverse myelopathy resulted in ambulation and normal bladder function.[94]

Hematomas that cause compressive mononeuropathies or plexopathies are infrequent.[33] The relative infrequency may also suggest that these conditions are overlooked in the ICU and are overshadowed by systemic illness.

Femoral nerve compression in the psoas and iliac compartments has been well documented.† The anatomic relationship between the femoral nerve and the obturator nerve in the fascial compartments is outlined in Figure 10-3.

Clinically, femoral nerve paralysis is characterized by pain in the groin and thigh radiating into the patellar area. Weakness of the iliopsoas or quadriceps muscle, absent knee jerk, and sensory loss over the anteromedial region of the lower extremities are further hallmarks of this neuropathy. Many patients have an antalgic position of the hip (flexed, abducted, and externally rotated).

---

*References 6, 12, 22, 38, 41, 46, 61, 69, 71, 85, 91, 95, 109–111.
†References 13, 16, 21, 28, 32, 51, 59, 68, 74, 76, 84, 103, 120, 128–130.

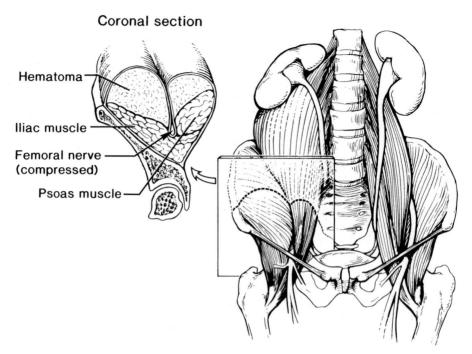

Figure 10-3. Anatomy of the femoral nerve in iliac and psoas muscles. The mechanism of compression in psoas hematoma is shown.

Computed tomography scanning[45,115] (Fig. 10-4) almost always demonstrates a retroperitoneal mass that may at times be bilateral.[103] Improvement after correction of the coagulopathy can be impressive with conservative measures. In patients with a coagulopathy, surgical evacuation of a psoas hematoma may lead to immediate recurrence of the hematoma or bleeding into the retroperitoneal space when the tamponade is released. In addition, mobilization of the colon and difficult identification of a displaced ureter make surgery a complicated task. Decompressive surgery may be indicated in patients who can undergo a major surgical procedure with minimal risk for postoperative complications, but in clinical practice this situation rarely occurs and conservative management is preferred.

Retroperitoneal hemorrhage is the most common anticoagulant-related hematoma, but hematoma in the gluteal muscles may cause severe hip pain and sudden weak foot from sciatic nerve compression. Outcome is excellent with conservative measures.[31,78,118]

Other compressive neuropathies are extremely rare. Two cases of acute carpal tunnel syndrome with anticoagulation have been reported.[20,75] Epineurolysis to release hematoma in the epineurium is often needed to relieve the excruciating pain. Generally, pain and diminished sensation in the wrist and fingers are experienced, and frank weakness of the opponens pollicis and abductor pollicis brevis is rare. Outcome of anticoagulation-associated neuropathies is summarized in Table 10-4.

THROMBOTIC THROMBOCYTOPENIC PURPURA

Moschcowitz's disease is viewed as unique because of the overwhelming systemic complications that accompany the disorder. Thrombotic throm-

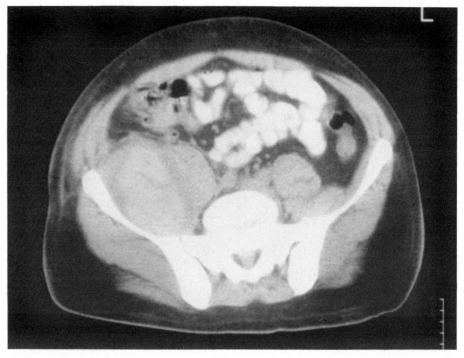

Figure 10–4. Psoas hematoma demonstrated on abdominal computed tomography scan.

bocytopenic purpura is not extremely rare (0.1 per 100,000 patients annually in the Rochester, Minnesota, area),[82] and the incidence may be increasing.[14] Treatment is complex, and mortality is substantial despite marked improvement after the introduction of plasma exchange. In this respect, many patients are cared for in medical ICUs, and neurologic manifestations are part of the triad of microangiopathic hemolytic anemia and thrombocytopenia.

Table 10–4 NERVE COMPRESSION DURING ANTICOAGULATION THERAPY

Nerve	Outcome
Femoral	Fair-good
Sciatic	Good
Median	Excellent
Brachial plexus	Poor-fair

Data from references 11, 118, and 129.

Clinical Features

The initial presentation of thrombotic thrombocytopenic purpura is abrupt, usually with bleeding and neurologic manifestations. Purpura is seldom the sole manifestation, and evidence of hemorrhage may include petechiae, ecchymoses, retinal hemorrhages, epistaxis, hemoptysis, and gastrointestinal hemorrhage. Of all the nonspecific symptoms, such as fatigue, arthralgia, and jaundice, fever is the most consistent, but it may be absent initially and at the time of neurologic manifestations.

Neurologic manifestations invariably punctuate the course of illness.[8,24,88,122] In a recent series of 102 patients, 64 had fluctuating neurologic signs at presentation, and neurologic abnormalities developed in 8 during the course of the illness.[89]

Many patients have changes in level of consciousness associated with delirium and restlessness. Headache is common. The most common clinical

Table 10-5 NEUROLOGIC MANIFESTATIONS OF THROMBOTIC THROMBOCYTOPENIC PURPURA

Headache
Behavior changes
Hemiparesis, hemisensory findings, aphasia, hemianopia, cortical blindness
Focal and generalized seizures
Ischemic optic neuropathy
Cauda equina syndrome

Data from references 8, 82, 88, 99, and 122.

presentations (Table 10-5) represent ischemic strokes from occlusion of small vessels. The waxing and waning of the neurologic deficits has been explained by brief ischemia caused by microthrombi composed of loose platelet aggregates occluding terminal arterioles and capillaries. Despite claims of complete recovery, permanent deficits are not uncommon, even in the plasma exchange era. Small cortical infarcts and multiple small subcortical infarcts that mimic lacunar disease have been described.

Occlusions of major arterial branches are uncommon but have been demonstrated on MRI. In addition, MRI or CT scan may demonstrate cerebral infarcts that are compatible with neurologic signs that have resolved, a suggestion of permanent damage rather than transient ischemic events.[88] Serial MRI scans in one patient (Fig. 10-5) may also show silent infarcts. Results of MRI, however, are most often normal in patients with waxing and waning level of consciousness alone. A 1991 study suggested that normal findings on CT scan predicted the potential for recovery in patients, including those with aphasia, hemiparesis, and visual field defects,[58] but in all likelihood, CT scan may not be sensitive enough to exclude cerebral infarcts when clinical findings are resolving.

Laboratory Findings and Treatment

Patients have moderately severe anemia, fragmented erythrocytes, increased blood levels of unconjugated bilirubin and lactic dehydrogenase, platelet counts close to 20,000/μL, and increased reticulocyte counts (75%). Proteinuria, hematuria, and abnormal results of liver function tests are also found.[62,90] The cerebrospinal fluid has only rarely been examined, because of obvious dangers and the possible deleterious effects of platelet transfusion on thrombotic thrombocytopenic purpura itself,[42] but xanthochromia and increased protein have been found.[96] The pathologic lesions of hyaline thrombi and occluded capillaries and arterioles may be demonstrated in 50% of gingiva biopsy specimens, but the finding is nonspecific.

Treatment is plasmapheresis (1.5 plasma volume removal in 4 days), which is more effective than plasma infusion.[89,90,96] Additional use of aspirin and dipyridamole or additional high doses of steroids are considered in patients with severe symptoms.

CONCLUSIONS

The addition of thrombolytic agents to the repertoire of the cardiologist has increased the incidence of hemorrhagic complications, in particular, intracranial hemorrhages. The troublesome systemic side effects of thrombolytic agents, often easily overcome, contrast sharply with the enormous morbidity and mortality of intracranial hemorrhages. Hemorrhages in multiple compartments and fluid levels inside the hematomas suggest continuing anticoagulation. Neurosurgical intervention is likely fruitless. In a localized hematoma with sedimented blood from inability of a firm clot to form, catheter placement or needle aspiration can be tried, but experience is anecdotal.

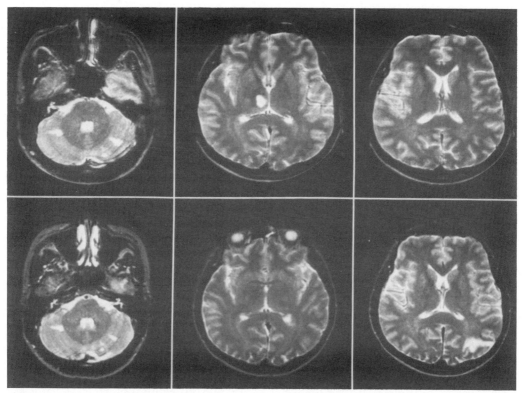

Figure 10–5. T2-weighted serial magnetic resonance images in patient with thrombotic thrombocytopenic purpura. *Upper row*, Multiple cerebral infarcts in cerebellar hemispheres and thalamus. *Lower row*, "Silent" occipital infarct 6 months later and resolution of thalamic infarct. (From Wijdicks,[122] with permission of the American Heart Association.)

The final common pathway of pathologic events is probably bleeding from severe amyloid angiopathy in patients who are overcoagulated. The increased risk of intracranial hematomas in the elderly confirms this hypothesis. This risk may also have resulted in diminished enthusiasm for the use of thrombolytic agents in the elderly. (Elderly patients with acute myocardial infarction are still six times less likely to receive these agents than are younger patients.) Invariably, heparin is used to prevent reocclusion of coronary arteries, and because similar CT scan findings have recently been reported in patients with increased bleeding time from warfarin alone, thrombolytic agents may not be the main instigators.

Another well-documented complication of anticoagulation is compression of the femoral nerve in the psoas and iliac compartments, which can be visualized on CT scan. The natural history can be good, so that a surgical approach to release compression is controversial.

REFERENCES

1. AIMS Trial Study Group: Long-term effects of intravenous anistreplase in acute myocardial infarction: Final report of the AIMS study. Lancet 335:427–431, 1990.
2. Anderson, JL, Karagounis, L, Allen, A, et al: Older age and elevated blood pressure are risk factors for intracerebral hemorrhage after thrombolysis. Am J Cardiol 68:166–170, 1991.
3. Anderson, JL, Sorensen, SG, Moreno, FL, et al: Multicenter patency trial of intravenous anistreplase compared with streptokinase in acute myocardial infarction. Circulation 83:126–140, 1991.
4. Asinger, RW, Mikell, FL, Elsperger, J, and Hodges, M: Incidence of left-ventricular thrombosis after acute transmural myocardial infarction: Serial evaluation by two-dimensional echocardiography. N Engl J Med 305:297–302, 1981.
5. Baker, WF Jr: Clinical aspects of disseminated intravascular coagulation: A clinician's point of view. Semin Thromb Hemost 15:1–57, 1989.
6. Bamford, CR: Spinal epidural hematoma due to heparin (letter). Arch Neurol 35:693–694, 1978.
7. Barnwell, SL, Higashida, RT, Halbach, VV, et al: Direct endovascular thrombolytic therapy for dural sinus thrombosis. Neurosurgery 28:135–142, 1991.
8. Ben-Yehuda, D, Rose, M, Michaeli, Y, and Eldor, A: Permanent neurological complications in patients with thrombotic thrombocytopenic purpura. Am J Hematol 29:74–78, 1988.
9. Bick, RL: Disseminated intravascular coagulation and related syndromes: A clinical review. Semin Thromb Hemost 14:299–338, 1988.
10. Bieger, R, Vreeken, J, Stibbe, J, and Loeliger, EA: Arterial aneurysm as a cause of consumption coagulopathy. N Engl J Med 285:152–154, 1971.
11. Blankenship, JC: Median and ulnar neuropathy after streptokinase infusion. Heart Lung 20:221–223, 1991.
12. Brandt, M: Spontaneous intramedullary haematoma as a complication of anticoagulant therapy. Acta Neurochir (Wien) 52:73–77, 1980.
13. Brantigan, JW, Owens, ML, and Moody, FG: Femoral neuropathy complicating anticoagulant therapy. Am J Surg 132:108–109, 1976.
14. Bukowski, RM: Thrombotic thrombocytopenic purpura: A review. Prog Hemost Thromb 6:287–337, 1982.
15. Buonanno, FS, Cooper, MR, Moody, DM, et al: Neuroradiologic aspects of cerebral disseminated intravascular coagulation. AJNR Am J Neuroradiol 1:245–250, 1980.
16. Butterfield, WC, Neviaser, RJ, and Roberts, MP: Femoral neuropathy and anticoagulants. Ann Surg 176:58–61, 1972.
17. Capistrant, T, Goldberg, R, Shibasaki, H, and Castle, D: Posterior fossa subdural haematoma associated with anticoagulant therapy. J Neurol Neurosurg Psychiatry 34:82–85, 1971.
18. Clark, JA, Finelli, RE, and Netsky, MG: Disseminated intravascular coagulation following cranial trauma: Case report. J Neurosurg 52:266–269, 1980.
19. Colman, RW and Rubin, RN: Disseminated intravascular coagulation due to malignancy. Semin Oncol 17:172–186, 1990.
20. Copeland, J, Wells, HG Jr, and Puckett, CL: Acute carpal tunnel syndrome in a patient taking coumadin. J Trauma 29:131–132, 1989.
21. Cranberg, L: Femoral neuropathy from iliac hematoma: Report of a case. Neurology 29:1071–1072, 1979.
22. Dahlin, PA and George, J. Intraspinal hematoma as a complication of anticoagulant therapy. Clin Pharmacol 3:656–661, 1984.
23. De Jaegere, PP, Arnold, AA, Balk, AH, and Simoons, ML: Intracranial hemorrhage in association with thrombolytic therapy: Incidence and clinical predictive factors. J Am Coll Cardiol 19:289–294, 1992.
24. De la Sayette, V, Gallet E, le Doze, F, et al: Purpura thrombotique thrombocy-

topénique: 1 cas avec imagerie par résonance magnétique. Rev Neurol (Paris) 147:314–317, 1991.

25. Einhäupl, KM, Villringer, A, Meister, W, et al: Heparin therapy in sinus venous thrombosis. Lancet 338:597–600, 1991.

26. Eleff, SM, Borel, C, Bell, WR, and Long, DM: Acute management of intracranial hemorrhage in patients receiving thrombolytic therapy: Case reports. Neurosurgery 26:867–869, 1990.

27. Eles, GR, Songer, JE, and DiPette, DJ: Neuroleptic malignant syndrome complicated by disseminated intravascular coagulation. Arch Intern Med 144:1296–1297, 1984.

28. Emery, S and Ochoa, J: Lumbar plexus neuropathy resulting from retroperitoneal hemorrhage. Muscle Nerve 1: 330–334, 1978.

29. Erbguth, F, Brenner, P, Schuierer, G, et al: Diagnosis and treatment of deep cerebral vein thrombosis. Neurosurg Rev 14:145–148, 1991.

30. Fisher, DF Jr, Yawn, DH, and Crawford, ES: Preoperative disseminated intravascular coagulation associated with aortic aneurysms: A prospective study of 76 cases. Arch Surg 118:1252–1255, 1983.

31. Fleming, RE Jr, Michelsen, CB, and Stinchfield, FE: Sciatic paralysis: A complication of bleeding following hip surgery. J Bone Joint Surg [Am] 61:37–39, 1979.

32. Galzio, R, Lucantoni, D, Zenobii, M, et al: Femoral neuropathy caused by iliacus hematoma. Surg Neurol 20:254–257, 1983.

33. Gilden, DH and Eisner, J: Lumbar plexopathy caused by disseminated intravascular coagulation. JAMA 237:2846–2847, 1977.

34. Gore, JM, Sloan, M, Price, TR, et al: Intracerebral hemorrhage, cerebral infarction, and subdural hematoma after acute myocardial infarction and thrombolytic therapy in the Thrombolysis in Myocardial Infarction study: Thrombolysis in Myocardial Infarction, Phase II, pilot and clinical trial. Circulation 83:448–459, 1991.

35. Grabowski, EF and Zimmerman, RD: Disseminated intravascular coagulation and the neuroradiologist. AJNR Am J Neuroradiol 12:344, 1991.

36. Gruppo Italiano per lo Studio della Streptochinasi nell'Infarto Miocardico (GISSI): Effectiveness of intravenous thrombolytic treatment in acute myocardial infarction. Lancet i:397–401, 1986.

37. Gruppo Italiano per lo Studio della Streptochinasi nell'Infarto Miocardico (GISSI): Long-term effects of intravenous thrombolysis in acute myocardial infarction: Final report of the GISSI study. Lancet ii:871–874, 1987.

38. Guthikonda, M, Schmidek, HH, Wallman, LJ, and Snyder, TM: Spinal subdural hematoma: Case report and review of the literature. Neurosurgery 5:614–616, 1979.

39. Hagner, G, Iglesias-Rozas, JR, Kölmel, HW, and Gerhartz, H: Hemorrhagic infarction of the basal ganglia: An unusual complication of acute leukemia. Oncology 40:387–391, 1983.

40. Hanley, DF, Feldman, E, Borel, CO, et al: Treatment of sagittal sinus thrombosis associated with cerebral hemorrhage and intracranial hypertension. Stroke 19:903–909, 1988.

41. Harik, SI, Raichle, ME, and Reis, DJ: Spontaneously remitting spinal epidural hematoma in a patient on anticoagulants. N Engl J Med 284:1355–1357, 1971.

42. Harkness, DR, Byrnes, JJ, Lian, EC-Y, et al: Hazard of platelet transfusion in thrombotic thrombocytopenic purpura. JAMA 246:1931–1933, 1981.

43. Haugland, JM, Asinger, RW, Mikell, FL, et al: Embolic potential of left ventricular thrombi detected by two-dimensional echocardiography. Circulation 70:588–598, 1984.

44. Hill, JB and Schwartzman, RJ: Cerebral infarction and disseminated intravascular coagulation with pheochromocytoma. Arch Neurol 38:395, 1981.

45. Hoyt, TE, Tiwari, R, and Kusske, JA: Compressive neuropathy as a compli-

cation of anticoagulant therapy. Neurosurgery 12:268–271, 1983.

46. Hurst, PG, Seeger, J, Carter, P, and Marcus, FI: Value of magnetic resonance imaging for diagnosis of cervical epidural hematoma associated with anticoagulation after cardiac valve replacement. Am J Cardiol 63:1016–1017, 1989.

47. The International Study Group: In-hospital mortality and clinical course of 20,891 patients with suspected acute myocardial infarction randomised between alteplase and streptokinase with or without heparin. Lancet 336:71–75, 1990.

48. The I.S.A.M. Study Group: A prospective trial of intravenous streptokinase in acute myocardial infarction (I.S.A.M.): Mortality, morbidity, and infarct size at 21 days. N Engl J Med 314:1465–1471, 1986.

49. ISIS-2 (Second International Study of Infarct Survival) Collaborative Group: Randomised trial of intravenous streptokinase, oral aspirin, both, or neither among 17,187 cases of suspected acute myocardial infarction: ISIS-2. Lancet ii:349–360, 1988.

50. ISIS-3 (Third International Study of Infarct Survival) Collaborative Group: A randomised comparison of streptokinase vs tissue plasminogen activator vs anistreplase and of aspirin plus heparin vs aspirin alone among 41,299 cases of suspected acute myocardial infarction. Lancet 339:753–770, 1992.

51. Jackson, S: Femoral neuropathy secondary to heparin induced intrapelvic hematoma: A case report and review of the literature. Orthopedics 10:1049–1052, 1987.

52. Kase, CS, O'Neal, AM, Fisher, M, et al: Intracranial hemorrhage after use of tissue plasminogen activator for coronary thrombolysis. Ann Intern Med 112:17–21, 1990.

53. Kase, CS, Pessin, MS, Zivin, JA, et al: Intracranial hemorrhage after coronary thrombolysis with tissue plasminogen activator. Am J Med 92:384–390, 1992.

54. Kase, CS, Robinson, RK, Stein, RW, et al: Anticoagulant-related intracerebral hemorrhage. Neurology 35:943–948, 1985.

55. Kaufman, HH, Hui, K-S, Mattson, JC, et al: Clinicopathological correlations of disseminated intravascular coagulation in patients with head injury. Neurosurgery 15:34–42, 1984.

56. Kaufman, HH, Moake, JL, Olson, JD, et al: Delayed and recurrent intracranial hematomas related to disseminated intravascular clotting and fibrinolysis in head injury. Neurosurgery 7:445–449, 1980.

57. Kawakami, Y, Ueki, K, Chikama, M, et al: Intracranial hemorrhage associated with nontraumatic disseminated intravascular coagulation — report of four cases. Neurol Med Chir (Tokyo) 30:610–617, 1990.

58. Kay, AC, Solberg, LA Jr, Nichols, DA, and Petitt, RM: Prognostic significance of computed tomography of the brain in thrombotic thrombocytopenic purpura. Mayo Clin Proc 66:602–607, 1991.

59. King, RB and Bechtold, DL: Warfarin-induced iliopsoas hemorrhage with subsequent femoral nerve palsy. Ann Emerg Med 14:362–364, 1985.

60. Komrad, MS, Coffey, CE, Coffey, KS, et al: Myocardial infarction and stroke. Neurology 34:1403–1409, 1984.

61. Krolick, MA and Cintron, GB: Spinal epidural hematoma causing cord compression after tissue plasminogen activator and heparin therapy. South Med J 84:670–671, 1991.

62. Kwaan, HC: Clinicopathological features of thrombotic thrombocytopenic purpura. Semin Hematol 24:71–81, 1987.

63. Longstreth, WT Jr, Grady, MS, and Schmer, G: Needle aspiration of an intracerebral hemorrhage complicating thrombolytic therapy for myocardial infarction (letter to the editor). Stroke 25:712–713, 1994.

64. Lubarsky, DA, Kaufman, B, and Turndorf, H: Anesthetic care of a patient with an intracranial hemorrhage after

thrombolytic therapy. J Clin Anesth 2:276–279, 1990.

65. Maggioni, AP, Franzosi, MG, Farina, ML, et al: Cerebrovascular events after myocardial infarction: Analysis of the GISSI trial. BMJ 302:1428–1431, 1991.

66. Maggioni, AP, Franzosi, MG, Santoro, E, et al: The risk of stroke in patients with acute myocardial infarction after thrombolytic and antithrombotic treatment. N Engl J Med 327:1–6, 1992.

67. Martin, VAF: Disseminated intravascular coagulopathy. Trans Ophthalmol Soc UK 98:506–507, 1978.

68. Mastroianni, PP and Roberts, MP: Femoral neuropathy and retroperitoneal hemorrhage. Neurosurgery 13:44–47, 1983.

69. Mayumi, T and Dohi, S: Spinal subarachnoid hematoma after lumbar puncture in a patient receiving antiplatelet therapy. Anesth Analg 62:777–779, 1983.

70. Mehta, B, Briggs, DK, Sommers, SC, and Karpatkin, M: Disseminated intravascular coagulation following cardiac arrest: A study of 15 patients. Am J Med Sci 264:353–363, 1972.

71. Metzger, G and Singbartl, G: Spinal epidural hematoma following epidural anesthesia versus spontaneous spinal subdural hematoma: Two case reports. Acta Anaesthesiol Scand 35:105–107, 1991.

72. More, RS and Vincent, R: Intracerebral haemorrhage after thrombolytic therapy for acute myocardial infarction. Postgrad Med J 68:800–803, 1992.

73. Nadel, L, Braun, IF, Kraft, KA, et al: MRI of intracranial sinovenous thrombosis: The role of phase imaging. Magn Reson Imaging 8:315–320, 1990.

74. Nielsen, BF: Haemorrhagic compression of the femoral nerve complicating anticoagulation therapy: Case eport. Acta Chir Scand 152:695–696, 1986.

75. Nkele, C: Acute carpal tunnel syndrome resulting from haemorrhage into the carpal tunnel in a patient on warfarin. J Hand Surg [Br] 11:455–456, 1986.

76. Olesen, LL: Femoral neuropathy secondary to anticoagulation. J Intern Med 226:279–280, 1989.

77. Olson, JD, Kaufman, HH, Moake, J, et al: The incidence and significance of hemostatic abnormalities in patients with head injuries. Neurosurgery 24:825–832, 1989.

78. Palliyath, S and Buday, J: Sciatic nerve compression: Diagnostic value of electromyography and computerized tomography. Electromyogr Clin Neurophysiol 29:9–11, 1989.

79. Papo, I and Luongo, A: Massive intramedullary hemorrhage in a patient on anticoagulants. J Neurosurg Sci 18:268–270, 1974.

80. Partanen, HJ and Nieminen, MS: Intracerebellar fatal haemorrhage after thrombolytic therapy of suspected non-Q-wave myocardial infarction (letter). Lancet 336:883, 1990.

81. Pendlebury, WW, Iole, ED, Tracy, RP, and Dill, BA: Intracerebral hemorrhage related to cerebral amyloid angiopathy and t-PA treatment. Ann Neurol 29:210–213, 1991.

82. Petitt, RM: Thrombotic thrombocytopenic purpura: A thirty year review. Semin Thromb Hemost 6:350–355, 1980.

83. Petty, GW, Lennihan, L, Mohr, JP, et al: Complications of long-term anticoagulation. Ann Neurol 23:570–574, 1988.

84. Piazza, I, Girardi, A, Giunta, G, and Pappagallo, G: Femoral nerve palsy secondary to anticoagulant-induced iliacus hematoma: A case report. Int Angiol 9:125–126, 1990.

85. Pisani, R, Carta, F, Guiducci, G, et al: Hematomyelia during anticoagulant therapy. Surg Neurol 24:578–580, 1985.

86. Pondaag, W: Disseminated intravascular coagulation related to outcome in head injury. Acta Neurochir Suppl (Wien) 28:98–102, 1979.

87. Ramsay, DA, Penswick, JL, and Robertson, DM: Fatal streptokinase-induced intracerebral haemorrhage in

cerebral amyloid angiopathy. Can J Neurol Sci 17:336–341, 1990.

88. Rinkel, GJE, Wijdicks, EFM, and Hené, RJ: Stroke in relapsing thrombotic thrombocytopenic purpura (letter). Stroke 22:1087–1089, 1991.

89. Rock, GA, Shumak, KH, Buskard, NA, et al: Comparison of plasma exchange with plasma infusion in the treatment of thrombotic thrombocytopenic purpura. N Engl J Med 325:393–397, 1991.

90. Ruggenenti, P and Remuzzi, G: Thrombotic thrombocytopenic purpura and related disorders. Hematol Oncol Clin North Am 4:219–241, 1990.

91. Russell, N, Maroun, FB, and Jacob, JC: Spinal subdural hematoma in association with anticoagulant therapy. Can J Neurol Sci 8:87–89, 1981.

92. Ryan, FP, Timperley, WR, Preston, FE, and Holdsworth, CD: Cerebral involvement with disseminated intravascular coagulation in intestinal disease. J Clin Pathol 30:551–555, 1977.

93. Schwartzman, RJ and Hill, JB: Neurologic complications of disseminated intravascular coagulation. Neurology 32:791–797, 1982.

94. Schwerdtfeger, K, Caspar, W, Alloussi, S, et al: Acute spinal intradural extramedullary hematoma: A nonsurgical approach for spinal cord decompression. Neurosurgery 27:312–314, 1990.

95. Senelick, RC, Norwood, CW, and Cohen, GH: "Painless" spinal epidural hematoma during anticoagulant therapy. Neurology 26:213–215, 1976.

96. Shepard, KV and Bukowski, RM: The treatment of thrombotic thrombocytopenic purpura with exchange transfusions, plasma infusions, and plasma exchange. Semin Hematol 24:178–193, 1987.

97. Siegal, T, Seligsohn, U, Aghai, E, and Modan, M: Clinical and laboratory aspects of disseminated intravascular coagulation (DIC): A study of 118 cases. Thromb Haemost 39:122–134, 1978.

98. Silverman, RA, Rhodes, AR, and Dennehy, PH: Disseminated intravascular coagulation and purpura fulminans in a patient with Candida sepsis. Biopsy of purpura fulminans as an aid to diagnosis of systemic Candida infection. Am J Med 80:679–684, 1986.

99. Silverstein, A: Thrombotic thrombocytopenic purpura. The initial neurologic manifestations. Arch Neurol 18:358–362, 1968.

100. Singh, R, Singh, MM, Hazra, DK, et al: A study of disseminated intravascular coagulopathy in hepatic coma complicating acute viral hepatitis. Angiology 34:470–479, 1983.

101. Sloan, MA and Price, TR: Intracranial hemorrhage following thrombolytic therapy for acute myocardial infarction. Semin Neurol 11:385–399, 1991.

102. Spallone, A, Mariani, G, Rosa, G, and Corrao, D: Disseminated intravascular coagulation as a complication of ruptured intracranial aneurysms: Report of two cases. J Neurosurg 59:142–145, 1983.

103. Stören, EJ: Bilateral iliacus haematoma with femoral nerve palsy complicating anticoagulant therapy. Acta Chir Scand 144:181–183, 1978.

104. Stratton, JR and Resnick, AD: Increased embolic risk in patients with left ventricular thrombi. Circulation 75:1004–1011, 1987.

105. Thompson, PL and Robinson, JS: Stroke after acute myocardial infarction: Relation to infarct size. Br Med J 2:457–459, 1978.

106. Thompson, RW, Adams, DH, Cohen, JR, et al: Disseminated intravascular coagulation caused by abdominal aortic aneurysm. J Vasc Surg 4:184–186, 1986.

107. Tikk, A and Noormaa, U: The significance of cerebral and systemic disseminated intravascular coagulation in early prognosis of brain injury. Acta Neurochir Suppl (Wien) 28:96–97, 1979.

108. The TIMI Study Group: Comparison of invasive and conservative strategies

after treatment with intravenous tissue plasminogen activator in acute myocardial infarction: Results of the Thrombolysis in Myocardial Infarction (TIMI) Phase II Trial. N Engl J Med 320:618–627, 1989.

109. Toledo, E, Shalit, MN, and Segal, R: Spinal subdural hematoma associated with anticoagulant therapy in a patient with spinal meningioma. Neurosurgery 8:600–603, 1981.

110. Tomarken, JL: Spinal subdural hematoma. Ann Emerg Med 14:261–263, 1985.

111. Tomarken, JL: Spinal subdural hematoma: A case report and literature review. Am J Emerg Med 5:123–125, 1987.

112. Turpie, AGG, Robinson, JG, Doyle, DJ, et al: Comparison of high-dose with low-dose subcutaneous heparin to prevent left ventricular mural thrombosis in patients with acute transmural anterior myocardial infarction. N Engl J Med 320:352–357, 1989.

113. Ugliette, JP, O'Connor, CM, Boyko, OB, et al: CT patterns of intracerebral hemorrhage complicating thrombolytic therapy for acute myocardial infarction. Radiology 181:555–559, 1991.

114. Ulmer, JL and Elster, AD: Physiologic mechanisms underlying the delayed delta sign. AJNR Am J Neuroradiol 12:647–650, 1991.

115. Uncini, A, Tonali, P, Falappa, P, and Danza, FM: Femoral neuropathy from iliac muscle hematoma induced by oral anticoagulation therapy: Report of three cases with CT demonstration. J Neurol 226:137–141, 1981.

116. Vaitkus, PT, Berlin, JA, Schwartz, JS, and Barnathan, ES: Stroke complicating acute myocardial infarction: A meta-analysis of risk modification by anticoagulation and thrombolytic therapy. Arch Intern Med 152:2020–2024, 1992.

117. Villringer, A, Seiderer, M, Bauer, WM, et al: Diagnosis of superior sagittal sinus thrombosis by three-dimensional magnetic resonance flow imaging (letter). Lancet i:1086–1087, 1989.

118. Wallach, HW and Oren, ME: Sciatic nerve compression during anticoagulation therapy: Computerized tomography aids in diagnosis. Arch Neurol 36:448, 1979.

119. Weber, MB: The neurological complications of consumption coagulopathies. Neurology 18:185–188, 1968.

120. Wells, J and Templeton, J: Femoral neuropathy associated with anticoagulant therapy. Clin Orthop 124:155–160, 1977.

121. White, HD, Norris, RM, Brown, MA, et al: Effect of intravenous streptokinase on left ventricular function and early survival after acute myocardial infarction. N Engl J Med 317:850–855, 1987.

122. Wijdicks, EFM: Silent cerebral infarcts in thrombotic thrombocytopenic purpura. Stroke 25:1297–1298, 1994.

123. Wijdicks, EFM and Jack, CR Jr: Intracerebral hemorrhage after fibrinolytic therapy for acute myocardial infarction. Stroke 24:554–557, 1993.

124. Wijdicks, EFM and Jack, CR Jr: Intracerebral hemorrhage after fibrinolytic therapy for acute myocardial infarction: Are fibrinolytic agents really the main instigators? Stroke 25:713–714, 1994.

125. Wijdicks, EFM, Silbert, PL, Jack, CR, et al: Subcortical hemorrhage in disseminated intravascular coagulation associated with sepsis. AJNR Am J Neuroradiol 15:763–765, 1994.

126. Wintzen, AR and Tijssen, JGP: Subdural hematoma and oral anticoagulant therapy. Arch Neurol 39:69–72, 1982.

127. Wolpert, SM, Bruckmann, H, Greenlee, R, et al, and the rt-PA Acute Stroke Study Group: Neuroradiologic evaluation of patients with acute stroke treated with recombinant tissue plasminogen activator. AJNR Am J Neuroradiol 14:3–13, 1993.

128. Wood, CL and Whang, R: Oral anticoagulation-induced femoral nerve en-

trapment. J Okla State Med Assoc 78:135–138, 1985.

129. Young, MR and Norris, JW: Femoral neuropathy during anticoagulant therapy. Neurology 26:1173–1175, 1976.

130. Zarranz, JJ, Simon, R, and Salisachs, P: Acute anticoagulant-induced com-pressive lumbar plexus neuropathy: A clinico-pathological study. Eur Neurol 20:469–472, 1981.

131. Zenteno-Alanis, GH, Corvera, J, and Mateos, JH: Subdural hematoma of the posterior fossa as a complication of an-ticoagulant therapy: Presentation of a case. Neurology 18:1133–1136, 1968.

Chapter 11

NEUROLOGIC COMPLICATIONS OF ACUTE VASCULITIC SYNDROMES

POLYARTERITIS NODOSA
CHURG-STRAUSS SYNDROME
WEGENER'S GRANULOMATOSIS
DRUG-INDUCED VASCULITIS

Medical intensive care units (ICUs) may have emergency admissions of patients with life-threatening vasculitic syndromes, although perhaps more commonly, the adverse consequences of long-term immunosuppressive therapy in patients with vasculitis may prompt sophisticated care.

In patients with systemic vasculitis, acute pulmonary, renal, and cardiac failure or acute bowel perforation accounts for a major proportion of ICU admissions and may occasionally be presenting features. Neurologic complications of acute vasculitis do not arise tangentially and, in fact, are in some clinical entities unique to the syndrome.

The vasculitic syndromes are very complex, consisting of a large group of heterogeneous disorders, and within the scope of this book are not dealt with in complete detail. The pathologic lesion in vasculitis can be characterized as destructive inflammatory disease of any size of blood vessel, including arterioles and venules. Some clinicians prefer a clinicopathologic classification based on size and type of vessel involvement (Table 11–1), and others classify vasculitis by whether an underlying disease is present. Lack of a cause in most patients with a vasculitic syndrome may indeed preclude classification, but in a 1990 review of 1337 patients with vasculitis, only 147 had a constellation of findings that could not be classified in one of the major histologic categories.[34] The disorders discussed in this chapter were chosen as typical of the problems that consulting neurologists may see in ICUs. Vasculitides whose clinical courses may become acutely life-threatening are Wegener's granulomatosis, Churg-Strauss syndrome, polyarteritis nodosa, and drug-induced vasculitis.[53–55]

POLYARTERITIS NODOSA

Polyarteritis is primarily a multisystem inflammatory disease of medium- and arteriolar-sized vessels. Pathologic examination characteristically shows infiltration of polymorphonuclear leukocytes, fibrinoid necrosis, and destruction of the media of the arterial wall. Aneurysm formation occurs at this stage and may lead to rupture, but vasculitis also results in circumferential proliferation of fibrous tissue and endothelial cells, eventually culminating in vascular occlusion and infarction. The most common reasons for ICU admission in patients with polyarteritis nodosa are perforation of the small or

Table 11–1 CLASSIFICATION OF VASCULITIS

Vasculitis	Vessel Size
Idiopathic vasculitides	
Polyarteritis nodosa	M, S
Wegener's granulomatosis	M, S
Churg-Strauss syndrome	M, S
Giant cell arteritis	L, M, S
Takayasu's arteritis	L, M, S
Behçet's disease	M, S
Primary CNS vasculitis	L, M, S
Kawasaki's disease	M, S
Cogan's syndrome	M, S
Henoch-Schönlein purpura	S
Buerger's disease	M, S
Secondary vasculitis	
Infectious angiitis (e.g., spirochetal, mycobacterial, pyogenic)	L, M, S
Vasculitis of collagen-vascular disease (rheumatoid arthritis, SLE, Sjögren's syndrome)	M, S
Cryoglobinemic vasculitis	S
Drug-induced, malignancy-associated, and transplant vasculitis	S
Vasculitis in sarcoid	M, S
Miscellaneous vasculitis	L, M, S

Data from Churg, A and Churg, J (eds): Systemic Vasculitides. Igaku-Shoin, New York, 1991.

CNS = central nervous system; L = large; M = medium; S = small; SLE = systemic lupus erythematosus.

large bowel, gastrointestinal hemorrhage from aneurysmal rupture, and congestive heart failure from coronary artery vasculitis and hypertension.

Clinical Features

The frequency of organ involvement is variable and wide-ranging. In some patients, only one organ is involved (Table 11–2). Typical clinical findings in polyarteritis are palpable purpuric lesions, livedo reticularis, infarcted skin lesions, and necrotic digital tips.[11] Nodules along the course of arteries (from which the name "polyarteritis nodosa" is derived) represent local inflammatory exudates and are seen mostly, if ever, in fulminant cases.

Gastrointestinal involvement is commonly a reason for admission to the ICU and, unfortunately, is catastrophic. Abdominal pain and persistent vomiting and diarrhea may indicate pancreatitis or ischemic necrosis of the appendix, gallbladder, or bowel. In some patients, multiple aneurysms may lead to bleeding in the intra-abdominal cavity. Gastrointestinal bleeding or bowel infarction resulting in perforation often requires surgical intervention. After appropriate medical treatment, unruptured aneurysms in large arterial branches may completely disappear. Necrotizing glomerulonephritis is seldom fulminant but can in occasional patients produce malignant hypertension, and perhaps the early descriptions of stupor and papilledema in polyarteritis nodosa can be directly attributed to hypertensive encephalopathy. One third of patients have overt cardiac dis-

Table 11–2 ORGAN INVOLVEMENT IN VASCULITIDES

Organ	Frequency (%)			
	Polyarteritis Nodosa	Churg-Strauss	Wegener's Granulomatosis	Drug-induced
Lung	<1	95	95	10
Kidney	70	40	85	40
Heart	30	40	10	10
GI tract	40	40	<1	<1
Skin	40	70	45	100
CNS	15	<1	<1	5
PNS	60	30	15	<1

CNS = central nervous system; GI = gastrointestinal; PNS = peripheral nervous system.

ease caused by coronary artery vasculitis or pericarditis, but it seldom leads to myocardial infarction.

Polyarteritis remains a clinical diagnosis, and laboratory test results are nonspecific. Hepatitis B surface antigen, decreased concentration of C3 and C4 complement components, cryoglobulinemia, or the recently discovered antineutrophilic cytoplasmic antibodies may suggest vasculitis.[15] These laboratory tests may help in differentiating polyarteritis nodosa from other critical conditions that may strongly mimic polyarteritis. Infective endocarditis, left atrial myxoma resulting in multiple embolic showers, and cholesterol embolization (see Chapters 4 and 5) should be excluded.

Visceral angiography is the preferred procedure for confirming the diagnosis, but skin, rectum, kidney, skeletal muscle, and possibly, nerve biopsies can determine the diagnosis, more often if these organs are clinically involved.[47,56] Only 30% of muscle biopsy specimens taken from muscles that are not particularly painful are positive.[37] The same holds for any blind biopsy in other tissue; approximately one third of muscle, nerve, and skin biopsy specimens yield the diagnosis of vasculitis.

Kernohan and Woltman[27] noted in their seminal paper on periarteritis nodosa that neurologic involvement is one of the most consistent clinical features. Peripheral neuropathies usually evolve over weeks but may have an insidious course and become more prominent clinically when organ involvement reaches its nadir.

Peripheral Nervous System Involvement

Multiple mononeuropathies (mononeuritis multiplex) are traditionally associated with necrotizing angiitis.[4–7,19,24,29,41] Peripheral nerve involvement in polyarteritis nodosa is often heralded by transitory shooting pain and paresthesias in the toes and followed by sudden unilateral or bilateral footdrop.[11] Additional nerve involvement develops in many patients, predominantly in the radial or femoral nerve. Marked asymmetries during examination should point to multiple mononeuropathies rather than a polyneuropathy. Large hypesthetic patches in the distribution of cutaneous sensory nerves are often asymmetrically distributed over the body. Nevertheless, a distal but slightly asymmetrical sensory-motor polyneuropathy is more frequent than mononeuritis multiplex. In Castaigne and associates' series of 27 patients,[6] 8 had mononeuropathy or multiple neuropathy, 17 had distal mixed motor-sensory polyneuropathy more pronounced in the legs than in the arms, and 2 had primarily sensory findings. Paroxysmal face and nerve root shooting pains have been reported, but involvement of sensory ganglia is rare. Brachial plexopathy has been reported.[3] Cranial nerves may be involved, most often the sixth and third,[23] but involvement occurs mostly as part of a brain stem stroke. Isolated internuclear ophthalmoplegia has been reported as an isolated finding but with cerebellar signs almost certainly resulting from occlusive cerebrovascular disease of the brain stem.[28] Bilateral acoustic nerve involvement leading to sudden deafness is noted in one report.[31]

The extent of involvement of multiple mononeuropathies in polyarteritis nodosa varies greatly, but they may lead to a crippling and, especially, a painful state. In a few patients, the cephalad progression of paresthesias and motor weakness may suggest Guillain-Barré syndrome, but in most patients, frequent alternating sequential involvement of isolated nerves clearly suggests mononeuritis multiplex.

The tendency of the disorder to progress in exacerbation and remission is typified by the pathologic finding of different stages of vasculitis in biopsied tissue and may have a clinical counterpart in a fluctuating course of sensory and motor deficits. Sural nerve biopsy has a high yield in patients with electro-

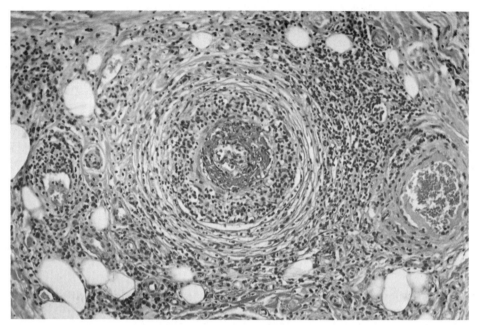

Figure 11-1. Photomicrograph of sural nerve. Large epineural artery with marked constriction, fibrinoid degeneration of intima, and cellular infiltration of media and adventitia, features typical of systemic necrotic vasculitis occurring in periarteritis nodosa, Churg-Strauss disease, Wegener's granulomatosis, and hypersensitivity angiitis. (Courtesy of Dr. P. Dyck, Peripheral Nerve Center, Mayo Clinic, Rochester, MN.)

diagnostic abnormalities and usually shows predominantly necrotizing vasculitis of the vasa vasorum with axonal and Wallerian degeneration[25] (Fig. 11-1).

The outcome of mononeuritis multiplex is difficult to predict, but recovery of the neuropathy often parallels control of the systemic vasculitis. Rapid remission of both mononeuritis multiplex and distal polyneuropathy occurs only in patients with limited involvement. Substantial recovery of nerve function, however, can be appreciated only after months and is less likely in patients with rapid onset and maximal deficits of the muscles innervated by the affected nerve. Unfortunately, many patients experience immense suffering from persisting pain and remain disabled from footdrop and wristdrop. Survival in patients with polyarteritis complicated by multiple mononeuropathies is not worse than that in patients whose nerves are relatively spared.[19]

Cyclophosphamide (1 to 2 mg/kg orally) and prednisone (40 to 60 mg) treatment is effective in patients with mononeuritis multiplex or distal polyneuropathy, but the individual response cannot be predicted.[17] In severe cases, additional treatment with plasma exchange, antiplatelet drugs, or azathioprine may have a rationale, but its efficacy is uncertain. Plasma exchange may be a consideration as a last resort for patients in whom signs and symptoms progress despite adequate immunosuppression.

Central Nervous System Involvement

Virtually any artery can be involved by polyarteritis, and necrotic vasculitic changes can be expected in large intracranial central arteries, small meningeal arteries, and, occasionally, the temporal artery but without the characteristic giant cells. Autopsy studies have reported well-documented cases of cerebral or brain stem infarction associated with occlusive vasculitic disease, in many already evident on cerebral angiograms. In Ford and Siekert's series,[18] 13% of the patients with polyarteritis nodosa had cerebral infarction or hemorrhage. Stroke occurred more often in patients with multiple organ failure but rarely as a presenting feature. Cerebral infarcts have been located in basal ganglia of patients with sudden Parkinson's syndrome,[38] in the posterior and middle cerebral arteries, and only occasionally in the brain stem circulation.

Intracerebral hemorrhage, most often localized in the putamen, is almost certainly from acute hypertension from renal failure. Subarachnoid hemorrhage may be caused by dissection through necrotic media.[20] Other patients may have global confusion, blurred vision, and generalized tonic-clonic seizures that can be attributed to malignant hypertension. A recently reported case with transient magnetic resonance imaging (MRI) abnormalities in the white matter can be fully explained by coexisting malignant hypertension.[30]

Patients with sudden spinal cord syndrome should undergo emergency MRI because extradural hematoma that compresses the spinal cord has been reported in polyarteritis.[22] In other anecdotal cases, necrotizing arteritis of spinal cord arteries resulted in spinal cord infarction.[46]

CHURG-STRAUSS SYNDROME

Churg and Strauss[9] pathologically established a distinctive clinical syndrome with systemic vasculitis similar to polyarteritis nodosa but with tissue infiltration by eosinophils, a vasculitic process extending into venules and capillaries, and predominant pulmonary involvement.[8,32,33]

Clinical Features

Late-onset asthma (third decade) is a dominant feature in this disorder, although the systemic vasculitis may occur years after recurrent rhinorrhea, pansinusitis, and repeated nasal polypectomies. The diagnosis of Churg-Strauss syndrome can be made after renal, skin, and muscle biopsies. Unless the typical granulomas surrounded by eosinophils are seen, open lung biopsy is often nonspecific. Most of the laboratory evaluation is similar to that in polyarteritis nodosa.

Patients with Churg-Strauss disease may be admitted to the medical ICU because of an initially puzzling pulmonary disorder, or patients with congestive heart failure are seen in a coronary care unit. Respiratory failure from acute lung injury results in urgent need for mechanical ventilation in many patients and causes death in 10%. Chest radiographs may demonstrate bilateral confluent or nodular infiltrates with pleural effusions that contain massive numbers of eosinophils, but the clinical and radiographic presentation may resemble that of many of the infectious pneumonias.[12] Diffuse interstitial or miliary lesions have been reported, but without cavitary lesions. Alveolar hemorrhage may suddenly worsen gas exchange, but its occurrence is not specific for this disorder.[10]

Congestive heart failure is a major cause of death in Churg-Strauss disease from involvement of the epicardium and may be clinically detected by a loud friction rub. Other cardiac manifestations that have certainly been known to occur are eosinophilic myocarditis with restrictive cardiomyopathy and coronary arteritis with myocardial infarction. Renal disease and acute hypertension are less common in Churg-Strauss syndrome.

Peripheral Nervous System Involvement

Mononeuritis multiplex is less common in Churg-Strauss syndrome than in polyarteritis but nevertheless affects two thirds of patients. Asthma always antedates the onset of neuropathy, but the interval varies (average, 7 years).[52] The clinical manifestations are similar to those in polyarteritis nodosa, but involvement is more extensive, as reflected by a potential for recovery of only 50%. Sehgal and colleagues[52] reported the Mayo Clinic experience of 47 patients with Churg-Strauss syndrome. Of 25 patients with a polyneuropathy, 17 had evidence of multiple mononeuropathy, 7 had a distal symmetrical polyneuropathy, and 1 had generalized polyneuropathy with asymmetrical findings. Cramping in calf muscles, caused by myositis, may be an overwhelming complaint in some patients. Muscle biopsy examination is rarely diagnostic, although typical granulomas are occasionally found.

Treatment of Churg-Strauss syndrome is similar to that of polyarteritis. The response can be brisk, and remission is expected within weeks of corticosteroid therapy.[36] As noted previously, outcome in mononeuritis multiplex or distal polyneuropathy is less favorable. Long-term high-dose steroid therapy (3 to 6 months, 60 mg daily) is preferred in patients with mononeuritis multiplex, and tapering of the dose when the systemic manifestations subside should be postponed to allow for aggressive treatment of the neuropathy.

Central Nervous System Involvement

Patients with fulminant Churg-Strauss syndrome may have central nervous system manifestations, often with psychiatric features. Acute psychosis, agitation, and vivid hallucinations are most likely a result of high doses of corticosteroids, but early in the disease, both severe hypoxemia and hypercarbia will be important contributing factors as well. Intracerebral hemorrhage has been reported but without further clinical or computed tomography (CT) details. In Lanham and associates' series of 50 patients,[33] 16% had intracranial hemorrhage. Cerebral infarcts have been reported but without pathologic confirmation of vasculitis. Because cardiomyopathy develops in a sizable proportion of patients with Churg-Strauss disease, a cardiac embolic source should be considered as well.[52] Isolated cranial nerve involvement (II, III, VII, VIII) has been noted but without assessment by neurologists. Transient monocular blindness or permanent retinal infarcts[50] may be manifestations of vasculitis or artery-to-artery embolism. Bilateral optic neuropathy resulting in dramatic visual loss in rapid succession in both eyes with peripapillary hemorrhage has been reported.[2] Recovery in visual acuity is not expected despite aggressive treatment.

WEGENER'S GRANULOMATOSIS

Wegener's triad (simultaneous involvement of upper and lower respiratory tract and kidneys) often points to the diagnosis, but the lesions of Wegener's granulomatosis may, as can be expected in a systemic vasculitis, involve nearly any organ.[14,16,21]

Clinical Features

Pulmonary infiltrates and sinusitis initially characterize the disease. Involvement of the respiratory tract can become immediately life-threatening. Multiple nodular and cavitary infiltrates are classic radiologic features, but in some patients fulminant pulmonary hemorrhage with hemoptysis prompts intensive care admission. Other emergency conditions are spontaneous pneumothorax, severe subglottic stenosis from pseudotumors, and massive epistaxis.

Although necrotizing glomerulonephritis is commonly seen in classic Wegener's granulomatosis, it is seldom reported as a cause of acute progressive renal failure. The diagnosis of Wegener's disease is greatly facilitated by the finding of cytoplasm-staining antineutrophil cytoplasmic antibodies, which has a reported sensitivity of 66% and specificity in excess of 90%. Open lung biopsy often is needed for pathologic diagnosis, although granulomatous foci may be found in virtually any tissue. Unfortunately, despite the easy accessibility of nasal mucosa, the diagnostic yield of nasal tissue biopsies is low. In approximately one third of patients with Wegener's granulomatosis, a neurologic manifestation develops during the course of the illness. Wegener's granulomatosis may first be seen with a neurologic finding. In a review series of 324 cases from the Mayo Clinic, cranial neuropathy (usually ophthalmoplegia), temporal arteritis, and ischemic stroke were the conditions at presentation.[44] Typical severe headache, jaw claudication, and sudden loss of vision associated with arteritis with or without giant cells were noted in 5 of 345 patients in whom Wegener's granulomatosis later became more apparent.[43]

Peripheral Nervous System Involvement

Mononeuritis multiplex or asymmetrical sensory-motor polyneuropathy occurred in 16% of patients in the Mayo Clinic series, a remarkably lower incidence than that in other systemic vasculitides.[44] The interval between onset of Wegener's granulomatosis and diagnosis of neuropathy is approximately 1 year. The peroneal or tibial nerve is most commonly affected, followed in order by the ulnar, median, radial, and femoral nerves. Because glomerulonephritis significantly increases the chance of polyneuropathy, uremic polyneuropathy may be contributory in some patients with Wegener-associated neuropathies. The second, sixth, and seventh cranial nerves are often involved, but multiple cranial neuropathy may occur, is often unilateral, and is caused by local invasion by destructive granulomatous tumors.

Central Nervous System Involvement

Granulomatous masses arising in the paranasal sinuses may cause destruc-
tion of the cavernous sinus manifested by external ophthalmoplegia, but a large localized mass may eventuate in carotid occlusion and ischemic stroke. Noteworthy is cortical vein thrombosis.[39] Some plausible anecdotes indeed suggest that vasculitis of cerebral arteries may cause ischemic or hemorrhagic stroke in Wegener's disease.[35,58] When panarthritic vessels rupture, subarachnoid hemorrhage or intracerebral hemorrhage may be seen.[13,26] Extensive involvement of the anterior cerebral artery may lead to bilateral frontal infarcts,[51] but more commonly, MRI demonstrates multiple cerebral infarcts from vasculitic involvement of small arteries. Cerebral angiography in patients with cerebral infarcts in Wegener's disease is often nondiagnostic for this reason. Granulomas may be seen on MRI and may disappear with appropriate treatment. In a recent case report, Wegener's disease was accompanied by seizures and multiple granulomatous lesions that markedly diminished in size after treatment with cyclophosphamide, prednisone, trimethoprim, and sulfamethoxazole.[40,45,49]

DRUG-INDUCED VASCULITIS

Drug-induced vasculitis is occasionally seen in ICUs and is categorized together with other hypersensitivity vasculitides (postinfectious Henoch-Schönlein syndrome in children and mixed cryoglobulinemia). The evidence for an association with drugs remains circumstantial, but this explanation is often the most likely in otherwise healthy patients in whom a fulminant vasculitis suddenly develops 7 to 10 days after drug ingestion. Commonly implicated drugs are antibiotics, nonsteroidal anti-inflammatory agents, sulfonamides, and antiepileptic drugs.

Examination of tissue with a fully developed lesion shows leukoclastic (polymorphonuclear necrotizing and fragmentary nuclei) small veins, particularly the postcapillary venules in the dermis. The skin is most commonly involved, and virtually all types of lesions can occur. None is specific for one drug category. Frequently, palpable patches of purpura that can be nodular, urticarial, ulcerative, and vesicular are found on the legs, but in other patients, maculopapular or erythema multiforme rashes are more characteristic.[1] Nasal and oral mucosae may not be spared. Renal failure is common. Gastrointestinal abnormalities and lung and cardiac involvement are uncommon, although in some patients, multiorgan involvement may be a direct cause of death. Fortunately, the disorder is frequently self-limiting. Treatment is supportive, and patients are additionally treated with prednisone.

With the almost complete disappearance of acute serum sickness, which has traditionally been associated with encephalopathy, polyneuropathy, plexopathy, seizures, and coma,[48] neurologic manifestations of drug-induced vasculitis are rare but most likely underreported. Numbness and painful paresthesias are common, but pruritus and burning sensations may be caused by the skin lesion itself rather than by sensory-motor polyneuropathy or a developing mononeuritis multiplex. Nonetheless, in a review of case reports by Mullick and associates,[42] sensory-motor polyneuropathy was reported anecdotally in 4 of 70 patients. Well-documented cases with histologic or electrodiagnostic confirmation are not available.

Focal or generalized seizures have been reported, usually without known cause. In one patient with an allopurinol-associated vasculitis, seizures could be linked to vasculitis documented on CT scan and cerebral angiograms.[57]

CONCLUSIONS

The peripheral nervous system is often seriously involved in severe forms of acute vasculitis syndromes with acute respiratory or renal failure.

The principal goal is to achieve rapid remission of the neuropathy that may cause severe disability. In general, the efficacy of immunosuppressive medication (cyclophosphamide, 1 to 2 mg/kg, and prednisone, 40 to 60 mg) is best demonstrated in less severe and limited distal polyneuropathy and mononeuritis multiplex.

In Wegener's granulomatosis, cranial neuropathy, temporal arteritis, and ischemic stroke may be presenting features. Central nervous system involvement is more sporadic. Predominantly ischemic stroke and basal ganglia hemorrhages (from associated hypertension) are found in polyarteritis and Churg-Strauss syndrome. In Wegener's syndrome, vasculitis of cerebral vessels may produce intracranial hemorrhages or multiple territory cerebral infarcts.

REFERENCES

1. Aboobaker, J and Greaves, MW: Urticarial vasculitis. Clin Exp Dermatol 11:436–444, 1986.
2. Acheson, JF, Cockerell, OC, Bentley, CR, and Sanders, MD: Churg-Strauss vasculitis presenting with severe visual loss due to bilateral sequential optic neuropathy. Br J Ophthalmol 77:118–119, 1993.
3. Allan, SG, Smith, CC, Towla, HMA, et al: Painful brachial plexopathy: An unusual presentation of polyarteritis nodosa. Postgrad Med J 58:311–313, 1982.
4. Belsole, RJ, Lister, GD, and Kleinert, HE: Polyarteritis: A cause of nerve palsy in the extremity. J Hand Surg 3:320–325, 1978.
5. Bouche, P, Léger, JM, Travers, MA, et al: Peripheral neuropathy in systemic vasculitis: Clinical and electrophysiologic study of 22 patients. Neurology 36:1598–1602, 1986.
6. Castaigne, P, Brunet, P, Hauw, JJ, et al: Système nerveux périphérique et panartérite noueuse: Revue de 27 cas. Rev Neurol (Paris) 140:343–352, 1984.
7. Chang, RW, Bell, CL, and Hallett, M: Clinical characteristics and prognosis

of vasculitic mononeuropathy multiplex. Arch Neurol 41:618–621, 1984.

8. Chumbley, LC, Harrison, EG Jr, and DeRemee, RA: Allergic granulomatosis and angiitis (Churg-Strauss syndrome): Report and analysis of 30 cases. Mayo Clin Proc 52:477–484, 1977.

9. Churg, J and Strauss, L: Allergic granulomatosis, allergic angiitis, and periarteritis nodosa. Am J Pathol 27:277–301, 1951.

10. Clutterbuck, EJ and Pusey, CD: Severe alveolar haemorrhage in Churg-Strauss syndrome. Eur J Respir Dis 71:158–163, 1987.

11. Cohen, RD, Conn, DL, and Ilstrup, DM: Clinical features, prognosis, and response to treatment in polyarteritis. Mayo Clin Proc 55:146–155, 1980.

12. Degesys, GE, Mintzer, RA, and Vrla, RF: Allergic granulomatosis: Churg-Strauss syndrome. AJR Am J Roentgenol 135:1821–1822, 1980.

13. Drachman, DA: Neurological complications of Wegener's granulomatosis. Arch Neurol 8:145–155, 1963.

14. Fahey, JL, Leonard, E, Churg, J, and Godman, GC: Wegener's granulomatosis. Am J Med 17:168–179, 1954.

15. Falk, RJ and Jennette, JC: Antineutrophil cytoplasmic autoantibodies with specificity for myeloperoxidase in patients with systemic vasculitis and idiopathic necrotizing and crescentic glomerulonephritis. N Engl J Med 318:1651–1657, 1988.

16. Fauci, AS, Haynes, BF, Katz, P, and Wolff, SM: Wegener's granulomatosis: Prospective clinical and therapeutic experience with 85 patients for 21 years. Ann Intern Med 98:76–85, 1983.

17. Fauci, AS, Katz, P, Haynes, BF, and Wolff, SM: Cyclophosphamide therapy of severe systemic necrotizing vasculitis. N Engl J Med 301:235–238, 1979.

18. Ford, RG and Siekert, RG: Central nervous system manifestations of periarteritis nodosa. Neurology 15:114–122, 1965.

19. Frohnert, PP and Sheps, SG: Long-term follow-up study of periarteritis nodosa. Am J Med 43:8–14, 1967.

20. Gherardi, GJ and Lee, HY: Localized dissecting hemorrhage and arteritis: Renal and cerebral manifestations. JAMA 199:219–220, 1967.

21. Godman, GC and Churg, J: Wegener's granulomatosis: Pathology and review of the literature. Arch Pathol 58:533–553, 1954.

22. Haft, H, Finneson, BE, Cramer, H, and Fiol, R: Periarteritis nodosa as a source of subarachnoid hemorrhage and spinal cord compression: Report of a case and review of the literature. J Neurosurg 14:608–616, 1957.

23. Hagen, NA, Stevens, JC, and Michet, CJ Jr: Trigeminal sensory neuropathy associated with connective tissue diseases. Neurology 40:891–896, 1990.

24. Harati, Y and Niakan, E: The clinical spectrum of inflammatory-angiopathic neuropathy. J Neurol Neurosurg Psychiatry 49:1313–1316, 1986.

25. Hawke, SHB, Davies, L, Pamphlett, R, et al: Vasculitic neuropathy: A clinical and pathological study. Brain 114:2175–2190, 1991.

26. Hearne, CB and Zawada, ET Jr: Survival after intracerebral hemorrhage in Wegener's granulomatosis. West J Med 137:431–434, 1982.

27. Kernohan, JW and Woltman, HW: Periarteritis nodosa: A clinicopathologic study with special reference to the nervous system. Arch Neurol Psychiatry 39:655–686, 1938.

28. Kirkali, P, Topaloglu, R, Kansu, T, and Bakkaloglu, A: Third nerve palsy and internuclear ophthalmoplegia in periarteritis nodosa. J Pediatr Ophthalmol Strabismus 28:45–46, 1991.

29. Kissel, JT, Slivka, AP, Warmolts, JR, and Mendell, JR: The clinical spectrum of necrotizing angiopathy of the peripheral nervous system. Ann Neurol 18:251–257, 1985.

30. Koppensteiner, R, Base, W, Bognar, H, et al: Course of cerebral lesions in a patient with periarteritis nodosa studied by magnetic resonance imaging. Klin Wochenschr 67:398–401, 1989.

31. Lake-Bakaar, G: Polyarteritis nodosa presenting with bilateral nerve deafness. J R Soc Med 71:144–147, 1978.

32. Lanham, JG and Churg, J: Churg-Strauss syndrome. In Churg, A and Churg, J (eds): Systemic Vasculitides.

Igaku-Shoin Medical Publishers, New York, 1991, pp 101–120.

33. Lanham, JG, Elkon, KB, Pusey, CD, and Hughes, GR: Systemic vasculitis with asthma and eosinophilia: A clinical approach to the Churg-Strauss syndrome. Medicine (Baltimore) 63:65–81, 1984.

34. Lie, JT: Diagnostic histopathology of major systemic and pulmonary vasculitic syndromes. Rheum Dis Clin North Am 16:269–292, 1990.

35. Lucas, FV, Benjamin, SP, and Steinberg, MC: Cerebral vasculitis in Wegener's granulomatosis. Cleve Clin Q 43:275–281, 1976.

36. MacFadyen, R, Tron, V, Keshmiri, M, and Road, JD: Allergic angiitis of Churg and Strauss syndrome: Response to pulse methylprednisolone. Chest 91:629–631, 1987.

37. Maxeiner, SR Jr, McDonald, JR, and Kirklin, JW: Muscle biopsy in the diagnosis of periarteritis nodosa: An evaluation. Surg Clin North Am 1225–1233, Aug 1952.

38. Mayo, J, Arias, M, Leno, C, and Berciano, J: Vascular parkinsonism and periarteritis nodosa (letter). Neurology 36:874–875, 1986.

39. Mickle, JP, McLennan, JE, Chi, JG, and Lidden, CW: Cortical vein thrombosis in Wegener's granulomatosis: Case report. J Neurosurg 46:248, 1977.

40. Miller, KS and Miller, JM: Wegener's granulomatosis presenting as a primary seizure disorder with brain lesions demonstrated by magnetic resonance imaging. Chest 103:316–318, 1993.

41. Moore, PM and Cupps, TR: Neurological complications of vasculitis. Ann Neurol 14:155–167, 1983.

42. Mullick, FG, McAllister, HA Jr, Wagner, BM, and Fenoglio, JJ Jr: Drug related vasculitis: Clinicopathologic correlations in 30 patients. Hum Pathol 10:313–325, 1979.

43. Nishino, H, DeRemee, RA, Rubino, FA, and Parisi, JE: Wegener's granulomatosis associated with vasculitis of the temporal artery: Report of five cases. Mayo Clin Proc 68:115–121, 1993.

44. Nishino, H, Rubino, FA, DeRemee, RA, et al: Neurological involvement in We-

gener's granulomatosis: An analysis of 324 consecutive cases at the Mayo Clinic. Ann Neurol 33:4–9, 1993.

45. Oimomi, M, Suehiro, I, Mizuno, N, et al: Wegener's granulomatosis with intracerebral granuloma and mammary manifestation: Report of a case. Arch Intern Med 140:853–854, 1980.

46. Ojeda, VJ: Polyarteritis nodosa affecting the spinal cord arteries. Aust N Z J Med 13:287–289, 1983.

47. Panegyres, PK, Blumbergs, PC, Leong, AS-Y, and Bourne, AJ: Vasculitis of peripheral nerve and skeletal muscle: Clinicopathological correlation and immunopathic mechanisms. J Neurol Sci 100:193–202, 1990.

48. Park, AM and Richardson, JC: Cerebral complications of serum sickness. Neurology 3:277–283, 1953.

49. Payton, CD and Boulton Jones, JM: Cortical blindness complicating Wegener's granulomatosis. Br Med J [Clin Res] 290:676, 1985.

50. Rabinowitz Dagi, L and Currie, J: Branch retinal artery occlusion in the Churg-Strauss syndrome. J Clin Neuroophthalmol 5:229–237, 1985.

51. Satoh, J, Miyasaka, N, Yamada, T, et al: Extensive cerebral infarction due to involvement of both anterior cerebral arteries by Wegener's granulomatosis. Ann Rheum Dis 47:606–611, 1988.

52. Sehgal, M, Swanson, JW, and DeRemee, RA: Neurological manifestations of Churg-Strauss syndrome (abstr). Neurology 43:419A, 1993.

53. Specks, V and DeRemee, RA: Granulomatous vasculitis: Wegener's granulomatosis and Churg-Strauss syndrome. Rheum Dis Clin North Am 16:377–397, 1990.

54. Travers, RL, Allison, DJ, Brettle, RP, and Hudges, GRV: Polyarteritis nodosa: A clinical and angiographic analysis of 17 cases. Semin Arthritis Rheum 8:184–199, 1979.

55. Walker, GL: Neurological features of polyarteritis nodosa. Clin Exp Neurol 15:237–247, 1978.

56. Wees, SJ, Sunwoo, IN, and Oh, SJ: Sural nerve biopsy in systemic necrotiz-

ing vasculitis. Am J Med 71:525–532, 1981.

57. Weiss, EB, Forman, P, and Rosenthal, IM: Allopurinol-induced arteritis in partial HGPRTase deficiency: Atypical seizure manifestation. Arch Intern Med 138:1743–1744, 1978.

58. Yamashita, Y, Takahashi, M, Bussaka, H, et al: Cerebral vasculitis secondary to Wegener's granulomatosis: Computed tomography and angiographic findings. J Comput Tomogr 10:115–120, 1986.

Part III

NEUROLOGIC COMPLICATIONS IN THE SURGICAL INTENSIVE CARE UNIT

Chapter 12

NEUROLOGIC COMPLICATIONS OF ATHERO-SCLEROTIC AORTIC DISEASE

In surgical intensive care units (ICUs), ischemic events are indisputable in patients with extensive vascular repairs. After aortic reconstruction, ischemic colitis and renal failure predominate and may extend the ICU stay. Spinal cord infarction, however, is fortunately less frequent,[1,32,39,40,42,63] but in the largest series reported, 16% of 1509 patients who had elective surgery of the descending aorta were left with spinal cord damage.[56] The incidence of paraplegia after emergency repair for traumatic or acute spontaneous rupture is higher and ranges from 20% to 30%[4] (Table 12-1). Prevention of spinal cord injury during thoracoabdominal aneurysm repair remains a challenge to the skills of vascular surgeons and monitoring anesthesiologists.

To a large extent, the pathophysiology of spinal cord ischemia can be explained by altered blood flow mechanics. During aortic cross-clamping, the spinal cord is extremely sensitive to ischemia from reduced blood flow distal to the clamp. However, some patients awaken without any signs of paraplegia only to deteriorate in subsequent postoperative days. Loss of spinal perfusion caused by arterial spasm or progressive aortic dissection has been implicated in these patients with delayed paraplegia.

Spinal cord injury from aortic surgery is easy to recognize but immensely frustrating, because any therapeutic intervention is futile and the handicap is permanent and of major size. Any therapeutic window in this situation exists at the time of surgery and the first day after surgery. The diagnostic approach, opportunities for intraoperative monitoring, and therapeutic options are discussed in this chapter.

VASCULAR ANATOMY OF THE SPINAL CORD

Three longitudinal arterial trunks, the anterior spinal artery and both posterior spinal arteries, regulate the blood supply to the entire spinal cord[28,29,36,64] (Fig. 12-1). The anterior spinal artery supplies approximately 75% of the blood to the cord. From this major contributing artery, sets of arteries pass through the central sulcus to the middle part of the cord. Each so-called central artery supplies one side of the cord and

199

Table 12–1 INCIDENCE OF PARAPLEGIA IN RECENT SERIES WITH SPONTANEOUS TRAUMATIC AORTIC RUPTURE OR ELECTIVE REPAIR OF THE AORTA

Series (y)	Paraplegia (%)	
	Rupture	Elective Repair
Katz et al., 1981[34]	24	—
Sturm et al., 1985[55]	16	—
Crawford et al., 1991[11]	27	—
Carlson et al., 1983[7]	—	5
Svensson et al., 1993[56]	—	16

provides flow to the gray matter, which harbors the cells of the origin of the ventral root fibers, preganglionic cells for the autonomic nervous system, and the incoming posterior horn fibers. Zülch and Kurth-Schumacher[73] postulated that the posterior horn is situated in a watershed area between the central artery and a branch of the posterior spinal artery, but posterior horn infarcts are rare and neurons in the central region are much more vulnerable to episodes of hypoperfusion. The central artery also supplies most of the lateral corticospinal tract, including the hand and arm areas. More peripherally located tracts, however, may also receive blood of tributaries from the coronal arteries, which arise from the anterior spinal artery or branches of the posterior spinal artery.

The paired posterior spinal arteries supply parts of the posterior columns of the white matter. The lateral spinothalamic tracts, which convey pain and temperature sensation, receive their vascular supply through the coronal arteries and are therefore not spared in a typical spinal artery syndrome.

In the longitudinal plane, a fairly consistent pattern has been recognized, but anatomic variations at various levels are the rule. Three major segments of vascularization of the spinal cord have been defined. The cervicothoracic territory includes the cervical cord and first two or three thoracic segments. The anterior spinal artery and posterior spinal arteries are branches of the vertebral arteries and costocervical trunk. Below the T-3 level, the intercostal arteries from the aorta supply the thoracic segments and are highly variable in number. One recent human cadaver study found a range of 2 to 17 (mean, 8) intercostal lumbar arteries. At T-7, a large thoracic radicular artery frequently contributes to the anterior spinal artery. The thoracolumbar territory derives its supply from the artery of Adamkiewicz,[66] which typically originates between T-8 and L-2 but is frequently identified between T-9 and T-12. In 10% to 15% of patients, this crucial artery arises at higher levels, usually from T-5 to T-8. The terminal portions of the spinal cord and cauda equina depend on branches from the internal iliac or middle sacral artery.

Although the division of the vascularization of the spinal cord into three larger arterial areas implies that vulnerable watershed areas are present in the midthoracic region (T-4 to T-8), any level in the thoracic region may become affected.[18] The vulnerability of the thoracic region is plausible when one considers the scarce supply derived from one to three anterior radicular arteries more widely spaced in the thoracic area than in other regions. (Spinal cord perfusion depends on the number of radicular arteries and not on the number of intercostal arteries that arise from the aorta.) In addition, central arteries, although abundant in the cervical and lumbar regions, are poorly represented in the thoracic region.[29] Pathologic studies found that in some areas in the thoracic region, one segment was supplied by one central artery and another segment was supplied by small ascending and descending branches from adjacent segments. Thus, perfusion of the thoracic spinal cord is largely guaranteed by the great radicular artery of Adamkiewicz.

SCOPE OF THE PROBLEM

Familiarity with anesthetic techniques during grafting of the thoracoab-

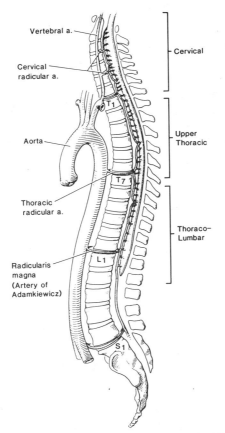

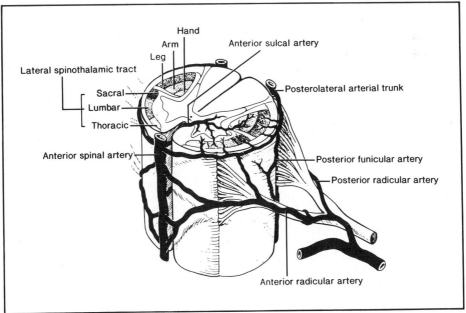

Figure 12–1. Vascularization of the spinal cord (see text for explanation).

dominal aorta is necessary to understand the risks of spinal cord injury from aortic surgery.

Immediately after aortic cross-clamping, arterial blood pressure increases, stroke volume and cardiac output decrease, and pulmonary artery occlusion pressure increases. Also during cross-clamping, cerebrospinal fluid pressure increases markedly,[27] probably from increased intraspinal venous blood volume that is a result of venous back pressure. Svensson and associates[60] evaluated cerebrospinal fluid alterations in 77 patients who underwent thoracic and thoracoabdominal aortic surgery and found that, in addition to significant increases during induction of general anesthesia and intubation, cerebrospinal fluid pressures correlated linearly with central venous pressures. This marked increase in cerebrospinal fluid pressure may result in decrease of the perfusion pressure of the spinal cord (perfusion pressure equals spinal cord arterial pressure minus cerebrospinal fluid pressure). Furthermore, a decrease in spinal cord arterial pressure resulting from exclusion of the aorta or use of vasodilators to overcome hypertension may significantly contribute to spinal cord ischemia.[60,62]

The spinal cord is particularly at risk for ischemic damage after aortic declamping. Release of the abdominal aortic cross-clamp may cause hypotension associated with reperfusion of the ischemic, vasodilated, and vasomotor-paralyzed lower extremity and pelvic arteries.[41] Volume loading before this procedure generally prevents this from happening, or if hypotension occurs, it responds to boluses of phenylephrine. Many anesthesiologists also reduce the concentration of inhalation agents before clamp release.

Many surgical series have reported risk factors for spinal cord injury. There is no doubt that repair of extensive abdominal aneurysms associated with long aortic cross-clamping (Table 12–2) increases the risk of postoperative spinal cord injury.

Many vascular surgeons routinely

Table 12–2 INCIDENCE OF PARAPLEGIA IN RELATION TO CROSS-CLAMP TIME

Time (min)	Patients (n)	Paraplegia (%)
0–15	8	0
16–30	142	3
31–45	90	10
46–60	16	13
>60	4	25

Modified from Livesay, et al.[38]

implant the intercostal arteries during aortic surgery, but others question whether the incidence of paraplegia with such a time-consuming procedure can be reduced. Aortic clamping time is probably the most important risk factor for postoperative spinal cord injury and emphasizes the nimbleness of the surgeon in this technically complex procedure. The vascular surgeon therefore is faced with the dilemma of reimplanting as many intercostal arteries as possible with the assumption that one or more critical radicular arteries are included or proceeding directly with replacing the aneurysm within a short clamping time.

The merit of preoperative localization of critical intercostal arteries, including the great radicular artery of Adamkiewicz, is controversial,[71] and there are patients who have sacrificed the artery of Adamkiewicz without paraplegia.[10] Early claims to have visualized the artery of Adamkiewicz in the vast majority of patients were offset by a more recent study of selective spinal arteriography in which the origin was found in a much lower percentage (55%).[71] The Baylor group recently perfected a new technique of intraoperative localization of segmental arteries important in spinal cord supply.[59] The method involves intrathecal placement of a platinum electrode that senses hydrogen. Saline saturated with hydrogen is injected into several segmental artery ostia, and "positive arteries" are reanastomosed. In a recent pilot study of eight patients, five did well despite long total clamp time. One patient died, and delayed paraplegia associated with hypotension developed in two patients.[59]

Revascularization resulted in a much lower incidence of paraplegia than that in historical controls. On the other hand, Williams and coworkers[71] hypothesized that patients with extensive aneurysm of the descending and abdominal aorta and a large patent great radicular artery arising from a large intercostal branch at the center of the aneurysm are at risk for spinal cord injury. Again, whether reimplantation results in better neurologic outcome is unsettled.

Most patients with spinal cord injuries awaken with paraplegia, but several large surgical series reported a fair number of patients in whom onset of a spinal cord lesion was delayed.[46] In Crawford and associates'[10] experience, this rather unusual presentation is transient, occurs up to 3 weeks after the operation, and is related to hypovolemia (e.g., hemorrhage from the gastrointestinal tract), low cardiac output during arrhythmias, or respiratory acidosis. Progressive aortic dissection or thrombosis in a graft limb has also been suggested as an alternative mechanism of delayed spinal cord injury. However, a recent study in rabbits documented that the incidence of delayed-onset paraplegia was significantly related to ischemia time and not to thrombosis or embolization in spinal arteries.[46] This finding has important implications for postoperative monitoring of patients with long aortic clamp times who awaken neurologically intact. Monitoring cerebrospinal fluid pressure in the postoperative period in patients with extensive bypass and long clamping time therefore makes logical sense, but its value has not been demonstrated.

NEUROLOGIC FEATURES OF SPINAL CORD INFARCTION

It has been well acknowledged that the incidence of paraplegia is very low in the aortic arch, in the high thoracic aorta, and in aortoiliac reconstructions but increases dramatically in thoracoabdominal aneurysmal repair, particularly in patients with extensive aneurysms. At the Mayo Clinic, the incidence of paraplegia after aortoiliac reconstruction was 0.1% (2 from 1901 patients) after elective repair and 1.4% (3 from 210 patients) after emergency repair.[26]

The typical clinical pattern of spinal cord injury after aortic surgery is flaccid paralysis, loss of deep tendon reflexes, severe bladder dysfunction, and analgesia caudal to the lesion. Very few patients recover from this devastating complication, which in most patients evolves to spastic paraplegia with eventually some improvement of lower extremity sensation. Intermittent catheterization continues to be needed for bladder control.

Total spinal cord infarction (Fig. 12–2I) is common, but other spinal cord syndromes with distinctive clinical features after aortic surgery have been described.

Anterior Spinal Artery Syndrome

If paired posterior spinal arteries with extensive collateral blood supply are present, clamping of the thoracic aorta may result in spinal cord infarction of the anterior two thirds of the spinal cord (Fig. 12–2II). Involvement of the corticospinal, pyramidal, and spinothalamic tracts and anterior horns results in flaccid paraplegia, decreased reaction to pin prick, and decreased reaction to hot and cold sensation. Light touch and position sense are preserved. Vibration sense may be decreased at the toes and ankles merely because the prevalence of diabetes is relatively high in patients undergoing vascular surgery (13% in a recent large series).[56] Many patients have fine fasciculations in the lower limbs that usually resolve within 1 or 2 days. The deep tendon reflexes and Babinski's signs are absent. Abdominal

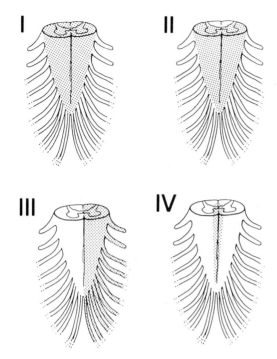

Figure 12–2. Patterns of spinal cord infarction after aortic repair: *I*, complete infarction; *II*, anterior spinal artery syndrome; *III*, Brown-Séquard syndrome; *IV*, central cord syndrome.

reflexes, often useful in localizing the level of damage in the rostrocaudal axis, are usually absent in these patients with large abdominal incisions and therefore not helpful. The rectal sphincters are usually paralyzed, and the genital reflexes are consistently lost. Because the descending thermoregulatory fibers supplying the sweat glands are closely localized to the corticospinal tracts, anhydrosis may be present. This may cause a marked increase in temperature and falsely suggest a postoperative infection. Lesions of the spinal cord after aortic surgery are very often located at the T-4 level, with an area of reduced sensation to the nipples, but sensory levels may range from T-10 to L-2.

Brown-Séquard Syndrome

A few instances of a Brown-Séquard–like syndrome (Fig. 12–2*III*) are on

record.[16] The classic presentation of this unilateral transverse lesion is ipsilateral limb weakness, loss of position and vibration sensation, and contralateral loss of pain and temperature sensation. At the level of the lesion, some patients have a small ipsilateral area of anesthesia. Occlusion of one central artery may explain this phenomenon. A Brown-Séquard syndrome may also develop during resolution of paraplegia.[24] In general, unilateral leg weakness is extremely rare after aortic surgery and may more frequently point to a possible plexopathy.

Central Cord Syndrome

A central cord–like syndrome (Fig. 12–2*IV*) has been clinically described and pathologically confirmed in patients after aortic surgery. These infarcts are located in the thoracolumbar spinal cord and produce a pencil-like softening.[73]

The clinical picture is similar to that of the anterior spinal artery syndrome, but the sacral dermatomes (S-3 to S-5) are spared.[6] The anal reflex is often preserved, and a reflex vesical contractility predominates. The only way to explain this anatomic lesion is embolization to both central sulcus arteries with collateral compensation through the arterial vasa corona. These proximal branches of the anterior spinal artery have their major supply zones in the periphery of the spinal cord and distribute blood to the spinothalamic tracts that represent the sacral dermatomes. Outcome in these incidentally reported patients is poor.

DIAGNOSTIC EVALUATION OF SPINAL CORD INJURY

Spinal cord injury remains a clinical diagnosis, and until recently there were no methods of confirming spinal cord ischemia other than postmortem examination.

Magnetic Resonance Imaging

Magnetic resonance imaging of the spinal cord is very helpful. Magnetic resonance images were recently described in a large series of patients in whom signs and symptoms of spinal cord ischemia developed.[42] They possibly may be used to predict the chance of recovery.

In 17 of 24 patients, magnetic resonance studies showed four patterns of signal abnormalities (Fig. 12–3). Twelve patients had a clinically completed spinal cord infarction, and T2-weighted images showed diffuse signal abnormality of the entire cross section of the spinal cord (Fig. 12–3D). Patients with focal abnormalities involving the anterior horns of the gray matter ("owl's eyes" pattern) (Fig. 12–3A) became ambulant.

These types of spinal cord involvement represent the range of severity of impact. Focal abnormalities (type A) have been linked to "spinal transient ischemic attack" and "spinal reversible ischemic neurologic deficit" without

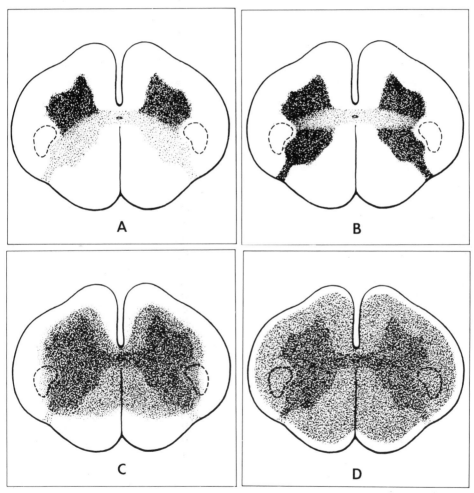

Figure 12–3. Schematic patterns of magnetic resonance images of spinal cord infarction: *type A*, anterior horn involvement (owl's eyes); *type B*, anterior and posterior horn involvement; *type C*, involvement of entire gray matter and adjacent central white matter; *type D*, diffuse signal abnormality of entire cross section of spinal cord. (From Mawad, et al,[42] by permission of the American Society of Neuroradiology.)

further clarification of symptoms. Focal abnormalities (type A) in an early postoperative episode may indicate a potential for recovery. Any other type seems to be associated with a permanent deficit.

Monitoring Techniques

Use of somatosensory evoked potentials (SSEPs) to monitor patients undergoing aortic surgery is not standard but is practiced in many institutions with high patient volumes of aortic repair. Enthusiasm has slightly diminished because a 1988 prospective study from Baylor College of Medicine showed that the incidences of false-negative and false-positive responses were considerable (Table 12–3). In addition, some investigators argue that the vulnerable lateral and ventral columns of the central gray matter are not primarily monitored by SSEPs, which are largely limited to stimulation of the dorsal columns.

Many studies have explored the value of SSEP recording in establishing potential ischemic damage.[12,19,33] The most detailed studies have been by Laschinger and colleagues[35] and Cunningham and associates.[14] Four SSEP responses were recognized.

Type I SSEP Response. This response, noted in some patients, is characterized by a gradual diminution of SSEP amplitude and increased latency 7 to 30 minutes after aortic cross-clamping. Usually, distal aortic perfusion pressure is less than 30 mm Hg. The incidence of paraplegia is considered to be extremely high (37.5%). Unclamping may restore conduction velocity and amplitude, but they may also fail to reappear.

Type II SSEP Response. Essentially, a normal SSEP associated with adequate distal aortic perfusion pressure is maintained throughout the clamping procedure. In the study by Cunningham and colleagues,[14] spinal cord infarction did not develop in these patients. In Crawford and associates' study[12] of a larger group of patients, 5% had immediate postoperative paraplegia.

Type III SSEP Response. Disappearance or significant decrease of the SSEP amplitude after placement of the distal aortic clamp has been linked to inclusion of critical intercostal vessels. Reimplantation of intercostal arteries may result in return of the SSEP response, even in patients in whom the SSEP response has been lost for more than 30 minutes. None of the patients with return of SSEP responses had neurologic deficits, but it is difficult to determine what would have happened if reconstruction had not been done.

Type IV SSEP Response. This response is characterized by gradual

Table 12–3 RELATION OF SPINAL CORD INFARCTION TO INTRAOPERATIVE SOMATOSENSORY EVOKED POTENTIAL (SSEP) RECORDING IN 99 PATIENTS

SSEP Response*	Patients (n)	Paraparesis and Paraplegia Patients, n (%)
No change	53	7 (13)
Change with return	11	3 (27)
Change with fluctuating return of response	10	2 (20)
Change with no return	25	8 (32)

Modified from Crawford, et al.[12]

*Change in SSEP response is defined as latency increase of not more than 10% and amplitude decrease of not more than 25% for 10 minutes. All patients had temporary bypass and distal perfusion pressure of 60 mm Hg or greater.

fade-out of SSEP tracings, sometimes associated with overzealous use of nitroprusside, and is associated with inadequate distal aortic perfusion pressure. Fade-out occurs in patients with long clamping times and often takes 1/2 hour to become clearly evident. Restoration of distal perfusion after unclamping results in a prompt return of SSEP but may falsely suggest normal cord function, because paraplegia may occur.

The current experience with SSEP recording may guide the vascular surgeon, but it has not been clearly demonstrated that measures taken to improve spinal cord flow will decrease the incidence of postoperative paraplegia. Whether catheter-type electrodes should be placed in the subarachnoid space for SSEP stimulation in unstable patients to monitor possible postoperative deterioration is unresolved.[50] Use of motor evoked potentials, an exciting new technique, deserves further study in this group of patients. Levy[37] noted that in a preliminary study of 45 spinal cord operations, motor evoked potentials correctly predicted spinal cord injury in all cases. Systematic data in thoracoabdominal aneurysmal surgery are not yet available. Preliminary animal data suggest that in prediction of spinal cord injury, loss of motor evoked potentials has a high specificity (100%) but a low sensitivity (16%).[20]

THERAPEUTIC OPTIONS

Numerous studies have claimed the potential usefulness of reimplantation of intercostal arteries, use of bypass or shunts, or, more recently, fractionated double-clamping to counteract steal from the spinal cord circulation. None of these studies has convincingly shown a decrease in the incidence of spinal cord infarction.[9,38,47,67,68] There is accumulating evidence that deep hypothermia (30°C), usually in association with atriofemoral bypass, decreases spinal cord injury. However, hypothermia is not generally used as a preventive measure.[3,57] Recently, attention has focused on cerebrospinal fluid drainage to prevent spinal cord injury with the reasoning that drainage may improve spinal perfusion pressure by decreasing the counteracting cerebrospinal fluid pressure.

A recent prospective study, however, did not demonstrate a reduction in the incidence of paraplegia with continuous drainage of lumbar spinal fluid and maintenance of normal to nearly normal cerebrospinal fluid pressures.[13] Multiple logistic regression analysis revealed that age (older than 64 years), aortic clamp time (over 44 minutes), and postoperative hypotension (less than 100 mm Hg systolic) were independent significant risk factors for postoperative paraplegia.[10]

The addition of intrathecally delivered papaverine to cause dilation of the anterior spinal artery and increased spinal cord blood flow had no marked effect in a preliminary study.[58,61] Intravenous administration of naloxone has shown promising results in reversal of neurologic deficits,[2] but prospective studies are not available. A high-dose methylprednisolone pulse of 30 mg/kg in patients with anticipated extensive repairs and long clamping times may be another therapeutic consideration. There is no evidence of benefit of methylprednisolone in aortic surgery, although one recent randomized trial in traumatic spinal cord injury demonstrated improved outcome in patients treated early (see Chapter 15). Therefore, both cerebrospinal fluid drainage and steroids in the perioperative and postoperative phases may protect the spinal cord.[72]

In summary, the postoperative management of patients with thoracoabdominal repairs may include monitoring of cerebrospinal fluid pressure for at least 24 hours, provision of adequate oxygenation and adequate systemic pulse pressure, and immediate action when these variables change. Methylprednisolone infusion can be considered when clamping times have been long.

PLEXOPATHIES

Unlike direct compression of the lumbosacral plexus by large aneurysms of the common iliac artery,[65,70] rupture of abdominal aneurysms may result in extensive retroperitoneal hematomas with damage to the femoral and obturator nerves.[5,43,51,53]

Recognition of the anatomic relationship between the intrapelvic parts of these nerves and the iliopsoas muscle is important.[49] The femoral nerve consists of the posterior portions of the L-2 through L-4 nerve roots and descends through the fibers of the psoas muscle. It usually lies in the groove between the psoas and the iliac muscles. It supplies the quadriceps, sartorius, and pectineal muscles. The anterofemoral cutaneous and saphenous sensory nerves supply the anteromedial thigh and calf.

The obturator nerve arises from the same divisions of the lumbar plexus as the femoral nerve and descends within the psoas, but it exits on the medial border to supply the adductor thigh muscles. Both nerves are located in the psoas and iliac muscles, which are tightly reinforced by fascial sheaths, and any hemorrhage in this pelvic muscle results in a compartment syndrome (see Chapter 10).

Other potential mechanisms for nerve damage may be hemorrhagic extension into the nerve sheath or compression of the distal femoral nerve segment against the inguinal ligament through enlarged anterior fascial pockets.

Computed tomography scan may demonstrate a hematoma in the psoas muscle, and in exceptional cases, it may even engulf the extraspinal segments of the second and third lumbar nerves. The classic presentation of a psoas muscle hematoma is a sudden onset of pain in the groin with occasional radiation down the anterior aspect of the leg. Pain is evident on hip flexion, and hyperesthesia may be noted in the cutaneous nerve distribution. The knee jerk and the adductor reflex are absent with involvement of the obturator nerve.

Fasciotomy may be indicated in the first 24 hours and may result in immediate resolution of weakness. Others, however, have noted spontaneous improvement, but only in patients with incomplete plexopathies. The approach in patients with coagulopathies is different and more likely to be conservative (see Chapter 10).

The clinical entity of unilateral or bilateral ischemic plexopathy after aortic repairs is poorly defined. It would appear virtually impossible to compromise plexus perfusion, because the vascular anatomy of the plexus is characterized by many collaterals. Nevertheless, patients may have unilateral leg weakness with electromyographic abnormalities that are very suggestive of a lumbosacral plexopathy. In general, these patients tend to have a more favorable outcome and a high probability of becoming ambulant within 1 year.[26]

AORTIC DISSECTION

Acute aortic dissection is a major vascular catastrophe.[44,54] A tear in the aortic intima allows blood to track into the aortic media, and dissection may extend into the entire length of the aorta, including the large arch arteries. Predisposing factors are hypertension, cannulation during cardiac surgery, angiographic catheterization, trauma, and cardiac valve replacement. Aortic dissections can be categorized according to DeBakey's classification (Fig. 12–4). Types I and II both originate in the ascending aorta, but type II terminates proximal to the origin of the innominate artery. In type III, the dissection begins distal to the origin of the left subclavian artery and may extend far into the iliac arteries (type IIIb).

Severe migrating chest pain is one of the salient features and may be associated with loss of a femoral pulse. Signs of aortic insufficiency or cardiac tamponade may be present.

The diagnosis may be confirmed with transesophageal echocardiography.[21,23,52] Echocardiography may di-

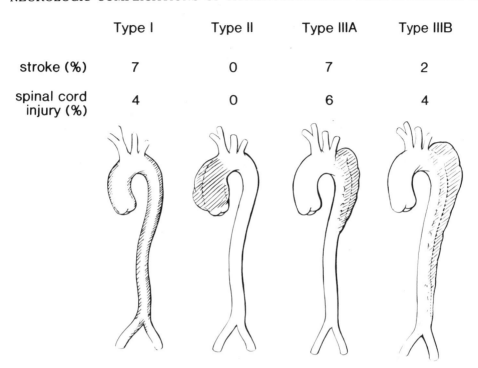

	Type I	Type II	Type IIIA	Type IIIB
stroke (%)	7	0	7	2
spinal cord injury (%)	4	0	6	4

Figure 12—4. Classification of dissection (DeBakey) and incidence of neurologic complications.

agnose aortic dissection with high accuracy. However, angiography remains the mainstay for confirming the diagnosis.

Acute dissections are treated medically with a regulated infusion of nitroprusside. Propranolol or labetalol is often also considered. Inability to control hypertension is an indication for surgery, but some vascular surgeons prefer emergency surgery in proximal dissections.

Neurologic complications are uncommon in acute aortic dissections[8,15,17,25,45] (Table 12—4). The reported incidences of stroke and spinal cord ischemia according to DeBakey's types are depicted in Figure 12—4.

Decreased level of consciousness, sometimes progressing to a state of stupor or coma, is frequent but reflects a marked decrease in systemic blood pressure, especially in patients with preexisting hypertension vigorously treated with antihypertensive agents. Focal signs, however, may occur when

the dissection extends into the common carotid artery. Inequality of the carotid pulses and unilateral tenderness over the left carotid may be helpful signs. Nissim[48] noted a unilateral reduplication in pulsations of the carotid artery (that is, two beats in quick succession on the right for every single beat on the left). This effect has been attributed to a difference in the velocity of the pulse wave through the lumen and through

Table 12—4 NEUROLOGIC MANIFESTATIONS OF AORTIC DISSECTION*

Findings	Patients, n (%)
Decreased level of consciousness or coma	26 (5)
Hemiplegia	10 (2)
Paraplegia	27 (5)
Transient blindness	4 (0.8)
Horner's syndrome	3 (0.6)

*Based on 505 cases from the literature compiled by Hirst and associates.[31]

the dissecting aneurysm. Carotid dissection may lead to Horner's syndrome and hypoglossal damage, but these characteristic signs may also be absent. Innominate occlusion may result in right hemispheric infarction and may be followed by paraparesis after extension of the dissection to the thoracic and abdominal portions of the aorta. Bilateral involvement of both left and right common carotids has been described, whereas dissection into the vertebral arteries has not.

Patients who present with acute ischemic stroke, often right-sided, and acute type A aortic dissection at the same time are particularly difficult to manage. Emergency replacement of the ascending aorta may produce reperfusion damage or hemorrhagic transformation. Indeed, this has been reported in two of seven patients who had emergency surgery in the face of a recent stroke.[22]

In their collection of 11 cases, Weisman and Adams[69] drew attention to ischemic necrosis of the peripheral nerves caused by obstruction of the iliac arteries. Most patients had a pulseless, cold extremity with weakness, anesthesia, and areflexia, but a shortcoming of all cases was that pathologic examination of the peripheral nerves was not done.

Very uncommon manifestations include putaminal hemorrhage, probably related to marked surges in blood pressure.[45] Transient blindness reported in older series may be a result of ophthalmic artery involvement from artery-to-artery embolism from occlusion of the common carotid.[69]

Spinal cord damage has been well recognized in many series, but it is generally not related to the extent of intercostal artery involvement in the dissection. The most common mechanism may be hypoperfusion of the spinal cord associated with shock. Concomitant infarction of the vertebral bodies that can be recognized on plain radiographs may accompany paraplegia.[30] Outcome of paraplegia in dissection is similarly poor.

CONCLUSIONS

Although statistically uncommon, neurologic complications of vascular reconstruction generally are most often associated with surgery of the aorta. Surgical repairs of thoracoabdominal aneurysm may result in paraplegia in 10% to 20% of patients after effective surgery; in acute spontaneous or traumatic rupture, the incidence doubles. Aortoiliac repair, however, is uncommonly complicated by spinal cord or plexus injury (less than 1%).

Several pathologic types of spinal cord infarction have been reported, but anterior spinal artery syndrome or complete spinal cord infarction at the midthoracic to low-thoracic level is most frequent. Magnetic resonance imaging can demonstrate signal changes in the spinal cord that not only confirm the ischemic damage but also predict recovery when only anterior horn abnormalities (owl's eyes) are present. Prevention of spinal cord injury begins in the operating suite, but some patients awaken neurologically intact only to deteriorate days later. Hypovolemia, hypotension, and respiratory acidosis have accompanied this delayed-onset paraplegia. This unfortunate affliction in critically ill surgical patients already at considerable risk for major postoperative complications may justify prolonged monitoring of cerebrospinal fluid pressures.

No study in humans has shown that measures such as hypothermia, cerebrospinal fluid drainage, intrathecally delivered papaverine, or combinations of treatments have actually decreased the incidence of paraplegia. An appropriate, but unproven, approach in patients with major risk factors (aged 64 years or older, aortic clamp time over 45 minutes) and abnormal SSEP responses during surgery is a high dose of methylprednisolone, 30 mg/kg, cerebrospinal fluid drainage, and very careful maintenance of adequate systemic blood pressure and normal acid-base balance. Drainage of cerebrospinal fluid (the increase in cerebrospinal fluid may result in a decrease of spinal cord perfusion pressure) should logically be the first action when leg function begins to deteriorate postoperatively. It remains imperative, however, that carefully designed studies be completed to establish justifiable recommendations.

Another major vascular emergency is aortic dissection. Neurologic complications appear to be related to extension of the dissection. Ischemic stroke, occurring in approximately 6%, may be related to extension into the carotid system. Management of ischemic stroke in aortic dissection is difficult because the neurologic deficit may worsen from vigorous antihypertensive treatment instituted to treat the aortic dissection and from hemorrhagic transformation when surgery is decided on.

REFERENCES

1. Adams, HD and van Geertruyden, HH: Neurologic complications of aortic surgery. Ann Surg 144:574–609, 1956.
2. Archer, CW, Wynn, MM, and Archibald, J: Naloxone and spinal fluid drainage as adjuncts in the surgical treatment of thoracoabdominal and thoracic aneurysms. Surgery 108:755–762, 1990.
3. Berguer, R, Porto, J, Fedoronko, B, and Dragovic, L: Selective deep hypothermia of the spinal cord prevents paraplegia after aortic cross-clamping in the dog model. J Vasc Surg 15:62–72, 1992.
4. Bolton, PM and Blumgart, LH: Neurological complications of ruptured abdominal aortic aneurysm. Br J Surg 59:707–709, 1972.
5. Boontje, AH and Haaxma, R: Femoral neuropathy as a complication of aortic surgery. J Cardiovasc Surg 28:286–289, 1987.
6. Byrne, TN and Waxman, SG: Spinal Cord Compression: Diagnosis and Principles of Management. FA Davis Company, Philadelphia, 1990, pp 21–65.
7. Carlson, DE, Karp, RB, and Kouchoukos, NT: Surgical treatment of aneurysms of the descending thoracic aorta: An analysis of 86 patients. Ann Thorac Surg 35:58–69, 1983.
8. Chase, TN, Rosman, NP, and Price, DL: The cerebral syndromes associated with dissecting aneurysm of the aorta: A clinicopathological study. Brain 91:173–190, 1968.
9. Colon, R, Frazier, OH, Cooley, DA, and McAllister, HA: Hypothermic regional perfusion for protection of the spinal cord during periods of ischemia. Ann Thorac Surg 43:639–643, 1987.
10. Crawford, ES, Crawford, JL, Safi, HJ, et al: Thoracoabdominal aortic aneurysms: Preoperative and intraoperative factors determining immediate and long-term results of operations in 605 patients. J Vasc Surg 3:389–404, 1986.
11. Crawford, ES, Hess, KR, Cohen, ES, et al: Ruptured aneurysm of the descending thoracic and thoracoabdominal aorta: Analysis according to size and treatment. Ann Surg 213:417–426, 1991.
12. Crawford, ES, Mizrahi, EM, Hess, KR, et al: The impact of distal aortic perfusion and somatosensory evoked potential monitoring on prevention of paraplegia after aortic aneurysm operation. J Thorac Cardiovasc Surg 95:357–367, 1988.
13. Crawford, ES, Svensson, LG, Hess, KR, et al: A prospective randomized study of cerebrospinal fluid drainage to prevent paraplegia after high-risk surgery on the thoracoabdominal aorta. J Vasc Surg 13:36–46, 1990.
14. Cunningham, JN Jr, Laschinger, JC, and Spencer, FC: Monitoring of somatosensory evoked potentials during surgical procedures on the thoracoabdominal aorta. IV. Clinical observations and results. J Thorac Cardiovasc Surg 94:275–285, 1987.
15. DeBakey, ME, McCollum, CH, Crawford, ES, et al: Dissection and dissecting aneurysms of the aorta: Twenty-year follow-up of five hundred twenty-seven patients treated surgically. Surgery 92:1118–1134, 1982.
16. Decroix, JP, Ciaudo-Lacroix, C, and Lapresle, J: Syndrome de Brown-Séquard dû a un infarctus spinal. Rev Neurol (Paris) 140:585–586, 1984.
17. DeSanctis, RW, Doroghazi, RM, Austen, WG, and Buckley, MJ: Aortic dissec-

tion. N Engl J Med 317:1060–1067, 1987.

18. Dommisse, GF: The blood supply of the spinal cord: A critical vascular zone in spinal surgery. J Bone Joint Surg [Br] 56:225–235, 1974.

19. Drenger, B, Parker, SD, McPherson, RW, et al: Spinal cord stimulation evoked potentials during thoracoabdominal aortic aneurysm surgery. Anesthesiology 76:689–695, 1992.

20. Elmore, JR, Gloviczki, P, Harper, CM, et al: Spinal cord injury in experimental thoracic aortic occlusion: Investigation of combined methods of protection (abstr). J Vasc Surg 14:422, 1991.

21. Erbel, R, Engberding, R, Daniel, W, et al: Echocardiography in diagnosis of aortic dissection. Lancet i:457–461, 1989.

22. Fann, JI, Sarris, GE, Miller, C, et al: Surgical management of acute aortic dissection complicated by stroke. Circulation 80 Suppl 1:I-257–I-263, 1989.

23. Farah, MG and Suneja, R: Diagnosis of circumferential dissection of the ascending aorta by transesophageal echocardiography. Chest 103:291–292, 1993.

24. Ferguson, LRJ, Bergan, JJ, Conn, J Jr, and Yao, JST: Spinal ischemia following abdominal aortic surgery. Ann Surg 181:267–272, 1975.

25. Gerber, O, Heyer, EJ, and Vieux, U: Painless dissections of the aorta presenting as acute neurologic syndromes. Stroke 17:644–647, 1986.

26. Gloviczki, P, Cross, SA, Stanson, AW, et al: Ischemic injury to the spinal cord or lumbosacral plexus after aorto-iliac reconstruction. Am J Surg 162:131–136, 1991.

27. Hantler, CB and Knight, PR: Intracranial hypertension following cross-clamping of the thoracic aorta. Anesthesiology 56:146–147, 1982.

28. Hassler, O: Blood supply to human spinal cord: A microangiographic study. Arch Neurol 15:302–307, 1966.

29. Herren, RY and Alexander, L: Sulcal and intrinsic blood vessels of human spinal cord. Arch Neurol Psychiatry 41:678–687, 1939.

30. Hill, CS Jr and Vasquez, JM: Massive infarction of spinal cord and vertebral bodies as a complication of dissecting aneurysm of the aorta. Circulation 25:997–1000, 1962.

31. Hirst, AE Jr, Johns, VJ Jr, and Kime, SW Jr: Dissecting aneurysm of the aorta: A review of 505 cases. Medicine (Baltimore) 37:217–279, 1958.

32. Hogan, EL and Romanul, FCA: Spinal cord infarction occurring during insertion of aortic graft. Neurology 16:67–74, 1966.

33. Kaplan, BJ, Friedmann, WA, Alexander, JA, and Hampson, SR: Somatosensory evoked potential monitoring of spinal cord ischemia during aortic operations. Neurosurgery 19:82–90, 1986.

34. Katz, NM, Blackstone, EH, Kirklin, JW, and Karp, RB: Incremental risk factors for spinal cord injury following operation for acute traumatic aortic transection. J Thorac Cardiovasc Surg 81:669–674, 1981.

35. Laschinger, JC, Izumoto, H, and Kouchoukos, NT: Evolving concepts in prevention of spinal cord injury during operations on the descending thoracic and thoracoabdominal aorta. Ann Thorac Surg 44:667–674, 1987.

36. Lazorthes, G, Gouaze, A, Zadeh, JO, et al: Arterial vascularization of the spinal cord: Recent studies of the anastomotic substitution pathways. J Neurosurg 35:253–262, 1971.

37. Levy, WJ Jr: Clinical experience with motor and cerebellar evoked potential monitoring. Neurosurgery 20:169–182, 1987.

38. Livesay, JJ, Cooley, DA, Ventemiglia, RA, et al: Surgical experience in descending thoracic aneurysmectomy with and without adjuncts to avoid ischemia. Ann Thorac Surg 39:37–46, 1985.

39. Lynch, C and Weingarden, SI: Paraplegia following aortic surgery. Paraplegia 20:196–200, 1982.

40. Lynch, DR, Dawson, TM, Raps, EC, and Galetta, SL: Risk factors for the neurologic complications associated with aortic aneurysms. Arch Neurol 49:284–288, 1992.

41. Marini, CP, Grubbs, PE, Toporoff, B, et al: Effect of sodium nitroprusside on spi-

nal cord perfusion and paraplegia during aortic cross-clamping. Ann Thorac Surg 47:379–383, 1989.

42. Mawad, ME, Rivera, V, Crawford, S, et al: Spinal cord ischemia after resection of thoracoabdominal aortic aneurysms: MR findings in 24 patients. AJNR Am J Neuroradiol 11:987–991, 1990.

43. Merchant, RF Jr, Cafferata, HT, and DePalma, RG: Ruptured aortic aneurysm seen initially as acute femoral neuropathy. Arch Surg 117:811–813, 1982.

44. Miller, DC, Stinson, EB, Oyer, PE, et al: Operative treatment of aortic dissections: Experience with 125 patients over a 16-year period. J Thoracic Cardiovasc Surg 78:365–382, 1979.

45. Moersch, FP and Sayre, GP: Neurologic manifestations associated with dissecting aneurysm of the aorta. JAMA 144:1141–1148, 1950.

46. Moore, WM and Hollier, LH: The influence of severity of spinal cord ischemia in the etiology of delayed-onset paraplegia. Ann Surg 213:427–432, 1991.

47. Murray, MJ, Werner, E, Oliver, WC Jr, et al: Anesthetic management of thoracoabdominal aortic aneurysm repair: Effects of CSF drainage and mild hypothermia (abstr). Anesthesiology 71 Suppl: 61A, 1989.

48. Nissim, JA: Dissecting aneurysm of the aorta: A new sign. Br Heart J 8:203–206, 1946.

49. Nobel, W, Marks, SC Jr, and Kubik, S: The anatomical basis for femoral nerve palsy following iliacus hematoma. J Neurosurg 52:533–540, 1980.

50. Okamoto, Y, Murakami, M, Nakagawa, T, et al: Intraoperative spinal cord monitoring during surgery for aortic aneurysm: Application of spinal cord evoked potential. Electroencephalogr Clin Neurophysiol 84:315–320, 1992.

51. Owens, ML: Psoas weakness and femoral neuropathy: Neglected signs of retroperitoneal hemorrhage from ruptured aneurysm. Surgery 91:363–366, 1982.

52. Petasnick, JP: Radiologic evaluation of aortic dissection. Radiology 180:297–305, 1991.

53. Razzuk, MA, Linton, RR, and Darling, RC: Femoral neuropathy secondary to ruptured abdominal aortic aneurysms with false aneurysms. JAMA 201:817–820, 1967.

54. Roberts, WC: Aortic dissection: Anatomy, consequences, and causes. Am Heart J 101:195–214, 1981.

55. Sturm, JT, Billiar, TR, Dorsey, JS, et al: Risk factors for survival following surgical treatment of traumatic aortic rupture. Ann Thorac Surg 39:418–421, 1985.

56. Svensson, LG, Crawford, ES, Hess, KR, et al: Experience with 1509 patients undergoing thoracoabdominal aortic operations. J Vasc Surg 17:357–370, 1993.

57. Svensson, LG, Crawford, ES, Patel, V, et al: Spinal oxygenation, blood supply localization, cooling, and function with aortic clamping. Ann Thorac Surg 54:74–79, 1992.

58. Svensson, LG, Grum, DF, Bednarski, M, et al: Appraisal of cerebrospinal fluid alterations during aortic surgery with intrathecal papaverine administration and cerebrospinal fluid drainage. J Vasc Surg 11:423–429, 1990.

59. Svensson, LG, Patel, V, Robinson, MF, et al: Influence of preservation or perfusion of intraoperatively identified spinal cord blood supply on spinal motor evoked potentials and paraplegia after aortic surgery. J Vasc Surg 13:355–365, 1991.

60. Svensson, LG, Rickards, E, Coull, A, et al: Relationship of spinal cord blood flow to vascular anatomy during thoracic aortic cross-clamping and shunting. J Thorac Cardiovasc Surg 91:71–78, 1986.

61. Svensson, LG, Stewart, RW, Cosgrove, DM III, et al: Intrathecal papaverine for the prevention of paraplegia after operation on the thoracic or thoracoabdominal aorta. J Thorac Cardiovasc Surg 96:823–829, 1988.

62. Svensson, LG, Von Ritter, CM, Groeneveld, HT, et al: Cross-clamping of the thoracic aorta: Influence of aortic shunts, laminectomy, papaverine, calcium channel blocker, allopurinol, and superoxide dismutase on spinal cord blood flow and paraplegia in baboons. Ann Surg 204:38–47, 1986.

63. Szilagyi, DE, Hageman, JH, Smith, RF, and Elliott, JP: Spinal cord damage in

surgery of the abdominal aorta. Surgery 83:38–56, 1978.

64. Turnbull, IM: Blood supply of the spinal cord: Normal and pathological considerations. Clin Neurosurg 20:56–84, 1973.

65. Vock, P, Mattle, H, Studer, M, and Mumenthaler, M: Lumbosacral plexus lesions: Correlation of clinical signs and computed tomography. J Neurol Neurosurg Psychiatry 51:72–79, 1988.

66. Wadouh, F, Lindemann, E-M, Arndt, CF, et al: The arteria radicularis magna anterior as a decisive factor influencing spinal cord damage during aortic occlusion. J Thorac Cardiovasc Surg 88:1–10, 1984.

67. Wadouh, F, Wadouh, R, Hartmann, M, and Crisp-Lindgren, N: Prevention of paraplegia during aortic operations. Ann Thorac Surg 50:543–552, 1990.

68. Wakabayashi, A and Connolly, JE: Prevention of paraplegia associated with resection of extensive thoracic aneurysms. Arch Surg 111:1186–1189, 1976.

69. Weisman, AD and Adams, RD: The neurological complications of dissecting aortic aneurysm. Brain 67:69–92, 1944.

70. Wilberger, JE: Lumbosacral radiculopathy secondary to abdominal aortic aneurysms: Report of three cases. J Neurosurg 58:965–967, 1983.

71. Williams, GM, Perler, BA, Burdick, JF, et al: Angiographic localization of spinal cord blood supply and its relationship to postoperative paraplegia. J Vasc Surg 13:23–35, 1991.

72. Woloszyn, TT, Marini, CP, Coons, MS, et al: Cerebrospinal fluid drainage and steroids provide better spinal cord protection during aortic cross-clamping than does either treatment alone. Ann Thorac Surg 49:78–83, 1990.

73. Zülch, KJ and Kurth-Schumacher, R: The pathogenesis of "intermittent spinovascular insufficiency" (spinal claudication of Dejerine) and other vascular syndromes of the spinal cord. Vasc Surg 4:116–136, 1970.

Chapter 13

NEUROLOGIC COMPLICATIONS OF CARDIAC SURGERY

GENERAL CONSIDERATIONS
STROKE AFTER CORONARY
  ARTERY BYPASS GRAFT SURGERY
NEUROPSYCHOLOGICAL
  ABNORMALITIES
NEURO-OPHTHALMOLOGIC
  COMPLICATIONS
PERIPHERAL NERVE DAMAGE

It has been well established that use of extracorporeal circulation in either coronary artery bypass grafting (CABG) or open heart surgery greatly increases the risk for neurologic complications.[36,39,89,90] Patients at particular risk for neurologic complications have been identified, but most of the risk factors cannot be modified. Equally important, the clinical profile of patients undergoing coronary bypass surgery is changing. There is a clear shift toward a greater prevalence of patients who are older than 70 years and a greater prevalence of diabetic patients; consequently, the frequency of acute neurologic events may increase along with other systemic perioperative complications.[53] Many of these insults considerably delay return to work or necessitate daily living assistance, all with enormous personal and social costs.

Occlusive disease of the carotid arteries and the ascending aorta is a risk factor for the development of stroke. Management of coexisting atherosclerotic disease in the aorta or carotid arteries is complicated. When formulating management guidelines, one should not be surprised to find an all-too-familiar pattern of (1) lack of well-designed randomized clinical trials and (2) evidence largely based on surgical expert opinion alone. This chapter reviews the major neurologic complications of cardiac surgery and highlights the possible pathophysiologic mechanism.

GENERAL CONSIDERATIONS

Comprehensive knowledge about the conditions and potential risks while the patient is on cardiopulmonary bypass is required for one to become familiar with the risks of neurologic complications after cardiac surgery. Monitoring of the central nervous system is limited during the procedure, and currently there is no evidence that cortical evoked responses or electroencephalographic (EEG) monitoring permits accurate evaluation of the patient's well-being. Also, if an abnormality is detected, the therapeutic options, if any, are limited.

The extracorporeal perfusion system is depicted in Figure 13–1. Essentially, venous return from two connecting catheters placed in the superior and inferior venae cavae passes through an oxygenator, and a nonocclusive roller pump returns blood to the ascending aorta. Additional left ventricular stenting is used in some institutions. Two types of oxygenators are commonly

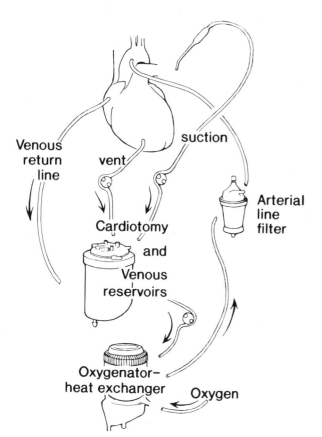

Figure 13–1. Extracorporeal circulation.

used: bubble oxygenators with very efficient oxygenation at low cost, and membrane oxygenators with the additional advantages of prolonged use and virtual absence of blood cell disruption that is otherwise created by gas bubbling. Filters may be placed on both sides of the system to ensure a low risk of infusing debris and air bubbles into the circulation. The extracorporeal system is primed with a heparinized and buffered physiologic salt solution, which is followed by administration of a cold cardioplegia solution through one of the roller heads on the pump oxygenator. Usually, a large dose of potassium cardioplegia solution is used.

Hypothermia permits adequate myocardial preservation and central nervous system protection.[95] Nevertheless, many physiologic changes occur that can result in significant risks. One of the most important changes—the decreased response of insulin to hypothermia—potentially causes hyperglycemia, but hyperglycemia may also be associated with the stress response of the procedure itself, use of pressor agents, and infusion of large volumes of dextrose solutions. Other serious problems with a potential for central nervous system injury are bubble expansion and subsequent air embolism during the cooling phase of bypass, hypotension during the procedure, increased intracranial pressure resulting from obstruction of the vena cava cannula, and decrease in hematocrit. Increase in blood viscosity may also occur from the effect of hypothermia or from infusion of hyperosmolar solutions. Warm heart surgery is a promising new technique that recently was evaluated by a randomized trial.[27] The advantages of warm blood cardioplegia are related to myocardial protection, particularly in complex cardiac procedures.

Despite many promising technical developments, hemodynamic threats and danger of microemboli remain major problems during cardiac surgery. During cardiopulmonary bypass, cerebral blood flow is altered by shifts in temperature, hemodynamic changes induced by anesthetic pharmacologic agents, and changes in PCO_2.[60–62,77] Cerebral autoregulation, however, remains intact. A scholarly account of cerebrovascular physiology and pharmacology can be found in a review by Schell and associates.[86]

A history of stroke or transient ischemic attacks indicates a predisposition for stroke after cardiac surgery. Whether a possible hemodynamic compromise exists in patients with unilateral or bilateral carotid stenosis has not been systematically studied. A transcranial Doppler study done at the time of bypass found that blood flow velocity may decrease just after the onset of cardiopulmonary bypass ipsilateral to a carotid stenosis, but reduced cerebral perfusion was not observed despite a marked drop in arterial blood pressure to less than 50 mm Hg during the first minutes of bypass.[106]

The pathophysiology of cerebral injury in cardiopulmonary bypass is not elucidated. Factors associated with increased incidence of cognitive deficits are intracardiac procedures, duration of bypass, use of bubble oxygenation,[72] and absence of arterial filters.[71] Certainly, hemodynamic hazards during the various stages of cardiopulmonary bypass may contribute to cerebral injury, but recent evidence suggests that microemboli may be more relevant.

Interposition of a filter in the arterial line of the extracorporeal circuit (Fig. 13–1) may diminish but not eliminate neurologic complications.[45] Pugsley and associates,[78] in a small group of patients who randomly received filtered (40-μm self-venting blood filter) or nonfiltered cardiopulmonary bypass grafts, assessed the effects with a battery of neuropsychologic tests and transcranial Doppler (TCD) ultrasonography. Significantly fewer microembolic events were detected by TCD examination in the patients in the filtered group, who also had significantly better neuropsychologic performance. In contrast, a randomized study from Spain in which 20-μm screen filters were used in the arterial line could not demonstrate any change in postoperative cerebral impairment.[5]

Microemboli may come from several sources: ventricular air,[66] atheromatous debris dislodged during insertion of the cannula, fat globules, platelet aggregates, atheromatous debris from large arteries,[73] and perhaps also particulate emboli from glove powder, foam products, and the lining of tubes.

Transcranial Doppler examination of the middle cerebral artery during bypass has greatly improved the recognition of these particles, but TCD cannot differentiate between particulate and gaseous emboli.[72] TCD monitoring of the middle cerebral artery blood velocities during bypass may identify high-amplitude flow disturbance signals that produce a chirping sound superimposed on a band created by nonpulsatile flow.

The end of bypass has been identified as the most critical period for embolization.[104] The number of embolic events significantly increases during filling of the beating heart rather than immediately after declamping of the aorta (Fig. 13–2). The clinical value of this finding may remain uncertain, but meticulous draining before filling of the empty heart may reduce this complication. Prospective studies that correlate the prevalence of embolic showers with postoperative stroke or neuropsychologic deficit are needed, but as pointed out recently, the actual "hit rate" (frequency of embolic rather than symptomatic ischemia) may be low.[20]

The neuropathologic counterpart of microemboli has recently been described. Neuropathologic investigation of patients who died after the procedure revealed many focal small capillary and arteriolar dilatations in the cortical and

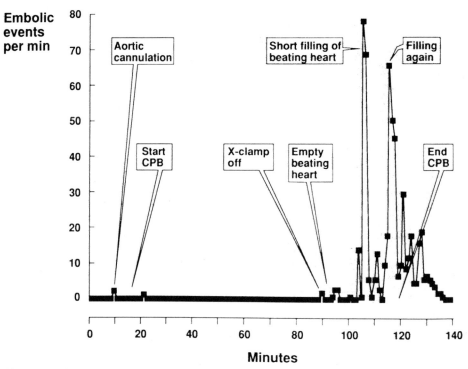

Figure 13–2. Transcranial Doppler recording of emboli during open heart surgery, indicating maximal embolic events during redistribution of blood when the heart is beginning to eject. CPB = cardiopulmonary bypass. (From van der Linden and Casimir-Ahn,[104] with permission of the Society of Thoracic Surgeons.)

deep nuclear gray matter.[67] These abnormalities have not been found in patients without bypass procedures and represent microgaseous or, perhaps more likely, lipid microemboli. In one patient, more than 1500 dilatations were found at the level of the basal ganglia. Serial magnetic resonance images have not detected abnormalities linked to neuropsychologic deficits,[87] but correlative studies with TCD ultrasonography have not been performed.

Monitoring during bypass graft surgery offers the possibility of recognizing damage to the cerebral cortex. Except for numerous studies that have tried to correlate EEG abnormalities with postoperative neuropsychologic or neurologic complications, convincing data are not available to support routine use of monitoring. Part of the question is whether aggressive intervention after detection of abnormalities during cardiac surgery can be successful. Indeed,

Arom and associates[6] carefully correlated computed EEG recordings with postoperative deficits and found that intervention (consisting of increase in cerebral perfusion pressure, increase in bypass pump flow, and use of pressors) resulted in improvement of EEG variables and, more important, decreased the incidence of postoperative neuropsychologic deficits; however, this sophisticated technology may not be widely available. Somatosensory evoked potentials may have no application, because marked hypothermia attenuates or may even abolish the cortical response.[4,29]

Few clinical trials have assessed the neurologic outcome with agents that may protect the brain during cardiopulmonary bypass surgery. Much of the gathered data are from animal studies. Reports of two large trials, both with thiopental loading, have been published thus far (Table 13–1). Nussmeier and

Table 13-1 BARBITURATE CEREBRAL PROTECTION STUDIES

Characteristics	Nussmeier, et al. Study[70]	Zaidan, et al. Study[110]
Patients (n)	182	300
Procedure	Open chamber	CABG
History of stroke	No	No
Oxygenation	Bubble	Membrane
Arterial filter	No	Yes
Temperature (°C)	>34	28
Duration of CPB (min)	50	90
Pump flow rate (L/min)	3.0-4.4	2.5
Thiopental dose (mg/kg)	39 ± 8	33 ± 11
EEG burst suppression	Yes	Yes
Mean arterial pressure (mm Hg)	40-90	50-100
Priming	5% dextrose	Plasmalyte
Stroke, TH/P	0/6	5/2

CABG = coronary artery bypass grafting; CPB = cardiopulmonary bypass; EEG = electroencephalographic; P = placebo; TH = thiopental.

associates' study[70] found a significantly lower incidence of stroke and neuropsychologic deficits in patients treated with thiopental loading, but a more recent study[110] reached the opposite conclusion. Important differences in patient selection (open heart or coronary artery bypass grafting) and cardiopulmonary bypass conditions (normothermic or hypothermic, arterial filters or no arterial filter, glucose priming or Plasmalyte primer) may have accounted for some of the differences but are not likely to explain the major differences in results. There is a compelling need for more detailed data before barbiturate use can be recommended.

The most important complications and their relevance to clinical practice and management will be reviewed. Although there have been several major advances in our understanding of the mechanism of neurologic complications, therapeutic options are limited.

STROKE AFTER CORONARY ARTERY BYPASS GRAFT SURGERY

The incidence of ischemic stroke after CABG may approach 3% to 5%.[18,28,40] After open heart surgery, the risk of stroke is markedly higher (up to 10%).[36] The risk of perioperative stroke is significantly increased in warm blood cardioplegia. In a recently published trial,[64] perioperative stroke was 3.1% in "warm blood cardioplegia" as opposed to 1.0% in "cold blood cardioplegia." No significant difference was found in delayed-onset stroke. This trial has been criticized for poor definition of neurologic events.

Fortunately, permanent stroke of marked severity occurs in less than 2% of the patients, and only a minority of the patients actually die from herniation. Many risk factors have been identified. Two large studies (Table 13-2) found that previous history of stroke, prolonged bypass time (often over 2 hours), and postoperative atrial fibrillation were significantly more common in patients who had an ischemic stroke after CABG.[98] Gardner and associates[38] emphasized that atherosclerosis of the ascending aorta may predispose patients to stroke. Although the diagnosis of a "shaggy aorta" ideally should be made by transesophageal echocardiography, this examination is not routinely done, and more often the condition is revealed at the time of insertion of extracorporeal circulation cannulae. The value of preoperative transesophageal echocardiography has not been studied but can be expected to be low. A 1981 study from Massachusetts General Hospital again stressed the risk of stroke in patients with carotid bruit, a major con-

Table 13-2 RISK FACTORS FOR STROKE AFTER CORONARY ARTERY BYPASS GRAFTING

Factors	Gardner, et al.[38]	Reed, et al.[80]
Age > 60 y	+	+
History of		
Myocardial infarction	−	+
Cardiac failure	NA	+
Diabetes mellitus	−	−
Stroke or TIA	+	+
Atherosclerosis of ascending aorta and arch	+	NA
Carotid bruits	NA	+
Aorta clamp time	NA	−
Protracted bypass time	+	+
Perioperative hypotension	+	−
Perioperative flow rates	−	NA
Postoperative		
Atrial fibrillation	NA	+
Hematocrit	NA	−
Platelet count	NA	−

+ = significant increased risk; − = no increased risk: NA = not assessed; TIA = transient ischemic attack.

troversy for years.[82] Atherosclerosis of the major vessels is not limited to coronary artery disease, and a small but significant proportion of patients scheduled for CABG have severe carotid disease. Conversely, patients with asymptomatic carotid disease have severe coronary artery disease. A study from the Cleveland Clinic prospectively evaluated coronary artery disease in patients with extracranial carotid atherosclerosis and convincingly demonstrated that 65% of 506 patients had advanced coronary artery disease.[47] (Eighteen percent of these patients had severe, uncorrectable coronary artery disease that had remained asymptomatic before discovery.)

The true proportion of patients with significant carotid artery disease is approximately 10% in an unselected series of CABG patients (Table 13-3). Other studies usually based their incidences of severe carotid disease on non-invasive angiographic studies in patients selected because they had carotid bruits or a history of transient ischemic attack or stroke.[52,54] A carotid bruit is poorly related to the severity of carotid stenosis whether evaluated by duplex ultrasonography[25,44] or angiography. Approximately two thirds of patients

Table 13-3 SEVERE ASYMPTOMATIC STENOSIS IN UNSELECTED SERIES OF CORONARY ARTERY BYPASS GRAFTING

Series (y)	Patients (n)	Method of Assessment	Patients with Carotid Stenosis, n (%)	Definition of Severe Carotid Stenosis
Turnipseed, et al., 1980[102]	170	Doppler	20 (12)	"Severe"
Barnes, et al., 1981[9]	324	Doppler	40 (12)	>50%
Breslau, et al., 1981[16]	78	Doppler	5 (6)	>50%
Balderman, et al., 1983[8]	500	OPG, angiography	9 (2)	≥80%
Brener, et al., 1987[15]	4047	OPG, Doppler	153 (4)	>50%
Faggioli, et al., 1990[35]	539	Doppler	47 (9)	>75%

OPG = oculoplethysmography.

scheduled for CABG who have severe carotid stenosis (defined as more than 50% on angiography) probably do not have carotid bruits (Fig. 13–3).

With the current data, it is difficult to give strong recommendations for management of carotid stenosis in CABG patients. Previous studies have not identified patients whose risk is sufficiently high to justify a trial of prophylactic endarterectomy.[10] Many prospective studies of CABG could not substantiate an increased risk of stroke in patients with asymptomatic stenosis.[37] Nonetheless, asymptomatic carotid disease significantly increases the risk of perioperative deaths, including those caused by myocardial infarction. A 1988 retrospective study found that older patients (aged 60 years or older) with severe carotid stenosis are at risk.[80] It is not known whether prophylactic carotid endarterectomy, staged or combined, will decrease the overall risk of stroke. Ideally, one should conduct a clinical trial in which all patients undergo noninvasive testing before cardiac surgery and randomly receive prophylactic carotid endarterectomy when severe unilateral or bilateral disease has been identified. The logistic problems of such a trial with an estimated initial patient pool of 20,000 to 30,000 are enormous (these large numbers are needed to recruit sufficient patients with severe stenosis and to demonstrate a significant reduction in postoperative stroke). Currently, no evidence supports prophylactic carotid repair in patients scheduled for cardiac surgery.

The management of symptomatic carotid stenosis, however, is another major controversy. Typically, 2% to 5% of all patients undergoing CABG have a history of stroke. Previous studies have indicated that the risk of postoperative stroke in symptomatic carotid stenosis is significantly higher. In a 1990 study of 126 patients with a history of stroke who underwent CABG, 13% had a new stroke or worsening of previous deficits.[83] Worsening of hemiparesis usually occurred in patients with recent strokes (within 3 months before open

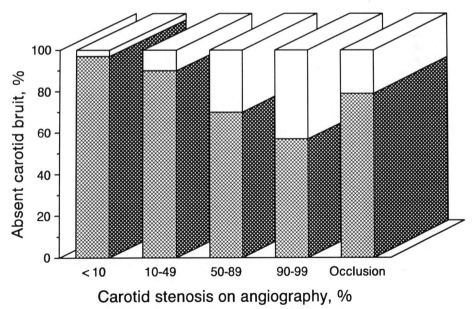

Figure 13–3. Relation of carotid bruit to severe carotid stenosis. Shaded areas, carotid bruit absent; unshaded areas, carotid bruit present. (Modified from Ingall, TJ, Homer, D, Whisnant, JP, et al: Predictive value of carotid bruit for carotid atherosclerosis. Arch Neurol 46:418–422, 1989.)

heart surgery). Symptoms persisted for 2 weeks in some patients but cleared within a few days in many others. It is unknown whether prophylactic carotid endarterectomy, proven to be effective in prevention of stroke in selected patients with severe symptomatic stenosis (70% to 99% in diameter on carotid angiograms),[34,69] decreases the incidence of stroke after cardiac surgery.

Postoperative strokes or transient ischemic attacks are not always evident on the first postoperative day. In a large series from Massachusetts General Hospital, ischemic stroke developed in less than half the patients on the first postoperative day. The remaining patients had manifestations up to 12 days after cardiac surgery. Postoperative atrial fibrillation has been significantly associated with late-onset stroke. At the Mayo Clinic, 21 of 25 patients with CABG associated with stroke had signs of new onset at least 2 days after surgery.[109]

In conclusion, it seems reasonable to consider carotid endarterectomy in symptomatic patients with severe carotid stenosis who are eligible for cardiac surgery. However, aside from increased risk of postoperative stroke, there is a considerable risk for postoperative cardiac failure and life-threatening myocardial infarction after carotid surgery in patients with still uncorrected triple coronary artery disease. Fatal myocardial infarction or cardiac death after carotid endarterectomy was about 1% in recent large series of carotid endarterectomy, but patients with severe cardiac disease were generally excluded.[34,50,69] Therefore, it seems safer to proceed with carotid endarterectomy after coronary reconstruction, but other cardiovascular surgeons disagree and favor combined repair.[19,30,31,46]

There is a widely held dictum that cardiac surgery after a recent stroke may significantly exacerbate the neurologic deficit. The problem of management in this subset of patients has been addressed in only a few studies. One review found no marked differences in patients with remote or recent strokes (defined as 3 months before the day of open heart surgery).[83] Zisbrod and associates[111] operated on 15 patients with recent strokes (within 2 to 28 days), and no patient's condition deteriorated after the procedure. Most patients recovered partially or completely despite the attendant risk of hemorrhagic transformation during anticoagulation. In a 1993 study of 41 patients with coronary artery bypass and previous stroke, new focal signs from ischemic stroke developed in only one patient,[11] a result suggesting that heparinization during bypass is not harmful in this subset of patients.

Large territory cerebral infarcts, particularly those in patients with early hypodensity on computed tomography (CT) scan, may transform into hemorrhagic infarcts, but often without any clinical worsening.[22] CT scanning in 36 patients in whom hemorrhagic infarction developed found that early hypodensity on CT involved the lentiform nucleus and cortex but not the lentiform nucleus alone.[14] The true incidence of hemorrhagic transformation is not known but may reach 25% in patients with large territory infarcts and may still be seen up to 20 days after the ictus.[58] Heparinization during cardiopulmonary bypass surgery may predispose the patient to hemorrhagic infarction and, more importantly, result in a massive hematoma in the infarcted area. Other surgeons have not found this to be true, finding instead that hemorrhagic infarction resolved in patients who received heparin or warfarin or both.[75] The risk of recurrent cardioembolic stroke is estimated to be up to 20% within the first 3 weeks.[57] Therefore, it has been proposed that reducing anticoagulation or holding the dosage for 1 to 2 days may be a better approach than complete discontinuation if a cerebral infarct becomes hemorrhagic.[75] Uniform management guidelines are difficult to give in patients with a recent ischemic stroke, but it seems prudent to defer cardiac surgery, if feasible, for 6 to 8 weeks.

Clinicoanatomic Correlations of Cardiogenic Brain Infarctions

When sudden focal signs occur in a patient after cardiac surgery, there is good reason to believe that a cardiac embolus is the cause. However, many patients undergoing cardiac surgery or invasive diagnostic procedures have severe atheromatous extracranial vascular lesions from which embolic material also may arise.

Cardiogenic embolus can be predicted from its clinical presentation. On the basis of a synthesis of the literature, the Cerebral Embolism Task Force recently provided guidelines for diagnosing cardiogenic embolus.[23,24] These guidelines (Table 13–4) must be interpreted with caution but may prove useful in differentiating cardiogenic stroke from other causes of ischemic brain injury.

Typically, the clinical course in a patient with a cardiogenic brain embolus is marked by a maximal sudden and unheralded neurologic deficit. The level of consciousness is often diminished at onset. This clinical sign is generally related not to horizontal displacement by edematous infarcted tissue but more likely to bilateral hemispheric dysfunction associated with either arrhythmia-induced hypotension or, as suggested by others, multiple emboli. A gradually progressive or stuttering clinical course

over hours or days is very unusual but may occur in patients with ischemic strokes in the posterior cerebral artery. Aldrich and associates[2] found gradual visual deterioration in 6 of 25 patients with cortical blindness after cardiac surgery.

A 1990 review of stroke data bank information on a large series of patients with a cardiac source of embolus suggested three significant discriminating features for cardiac embolic stroke: (1) recent systemic embolism, (2) abrupt onset, defined as a neurologic deficit occurring during the first 10 minutes and no subsequent deterioration for the first 24 hours, and (3) decreased level of consciousness.[56]

Why ischemic strokes occur several days after the procedure remains obscure. Postoperative atrial fibrillation after CABG has been significantly associated with ischemic stroke. Unfortunately, however, a 1990 prospective study in 418 consecutive patients admitted for elective CABG failed to identify predictive factors for atrial fibrillation after CABG.[32] Therefore, therapeutic measures cannot be tailored to individual patients and preventive measures are questionable.

The second potential source of cardiac embolus is left ventricular thrombi in patients undergoing open heart surgery. A restrospective study from the Cleveland Clinic found that the incidence of stroke was approximately 10% in patients with intraluminal defects on left ventriculography but only 2% in patients without left ventricular thrombi.[17] The chance of ventricular thrombi is comparatively small. Therefore, these data do not resolve the cause in the vast majority of patients with postoperative stroke.

As alluded to previously, atherosclerosis of the ascending aorta[38] may be an equally important source for CABG-associated stroke. The incidence of moderate-to-severe atherosclerosis of the aorta (defined as circumferential involvement of most of the ascending aorta and protruding atheroma) was 20% in an unselected series of cardiac

Table 13–4 CLINICAL FEATURES SUGGESTIVE OF CARDIOGENIC BRAIN EMBOLISM

Abrupt onset of maximal deficit
Decreased level of consciousness at onset
Recent history of systemic emboli
Additional evidence
  No atherosclerotic vascular disease
  Evidence of cardiac thrombi
    (echocardiography, CT, or MRI)
  Hemorrhagic infarct or multiple brain
    infarcts in multiple vascular territories

Data from Cerebral Embolism Study Group,[22] Cerebral Embolism Task Force,[23,24] and Kittner, et al.[56]

CT = computed tomography; MRI = magnetic resonance imaging.

surgical patients.[107] This finding prompted one group to replace this aortic segment, and there were no postoperative ischemic complications in a preliminary series of 27 patients.[107]

Although hemodynamic changes are frequently encountered during the operation or in the immediate postoperative course, true cerebral infarctions associated with hypotension are rare after cardiac surgery. Border zone infarcts between major vascular territories occur in a minority of the patients only, and territorial types of infarction in single territories are far more frequent.

In summary, several mechanisms may be involved in early postoperative stroke, and manipulation during surgery and sudden marked hypotensive episodes are the most likely ones. In delayed ischemic stroke, the type of stroke suggests embolization of retained emboli in the heart, probably associated with cardiopulmonary bypass surgery.

Computed Tomography Scan Patterns

The limited data available do not identify CT patterns that are highly specific for cardiogenic embolization,[49,81] although infarction in the posterior cerebral artery territory has commonly been associated with emboli from cardiac sources, particularly cardiac surgery. Localization of the occipital infarct in the calcaneal area suggests posterior branch occlusion or a watershed infarction, but most patients have large unilateral or bilateral parietal occipital infarcts on CT scan.

Visual field defects are usually the only neurologic abnormality. Occasionally, patients awake after cardiac surgery with blindness.[2] Denial of blindness is uncommon, but denial often is accompanied with confabulations. Some patients have partial seizures resulting in hallucinations of flashing red lights or vivid, detailed images of persons.[76] Macular sparing is common in patients with large infarcts involving the upper and lower calcarine cortex or optic radiations. Prognosis in patients with cortical blindness is poor.

Watershed cerebral infarcts occur in the border zones between two large cerebral artery territories and have traditionally been linked to a hemodynamic compromise during cardiac surgery. CT scan documentation of bilateral or unilateral infarcts is rare. The exact mechanism is not clearly understood, and some investigators have taken an opposing view in explaining bilateral border zone infarction by showers of microemboli.[101]

An interesting phenomenon is the occurrence of unilateral watershed cerebral infarcts. Recent positron emission tomography studies found no evidence for selective border zone impairment in patients with severe (more than 75%) stenosis of the carotid artery,[21] although others found that unilateral watershed infarcts were associated with severe carotid stenosis.[13]

Multiple emboli may also occur and have traditionally been linked to a cardiogenic source.[81] Recently, infarcts in the superior cerebellar artery territory have been specifically linked to a cardiogenic source.[3] To address some of the gaps in knowledge, we recently reviewed 25 ischemic strokes occurring after coronary bypass surgery. As expected, most ischemic infarcts were located in the middle cerebral artery territory. Purely watershed infarcts were not found[109] (Table 13–5). Not awakening was most often associated with multiple territory strokes. Late strokes (more than 2 days), however, occurred mostly in single territories.[104]

NEUROPSYCHOLOGICAL ABNORMALITIES

When extensive testing is done, neuropsychological impairment after CABG operation may be found in 30% of patients.[1,10,92–94] Intellectual deterioration may vary from overt memory deficits to difficulties in attention and concentration in more demanding tasks. In

Table 13–5 COMPUTED TOMOGRAPHY SCAN FINDINGS IN 25 PATIENTS WITH ISCHEMIC STROKE ASSOCIATED WITH CORONARY ARTERY BYPASS GRAFTING

Type of Ischemic Stroke	Patients (n)
SINGLE TERRITORY	
MCA Anterior division	3
Posterior division	0
Subcortical	4
Complete	5
PCA Thalamus	2
Occipital	2
ACA Frontal (distal branch)	4
MULTIPLE TERRITORIES	
Bilateral MCA and PCA occlusion	1
Multiple subcortical infarcts	4

Data from Wijdicks and Jack.[109]
ACA = anterior cerebral artery; MCA = middle cerebral artery; PCA = posterior cerebral artery.

most series, patients have decreased attention span, decreased motor speed, and problems with immediate retrieval of memory. Savageau and associates[84,85] found no definite risk factors for neuropsychological involvement, but patients older than 60 years with enlarged heart, long aortic cross-clamp time, or extensive postoperative blood loss appeared to be significantly more at risk. A follow-up study 6 months later found that in more than 80% of the patients with abnormal performance, these abnormalities subsided. A long-term outcome study[94] found marked improvement in the first year and gradual further improvement up to 5 years in all neuropsychological dimensions. Fatigue and depression may strongly influence test results, but psychological abnormalities were consistently absent in a control group of patients undergoing major vascular surgical procedures without the concomitant use of cardiopulmonary bypass. Therefore, the procedure of cardiopulmonary bypass itself has a transient and, less likely, permanent deleterious effect on cognition. Whether warm blood cardioplegia increases the risk of neuropsychological abnormalities is not known. A subgroup analysis of 150 patients of the study at Emory University found no differences between warm and cold blood cardioplegia.[64]

NEURO-OPHTHALMOLOGIC COMPLICATIONS

The proportion of patients with neuro-ophthalmologic sequelae after cardiopulmonary bypass may be as high as 25%[88,91] (Table 13–6). In a prospective study in which bedside neurologic assessment was done in patients who underwent CABG surgery, areas of retinal infarction were most frequently found.[91]

Cotton-wool spots, produced by occlusion of small vessels supplying the inner nerve layer of the retina, occurred in 54 of 312 (17%) patients. Only half the patients, including those with multiple lesions, were aware of visual symptoms, most likely because of the spottiness of these tiny foci. Usually, retinal infarcts are manifested by blurred vision, haziness in the peripheral parts of the visual field, or difficulty reading, and a lodged embolus may be seen by direct ophthalmoscopy. This ocular complication, found specifically in patients after nonpulsatile cardiopulmonary bypass, may have several possible explanations. Both platelet-fibrin microaggregates and gaseous microbubbles could produce this retinal damage, but theoretically this phenomenon may also be the result of a regional maldistribution of perfusion. An elegant study in patients undergoing elective

Table 13–6 NEURO-OPHTHALMOLOGIC FINDINGS AFTER CARDIOPULMONARY BYPASS

Retinal cotton-wool spots
Ischemic optic neuropathy
Transient macular edema
Cortical blindness
Homonymous hemianopia
Altitudinal hemianopia
Isolated quadrantanopia

coronary operation with bubble oxygenators found retinal abnormalities in all patients serially studied with retinal fluorescein angiography.[12] New cotton-wool spots, however, were noted in only 10% of the patients. The clinical significance is uncertain. Most patients did not experience visual loss, and neuropsychological and neurologic complications were similar in patients with massive occlusions. This condition is considered to be benign, with few, if any, persistent residual deficits. Return to normal usually takes at least a few weeks.

Visual field defects are less common but may be substantial and often are permanent.[97] Partial or complete occipital infarction is often recognized, but quadrantanopia that reflects infarction in more distal parts of the radiation optica may go unnoticed by the patient and physician.

Unilateral altitudinal field defect is an uncommon visual field deficit.[43] In the Cleveland Clinic experience,[96] 7 of 7685 patients were found to have bilateral involvement. In each patient, a swollen and pale optic nerve disc could be demonstrated. This ischemic optic neuropathy was caused by infarction in the laminar anterior portion of the optic nerve. Most of the patients had considerable blood loss from hemorrhage and shock.[99]

PERIPHERAL NERVE DAMAGE

Most cardiovascular surgeons are primarily concerned with the potential deleterious effects on the central nervous system, but damage to peripheral nerves is equally important.[51,54,59,68] Many of the mononeuropathies can be explained by malpositioning during surgery.

The incidence of brachial plexus injury is less than 10% in major series (Table 13–7). Its cause is not clearly understood. Usually, the lower trunk or medial cord fibers are involved. Burning pain and numbness are present in the C-8 and T-1 to T-2 segments, and many patients have profound weakness of the intrinsic hand muscles and long finger flexors. The myotatic reflexes are usually normal, but finger flexion and triceps jerks may be reduced. Horner's syndrome may accompany this type of lesion, but it has also been reported as an isolated finding. Approximately half of the patients with postsurgical plexopathy have disabling dysesthesias and pain or marked weakness at onset.[103] Outcome is generally good, and the neurologic deficits resolve within 3 to 4 months. Only a few patients have persistent weakness.

The mechanism of brachial plexus injury has been actively studied and is thought to be related to the position of the sternal retractors and the extent to which the halves are opened. An autopsy study postulated that when the retractor is opened to its fullest extent (which may occur in patients with grafting of an internal mammary artery), the lower trunk of the brachial plexus is pinched between the first rib and the clavicle[55] (Fig. 13–4). Vander Salm and associates[105] suggested that fractures of the first rib related to placement of the

Table 13–7 INCIDENCE OF UNILATERAL BRACHIAL PLEXUS INJURY AFTER CARDIAC SURGERY

Series (y)	Patients (n)	Brachial Plexus Injury, n (%)
Vander, Salm et al., 1980[105]	188	35 (19)
Morin, et al., 1982[68]	958	10 (1)
Hanson, et al., 1983[42]	531	25 (5)
Shaw, et al., 1985[89]	312	21 (7)
Tomlinson, et al., 1987[100]	335	16 (5)
Vahl, et al., 1991[103]	1000	27 (3)

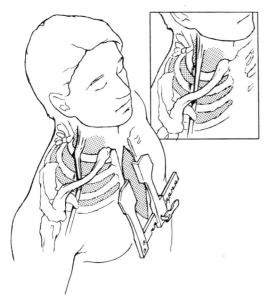

Figure 13–4. Possible mechanism of brachial plexus injury after use of retractors during cardiac surgery (inset shows normal anatomy).

cephalad blade of the retractor at the level of the second intercostal space may contribute to nerve damage. No fractures were seen after a more caudal placement of the retractor. Rib fractures may not be evident on conventional chest roentgenograms but may be visualized by bone scans.[7] In some patients with persisting complaints, transaxillary resection of the first rib may result in resolution of the nerve injury. Intraoperative somatosensory evoked potential may predict brachial plexopathy, but as mentioned previously, recovery can be expected in most patients in the first postoperative week. The magnitude of sternal separation in a small study was not related to changes in somatosensory evoked potential.[48] Traction on the brachial plexus, however, remains the most likely mechanism and is preventable. In a prospective study using asymmetrical traction with Favaloro retractors for harvesting of the internal mammary artery as a graft for CABG, the incidence of brachial plexopathy increased to 10%.[103]

Mononeuropathy may be more frequent than previously appreciated. In a prospective study, mononeuropathies were found in 17 of 312 patients (5%) who underwent elective coronary artery bypass.[108] Ulnar and lateral femoral cutaneous nerves were most frequently affected, and all instances might have been preventable. Ulnar nerve palsy is common after cardiac surgery, and compression at the cubital tunnel can be remarkably diminished, as shown in nerve conduction studies, by placing the patient's arms above the head with the elbows flexed.[108] A 1991 report suggested that meralgia paresthetica was not associated with vein harvesting but rather was caused by placing the thighs in the frog leg position during this procedure.[74]

Saphenous neuropathy, vocal cord paralysis, and peroneal neuropathy have also been repeatedly reported to occur after cardiac surgery but may not be specific for this type of procedure. Direct injury is probably the most plausible explanation, but hypothermia and ischemic damage to peripheral nerves caused by inadequate perfusion of the vasa nervorum may also be significant risk factors. A preventable wrist-drop from radial nerve damage was reported in two obese patients.[41,79] The supporting post of the retractor presumably compressed the upper arm in both patients. Outcome was good.

Another important hazard of hypothermia during open heart surgery is bilateral diaphragmatic paralysis. In a 1993 prospective study that used phrenic nerve conduction, ultrasonography of the diaphragm, and chest radiographs, 24 of 92 patients (26%) had phrenic neuropathy but none required prolonged mechanical ventilation and most had resolution within 1 year.[33] In another study, the incidence of this complication was only 2%.[26,33,63,65] Electrophysiologic evaluation of the function of the phrenic nerve and diaphragm showed that no marked changes in nerve conduction occurred during surgery. The lowest myocardial temperature recorded in patients with phrenic nerve palsy was similar to that in the other patients, but the duration of cardiopulmonary bypass was significantly longer. These findings suggested that prolonged pericardial stretch during the operation was the main cause.

Local hypothermia may also be a contributing factor, because filling of the pericardial sac with ice and saline to protect the myocardium during periods of ischemic arrest was strongly linked to bilateral diaphragmatic paralysis and compromised recovery in many patients.

CONCLUSIONS

For many patients, CABG is a surgical procedure without frequent neurologic complications, but many patients (estimated in prospective series to be up to 50%) have a worse functional status after the operation than before. Rather than substantial intellectual deterioration, problems with executive functions, such as decision-making, are common and almost certainly pass unnoticed in the postoperative days. Fortunately, despite contradictory reports, these abnormalities subside in 6 months in the vast majority of patients. (These observations may need reevaluation as data from normothermic bypass procedures become available.)

Coexisting carotid disease is often found in patients scheduled for CABG surgery. The risk of stroke is increased in patients with carotid bruit. The lack of a prospective randomized study of prophylactic carotid endarterectomy hampers our ability to give sound scientific advice. The incidence of stroke after CABG surgery is very low (probably less than 1%), and occurrence commonly is days after surgery. A recent clinical and neuroradiologic study found evidence of an embolic mechanism (single-territory and mostly in the middle cerebral artery territory) rather than a flow-related mechanism, which would result in watershed-type cerebral infarcts. In contrast, the risk of perioperative stroke after carotid endarterectomy is 3% to 5%, and a patient with uncorrected triple coronary artery disease has a 1% risk of fatal myocardial infarc-

tion, not a very favorable net clinical benefit.

In patients with proven carotid disease who have symptoms, it seems reasonable to proceed with carotid endarterectomy, most likely after coronary reconstruction. If a stroke occurs after CABG in a patient with an asymptomatic carotid stenosis, one should still be reluctant to attribute this to carotid disease. Much more commonly, thrombi retained in the heart or thrombi from damage to the aorta associated with clamping or postoperative atrial fibrillation are the main culprits.

Brachial plexopathy from use of sternal retractors is occasionally observed in the intensive care unit. Recovery to full function can be expected after conservative management.

REFERENCES

1. Åberg, T, Ronquist, G, Tydén, H, et al: Adverse effects on the brain in cardiac operations as assessed by biochemical, psychometric, and radiologic methods. J Thorac Cardiovasc Surg 87:99–105, 1984.
2. Aldrich, MS, Alessi, AG, Beck, RW, and Gilman, S: Cortical blindness: Etiology, diagnosis, and prognosis. Ann Neurol 21:149–158, 1987.
3. Amarenco, P, Roullet, E, Goujon, C, et al: Infarction in the anterior rostral cerebellum (the territory of the lateral branch of the superior cerebellar artery). Neurology 41:253–258, 1991.
4. Arén, C, Badr, G, Feddersen, K, and Rådegran, K: Somatosensory evoked potentials and cerebral metabolism during cardiopulmonary bypass with special reference to hypotension induced by prostacyclin infusion. J Thorac Cardiovasc Surg 90:73–79, 1985.
5. Aris, A, Solanes, H, Cámara, ML, et al: Arterial line filtration during cardiopulmonary bypass: Neurologic, neuropsychologic, and hematologic studies. J Thorac Cardiovasc Surg 91:526–533, 1986.
6. Arom, KV, Cohen, DE, and Strobl, FT:

Effect of intraoperative intervention on neurological outcome based on electroencephalographic monitoring during cardiopulmonary bypass. Ann Thorac Surg 48:476–483, 1989.

7. Baisden, CE, Greenwald, LV, and Symbas, PN: Occult rib fractures and brachial plexus injury following median sternotomy for open-heart operations. Ann Thorac Surg 38:192–194, 1984.

8. Balderman, SC, Gutierrez, IZ, Makula, P, et al: Noninvasive screening for asymptomatic carotid artery disease prior to cardiac operation. J Thorac Cardiovasc Surg 85:427–433, 1983.

9. Barnes, RW, Liebman, PR, Marszalek, PB, et al: The natural history of asymptomatic carotid disease in patients undergoing cardiovascular surgery. Surgery 90:1075–1083, 1981.

10. Barnes, RW and Marszalek, PB: Asymptomatic carotid disease in the cardiovascular surgical patient. Is prophylactic endarterectomy necessary? Stroke 12:497–500, 1981.

11. Beall, AC Jr, Jones, JW, Guinn, GA, et al: Cardiopulmonary bypass in patients with previously completed stroke. Ann Thorac Surg 55:1383–1385, 1993.

12. Blauth, CI, Arnold, JV, Schulenberg, WE, et al: Cerebral microembolism during cardiopulmonary bypass: Retinal microvascular studies in vivo with fluorescein angiography. J Thorac Cardiovasc Surg 95:668–676, 1988.

13. Bogousslavsky, J and Regli, F: Unilateral watershed cerebral infarcts. Neurology 36:373–377, 1986.

14. Bozzao, L, Angeloni, U, Bastianello, S, et al: Early angiographic and CT findings in patients with hemorrhagic infarction in the distribution of the middle cerebral artery. AJNR Am J Neuroradiol 12:1115–1121, 1991.

15. Brener, BJ, Brief, DK, Alpert, J, et al: The risk of stroke in patients with asymptomatic carotid stenosis undergoing cardiac surgery: A follow-up study. J Vasc Surg 5:269–279, 1987.

16. Breslau, PJ, Fell, G, Ivey, TD, et al: Carotid arterial disease in patients undergoing coronary artery bypass operations. J Thorac Cardiovasc Surg 82:765–767, 1981.

17. Breuer, AC, Franco, I, Marzewski, D, and Soto-Velasco, J: Left ventricular thrombi seen by ventriculography are a significant risk factor for stroke in open-heart surgery (abstract). Ann Neurol 10:103–104, 1981.

18. Breuer, AC, Furlan, AJ, Hanson, MR, et al: Central nervous system complications of coronary artery bypass graft surgery: Prospective analysis of 421 patients. Stroke 14:682–687, 1983.

19. Cambria, RP, Ivarsson, BL, Akins, CW, et al: Simultaneous carotid and coronary disease: Safety of the combined approach. J Vasc Surg 9:56–64, 1989.

20. Caplan, LR: Brain embolism, revisited. Neurology 43:1281–1287, 1993.

21. Carpenter, DA, Grubb, RL Jr, and Powers, WJ: Borderzone hemodynamics in cerebrovascular disease. Neurology 40:1587–1592, 1990.

22. Cerebral Embolism Study Group: Cardioembolic stroke, early anticoagulation, and brain hemorrhage. Arch Intern Med 147:636–640, 1987.

23. Cerebral Embolism Task Force: Cardiogenic brain embolism. Arch Neurol 43:71–84, 1986.

24. Cerebral Embolism Task Force: Cardiogenic brain embolism: The second report of the Cerebral Embolism Task Force. Arch Neurol 46:727–743, 1989.

25. Chambers, BR and Norris, JW: Outcome in patients with asymptomatic neck bruits. N Engl J Med 315:860–865, 1986.

26. Chandler, KW, Rozas, CJ, Kory, RC, and Goldman, AL: Bilateral diaphragmatic paralysis complicating local cardiac hypothermia during open heart surgery. Am J Med 77:243–249, 1984.

27. Christakis, GT, Koch, JP, Deemar, KA, et al: A randomized study of the systemic effects of warm heart surgery. Ann Thorac Surg 54:449–459, 1992.

28. Coffey, CE, Massey, EW, Roberts, KB, et al: Natural history of cerebral complications of coronary artery bypass

graft surgery. Neurology 33:1416–1421, 1983.

29. Coles, JG, Taylor, MJ, Pearce, JM, et al: Cerebral monitoring of somatosensory evoked potentials during profoundly hypothermic circulatory arrest. Circulation 70 Suppl 1:I-96–I-102, 1984.

30. Cosgrove, DM, Hertzer, NR, and Loop, FD: Surgical management of synchronous carotid and coronary artery disease. J Vasc Surg 3:690–692, 1986.

31. Crawford, ES, Palamara, AE, and Kasparian, AS: Carotid and noncoronary operations: Simultaneous, staged, and delayed. Surgery 87:1–7, 1980.

32. Crosby, LH, Pifalo, WB, Woll, KR, and Burkholder, JA: Risk factors for atrial fibrillation after coronary artery bypass grafting. Am J Cardiol 66:1520–1522, 1990.

33. DeVita, MA, Robinson, LR, Rehder, J, et al: Incidence and natural history of phrenic neuropathy occurring during open heart surgery. Chest 103:850–856, 1993.

34. European Carotid Surgery Trialists' Collaborative Group: MRC European Carotid Surgery Trial: Interim results for symptomatic patients with severe (70–99%) or with mild (0–29%) carotid stenosis. Lancet 337:1235–1243, 1991.

35. Faggioli, GL, Curl, GR, and Ricotta, JJ: The role of carotid screening before coronary artery bypass. J Vasc Surg 12:724–731, 1990.

36. Furlan, AJ and Breuer, AC: Central nervous system complications of open heart surgery. Stroke 15:912–915, 1984.

37. Furlan, AJ and Craciun, AR: Risk of stroke during coronary artery bypass graft surgery in patients with internal carotid artery disease documented by angiography. Stroke 16:797–799, 1985.

38. Gardner, TJ, Horneffer, PJ, Manolio, TA, et al: Stroke following coronary artery bypass grafting: A ten-year study. Ann Thorac Surg 40:574–581, 1985.

39. Gilman, S: Cerebral disorders after open-heart operations. N Engl J Med 272:489–498, 1965.

40. Gonzáles-Scarano, F and Hurtig, HI: Neurologic complications of coronary artery bypass grafting: Case-control study. Neurology 31:1032–1035, 1981.

41. Guzman, F, Naik, S, Weldon, OGW, and Hilton, CJ: Transient radial nerve injury related to the use of a self retaining retractor for internal mammary artery dissection. J Cardiovasc Surg 30:1015–1016, 1989.

42. Hanson, MR, Breuer, AC, Furlan, AJ, et al: Mechanism and frequency of brachial plexus injury in open-heart surgery: A prospective analysis. Ann Thorac Surg 36:675–679, 1983.

43. Hayreh, SS: Anterior ischemic optic neuropathy. VIII. Clinical features and pathogenesis of post-hemorrhagic amaurosis. Ophthalmology 94:1488–1502, 1987.

44. Hennerici, M, Hülsbömer, H-B, Hefter, H, et al: Natural history of asymptomatic extracranial arterial disease: Results of a long-term prospective study. Brain 110:777–791, 1987.

45. Henriksen, L and Hjelms, E: Cerebral blood flow during cardiopulmonary bypass in man: Effect of arterial filtration. Thorax 41:386–395, 1986.

46. Hertzer, NR, Loop, FD, Taylor, PC, and Beven, EG: Combined myocardial revascularization and carotid endarterectomy: Operative and late results in 331 patients. J Thorac Cardiovasc Surg 85:577–589, 1983.

47. Hertzer, NR, Young, JR, Beven, EG, et al: Coronary angiography in 506 patients with extracranial cerebrovascular disease. Arch Intern Med 145:849–852, 1985.

48. Hickey, C, Gugino, LD, Aglio, LS, et al: Intraoperative somatosensory evoked potential monitoring predicts peripheral nerve injury during cardiac surgery. Anesthesiology 78:29–35, 1993.

49. Hise, JH, Nipper, ML, and Schnitker, JC: Stroke associated with coronary artery bypass surgery. AJNR Am J Neuroradiol 12:811–814, 1991.

50. Hobson, RW II, Weiss, DG, Fields, WS, et al: Efficacy of carotid endarterec-

tomy for asymptomatic carotid stenosis. N Engl J Med 328:221–227, 1993.

51. Honet, JC, Raikes, JA, Kantrowitz, A, et al: Neuropathy in the upper extremity after open-heart surgery. Arch Phys Med Rehabil 57:264–267, 1976.

52. Ivey, TD, Strandness, DE, Williams, DB, et al: Management of patients with carotid bruit undergoing cardiopulmonary bypass. J Thorac Cardiovasc Surg 87:183–189, 1984.

53. Jones, EL, Weintraub, WS, Craver, JM, et al: Coronary bypass surgery: Is the operation different today? J Thorac Cardiovasc Surg 101:108–115, 1991.

54. Keates, JRW, Innocenti, DM, and Ross, DN: Mononeuritis multiplex: A complication of open-heart surgery. J Thorac Cardiovasc Surg 69:816–819, 1975.

55. Kirsh, MM, Magee, KR, Gago, O, et al: Brachial plexus injury following median sternotomy incision. Ann Thorac Surg 11:315–319, 1971.

56. Kittner, SJ, Sharkness, CM, Price, TR, et al: Infarcts with a cardiac source of embolism in the NINCDS Stroke Data Bank: Historical features. Neurology 40:281–284, 1990.

57. Koller, RL: Recurrent embolic cerebral infarction and anticoagulation. Neurology 32:283–285, 1982.

58. Laureno, R, Shields, RW Jr, and Narayan, T: The diagnosis and management of cerebral embolism and hemorrhagic infarction with sequential computerized cranial tomography. Brain 110:93–105, 1987.

59. Lederman, RJ, Breuer, AC, Hanson, MR, et al: Peripheral nervous system complications of coronary artery bypass graft surgery. Ann Neurol 12:297–301, 1982.

60. Lundar, T, Frøysaker, T, Lindegaard, K-F, et al: Some observations on cerebral perfusion during cardiopulmonary bypass. Ann Thorac Surg 39:318–323, 1985.

61. Lundar, T, Lindegaard, K-F, Frøysaker, T, et al: Cerebral perfusion during nonpulsatile cardiopulmonary bypass. Ann Thorac Surg 40:144–150, 1985.

62. Lundar, T, Lindegaard, K-F, Frøysaker, T, et al: Cerebral carbon dioxide reactivity during nonpulsatile cardiopulmonary bypass. Ann Thorac Surg 41:525–530, 1986.

63. Markand, ON, Moorthy, SS, Mahomed, Y, et al: Postoperative phrenic nerve palsy in patients with open-heart surgery. Ann Thorac Surg 39:68–73, 1985.

64. Martin, TD, Craver, JM, Gott, JP, et al: Prospective, randomized trial of retrograde warm blood cardioplegia: Myocardial benefit and neurologic threat. Ann Thorac Surg 57:298–304, 1994.

65. Mickell, JJ, Oh, KS, Siewers, RD, et al: Clinical implications of postoperative unilateral phrenic nerve paralysis. J Thorac Cardiovasc Surg 76:297–304, 1978.

66. Mills, NL and Ochsner, JL: Massive air embolism during cardiopulmonary bypass: Causes, prevention, and management. J Thorac Cardiovasc Surg 80:708–717, 1980.

67. Moody, DM, Bell, MA, Challa, VR, et al: Brain microemboli during cardiac surgery or aortography. Ann Neurol 28:477–486, 1990,

68. Morin, JE, Long, R, Elleker, MG, et al: Upper extremity neuropathies following median sternotomy. Ann Thorac Surg 34:181–185, 1982.

69. North American Symptomatic Carotid Endarterectomy Trial Collaborators: Beneficial effect of carotid endarterectomy in symptomatic patients with high-grade carotid stenosis. N Engl J Med 325:445–453, 1991.

70. Nussmeier, NA, Arlund, C, and Slogoff, S: Neuropsychiatric complications after cardiopulmonary bypass: Cerebral protection by a barbiturate. Anesthesiology 64:165–170, 1986.

71. Padayachee, TS, Parsons, S, Theobold, R, et al: The effect of arterial filtration on reduction of gaseous microemboli in the middle cerebral artery during cardiopulmonary bypass. Ann Thorac Surg 45:647–649, 1988.

72. Padayachee, TS, Parsons, S, Theobold, R, et al: The detection of microemboli in the middle cerebral artery during cardiopulmonary bypass: A

transcranial Doppler ultrasound investigation using membrane and bubble oxygenators. Ann Thorac Surg 44:298–302, 1987.

73. Parker, FB Jr, Marvasti, MA, and Bove, EL: Neurologic complications following coronary artery bypass: The role of atherosclerotic emboli. Thorac Cardiovasc Surg 33:207–209, 1985.

74. Parsonnet, V, Karasakalides, A, Gielchinsky, I, et al: Meralgia paresthetica after coronary bypass surgery. J Thorac Cardiovasc Surg 101:219–221, 1991.

75. Pessin, MS, Estol, CJ, Lafranchise, F, and Caplan, LR: Safety of anticoagulation after hemorrhagic infarction. Neurology 43:1298–1303, 1993.

76. Pessin, MS, Lathi, ES, Cohen, MB, et al: Clinical features and mechanism of occipital infarction. Ann Neurol 21:290–299, 1987.

77. Prough, DS, Rogers, AT, Stump, DA, et al: Hypercarbia depresses cerebral oxygen consumption during cardiopulmonary bypass. Stroke 21:1162–1166, 1990.

78. Pugsley, W, Klinger, L, Paschalis, C, et al: Microemboli and cerebral impairment during cardiac surgery. Vasc Surg 24:34–43, 1990.

79. Rao, S, Chu, B, and Shevde, K: Isolated peripheral radial nerve injury with the use of the Favaloro retractor. J Cardiothorac Anesth 1:325–327, 1987.

80. Reed, GL III, Singer, DE, Picard, EH, and DeSanctis, RW: Stroke following coronary artery bypass surgery: A case-control estimate of the risk from carotid bruits. N Engl J Med 319:1246–1250, 1988.

81. Ringelstein, EB, Koschorke, S, Holling, A, et al: Computed tomographic patterns of proven embolic brain infarctions. Ann Neurol 26:759–765, 1989.

82. Ropper, AH, Wechsler, LR, and Wilson, LS: Carotid bruit and the risk of stroke in elective surgery. N Engl J Med 307:1388–1390, 1981.

83. Rorick, MB and Furlan, AJ: Risk of cardiac surgery in patients with prior stroke. Neurology 40:835–837, 1990.

84. Savageau, JA, Stanton, B-A, Jenkins, CD, and Frater, RWM: Neuropsychological dysfunction following elective cardiac operation. II. A six-month assessment. J Thorac Cardiovasc Surg 84:595–600, 1982.

85. Savageau, JA, Stanton, B-A, Jenkins, CD, and Klein, MD: Neuropsychological dysfunction following elective cardiac operation. I. Early assessment. J Thorac Cardiovasc Surg 84:585–594, 1982.

86. Schell, RM, Kern, FH, Greeley, WJ, et al: Cerebral blood flow and metabolism during cardiopulmonary bypass. Anesth Analg 76:849–865, 1993.

87. Schmidt, R, Fazekas, F, Offenbacher, H, et al: Brain magnetic resonance imaging in coronary artery bypass grafts: A pre- and postoperative assessment. Neurology 43:775–778, 1993.

88. Shahian, DM and Speert, PK: Symptomatic visual deficits after open heart operations. Ann Thorac Surg 48:275–279, 1989.

89. Shaw, P, Bates, D, Cartlidge, NEF, et al: Early neurological complications of coronary artery bypass surgery. BMJ 291:1384–1387, 1985.

90. Shaw, PJ, Bates, D, Cartlidge, NEF, et al: Neurologic and neuropsychological morbidity following major surgery: Comparison of coronary artery bypass and peripheral vascular surgery. Stroke 18:700–707, 1987.

91. Shaw, PJ, Bates, D, Cartlidge, NEF, et al: Neuro-ophthalmological complications of coronary artery bypass graft surgery. Acta Neurol Scand 76:1–7, 1987.

92. Smith, PLC, Treasure, T, Newman, SP, et al: Cerebral consequences of cardiopulmonary bypass. Lancet i:823–825, 1986.

93. Sotaniemi, KA: Brain damage and neurological outcome after open-heart surgery. J Neurol Neurosurg Psychiatry 43:127–135, 1980.

94. Sotaniemi, KA, Mononen, H, and Hokkanen, TE: Long-term cerebral outcome after open-heart surgery: A five-year neuropsychological follow-up study. Stroke 17:410–416, 1986.

95. Swain, JA, McDonald, TJ Jr, Balaban,

RS, and Robbins, RC: Metabolism of the heart and brain during hypothermic cardiopulmonary bypass. Ann Thorac Surg 51:105–109, 1991.

96. Sweeney, PJ, Breuer, AC, Selhorst, JB, et al: Ischemic optic neuropathy: A complication of cardiopulmonary bypass surgery. Neurology 32:560–562, 1982.

97. Taugher, PJ: Visual loss after cardiopulmonary bypass. Am J Ophthalmol 81:280–288, 1976.

98. Taylor, GJ, Malik, SA, Colliver, JA, et al: Usefulness of atrial fibrillation as a predictor of stroke after isolated coronary artery bypass grafting. Am J Cardiol 60:905–907, 1987.

99. Tice, DA: Ischemic optic neuropathy and cardiac surgery (letter). Ann Thorac Surg 44:677, 1987.

100. Tomlinson, DL, Hirsch, IA, Kodali, SV, and Slogoff, S: Protecting the brachial plexus during median sternotomy. J Thorac Cardiovasc Surg 94:297–301, 1987.

101. Torvik, A and Skullerud, K: Watershed infarcts in the brain caused by microemboli. Clin Neuropathol 1:99–105, 1982.

102. Turnipseed, WD, Berkoff, HA, and Belzer, FO: Postoperative stroke in cardiac and peripheral vascular disease. Ann Surg 192:365–367, 1980.

103. Vahl, CF, Carl, I, Müller-Vahl, H, and Struck, E: Brachial plexus injury after cardiac surgery: The role of internal mammary artery preparation: A prospective study of 1000 consecutive patients. J Thorac Cardiovasc Surg 102:724–729, 1991.

104. van der Linden, J and Casimir-Ahn, H: When do cerebral emboli appear during open heart operations? A transcranial Doppler study. Ann Thorac Surg 51:237–241, 1991.

105. Vander Salm, TJ, Cereda, J-M, and Cutler, BS: Brachial plexus injury following median sternotomy. J Thorac Cardiovasc Surg 80:447–452, 1980.

106. von Reutern, G-M, Hetzel, A, Birnbaum, D, and Schlosser, V: Transcranial Doppler ultrasonography during cardiopulmonary bypass in patients with severe carotid stenosis or occlusion. Stroke 19:674–680, 1988.

107. Wareing, TH, Davila-Roman, VG, Daily, BB, et al: Strategy for the reduction of stroke incidence in cardiac surgical patients. Ann Thorac Surg 55:1400–1408, 1993.

108. Wey, JM and Guinn, GA: Ulnar nerve injury with open-heart surgery. Ann Thorac Surg 39:358–360, 1985.

109. Wijdicks, EFM, and Jack, CJ: CABG associated stroke: Clinical and radiologic features (submitted).

110. Zaidan, JR, Klochany, A, Martin, WM, et al: Effect of thiopental on neurologic outcome following coronary artery bypass grafting. Anesthesiology 74:406–411, 1991.

111. Zisbrod, Z, Rose, DM, Jacobowitz, IJ, et al: Results of open heart surgery in patients with recent cardiogenic embolic stroke and central nervous system dysfunction. Circulation 76 Suppl 5:V-109–V-112, 1987.

Chapter 14

NEUROLOGIC COMPLICATIONS OF ENVIRONMENTAL INJURIES

THERMAL BURNS
SMOKE INHALATION
ELECTRICAL BURNS
ACCIDENTAL HYPOTHERMIA
HEAT STROKE
NEAR-DROWNING

In children and young adults, environmental injuries are a leading cause of death and disability. These accidental injuries have a propensity for pulmonary, cardiovascular, and renal involvement and pose formidable problems in management. Certain types of environmental injuries can produce specific neurologic manifestations, and there are situations in which morbidity is determined by a neurologic insult. This chapter presents a condensed overview of the most common neurologic syndromes in accidental injuries.

THERMAL BURNS

The medical complexity of patients with major burns and the need for multidisciplinary physicians fit well into the definition of critical illness.[17] Patients with extensive burns often are managed in specialized burn centers, but major institutions are occasionally challenged with the intensive care management of thermal or electrical burns. One may expect neurologic complica-

tions of major thermal burns in a number of patients, but their recognition may be overshadowed by metabolic and infectious problems. Neurologic complications are frequently appreciated only after the patient's critical condition has subsided.

The morbidity and mortality in patients with major burns depend on the extent of third- or second-degree burn surface. The extent of the burn can be assessed by the rule of nine in adults. When the extent of injury approximates 50% of the total skin surface area, significant sequelae or early mortality can be expected (Fig. 14–1).

The neurologic presentation of patients with extensive burns is often associated with systemic factors, none of which is specific for burns (Table 14–1). Severe burns result in hypovolemic shock from fluid loss in the burn surface, and direct myocardial depression may result in decreased cardiac output. Both factors may cause a robust reduction in cerebral tissue perfusion and readily predispose to anoxic ischemic encephalopathy (see Chapter 6).

In other burn patients, a hypermetabolic response with tripled energy needs is seen. This hypermetabolic phase is characterized by fever, massive weight loss, and protein catabolism similar to sepsis syndrome (see Chapter 5). Nutrition, therefore, should be adequate and meet the demands, but many nutrition

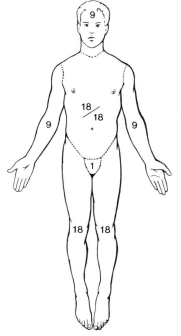

Data Obtained from Specialized Burn Facilities for Mean Survival Rate (%) Comparing Age and Burn Size

Burn size (%)	Age (yr)				
	5-34	35-49	50-59	60-74	> 75
0-10	> 95	> 95	> 95	95	90
10-20	> 95	> 90	> 85	80	50
20-30	95	90	75	50	25
30-40	90	80	60	30	< 10
40-50	80	60	40	10	< 5
50-60	60	45	30	< 10	< 5
60-70	40	20	15	< 5	0
70-80	25	10	5	0	0
80-90	10	< 10	< 5	0	0
90-100	< 5	< 5	0	0	0

Figure 14–1. Extent of burns assessed by the rule of nine and correlation with survival rate. The drawing shows the rule of nine and distribution over the body surface. The table can be used to assess survival rate when the percentage of burned skin surface has been calculated.

schedules include adequate vitamin supplements. Very occasionally, zinc deficiency may result in a decreased level of consciousness and in irritability.

Another life-threatening condition is wound infection resulting in sepsis, multiorgan failure, or endocarditis. *Staphylococcus aureus*, *Klebsiella pneumoniae*, and *Pseudomonas aeruginosa* infections may develop in burn

Table 14–1 NEUROLOGIC COMPLICATIONS OF BURN INJURY

Trigger	Manifestation
Hypovolemia, sepsis, shock	Anoxic-ischemic encephalopathy
Bacterial endocarditis, cardiac arrhythmias*	Embolic stroke
Hyponatremia, hyperosmolarity	Central pontine myelinolysis
Hypocalcemia	Seizures

*Electrical burns.

patients and may result in septic emboli to the brain. *Candida* infections have recently been recognized as well. Recently, central pontine myelinolysis has been reported in burns following correction of hyponatremia (see Chapter 7).[12,84] Failure to awaken was a common first presentation; in some reported patients, narcotic overdose was deemed likely until magnetic resonance imaging abnormalities and bulbar palsy appeared.

Perhaps one of the most important pathophysiologic changes in patients with major burns is the alteration of pharmacokinetics.[5,9] Predisposing factors are protein loss from the burn wound; hepatic failure from hypovolemic shock, sepsis, or toxic inhalation; and renal failure from myoglobinuria.

Martyn[45,46] pioneered the pharmacokinetic studies in burn patients at The Shriners Burn Institute. Important drug-binding proteins such as albumin may be reduced to 50% of baseline, although another, equally important, drug-binding protein, alpha$_1$-globulin, may increase considerably in the first weeks after burn injury. An acute decrease in the protein-binding capacity of drugs results in an increase in free drug concentration. In patients with signs of toxic levels, one should measure free drug concentrations rather than the more commonly measured total drug concentration, which includes the bound fraction (see Chapter 2).

A significant percentage of patients with major burns may have epilepsy. An overview of drugs that may interfere with neurologic assessment in the intensive care unit in patients with hypoalbuminemia is shown in Table 14–2.

Burn Encephalopathy

Severely burned patients tend to have fluctuating levels of consciousness.[32,51,65,68] In approximately 30% of

Table 14–2 CHANGE IN SERUM DRUG CONCENTRATIONS AFTER BURNS

Drug	Expected Change
Diazepam	Increase
Chlordiazepoxide	Increase
Lorazepam	Same
Phenytoin	Increase
Phenobarbital	Increase
Valproate	Increase
Morphine	Same
Meperidine	Decrease
Imipramine	Decrease
Pancuronium	Decrease
Suxamethonium	Increase

Data from Brown, TCK and Bell, B: Electromyographic responses to small doses of suxamethonium in children after burns. Br J Anaesth 59:1017–1021, 1987; Martyn;[45,46] Martyn, JAJ, Abernethy, DR, and Greenblatt, DJ: Plasma protein binding of drugs after severe burn injury. Clin Pharmacol Ther 35:535–539, 1984; Martyn, JAJ, Goldhill, DR, and Goudsouzian, NG: Clinical pharmacology of neuromuscular relaxants in patients with burns. J Clin Pharmacol 26:680–685, 1986; Pugh, CB: Phenytoin and phenobarbital protein binding alterations in a uremic burn patient. Drug Intell Clin Pharm 21:264–267, 1987; and Stanford and Pine.[77]

Table 14–3 DIFFERENTIAL DIAGNOSIS IN BURN ENCEPHALOPATHY

Wernicke's encephalopathy
Sinus thrombosis
Anoxic-ischemic encephalopathy
Osmotic demyelination syndrome
Nonketotic hyperosmolar hyperglycemia

the patients, agitation, visual hallucinations, and coarse tremor develop in association with burn delirium.[1,51,65,68] Systemic factors may initiate a delirious state, but in most patients, fever is already an important trigger in itself. Massive facial swelling and eye bandages to treat corneal damage may contribute to deprivation, and the long-term use of benzodiazepines may give rise to delirium as well.[77]

Burn encephalopathy is a poorly defined clinical entity and may occur more frequently in children.[2,51] Many other more common and certainly better defined circumstances should be excluded (Table 14–3). Nevertheless, neuropathologic findings consisting of small areas of demyelination and degeneration of axons with scattered annular hemorrhages have been found at autopsy in severely burned patients. In some patients with documented sepsis, bacterial colonies have been found in small vessels, but they may not necessarily explain the clinical manifestations. In others, massive cerebral edema with evidence of both temporal lobe and tonsillar herniation is prominent. If accepted as a neurologic manifestation, burn encephalopathy clinically is manifested by a flurry of generalized tonic-clonic seizures, drowsiness, or stupor with unpredictable onset. Onset may be weeks after the burn injury, even at times when fever and metabolic derangements have subsided. Seizures are often associated with hyponatremia, usually as a result of iatrogenic fluid loading.[34]

A fortunately rare but devastating complication of extensive burns is acute blindness.[61,67,83,85] Blindness in children and young adults commonly occurs in the second or third week after the ictus. Optic discs may be normal, pale, or edematous. Outcome is not necessarily poor, and complete recovery has been reported, sometimes in only one eye.

Central Nervous System Infections

Wound infection is common in patients with burns that cover more than 30% of total body surface area. S. aureus and P. aeruginosa should be considered first as causative organisms. The frequency of central nervous system infections in patients with systemic infection is not known, and most data are derived only from autopsy studies. Winkelman and Galloway's comprehensive autopsy series[84] noted that all patients with intracranial infections had systemic signs of sepsis syndrome, many with positive blood cultures (Table 14–4). The most common organisms causing both significant multiorgan failure and cerebral microabscesses, septic infarcts, and meningitis were Candida species, P. aeruginosa, and S. aureus. All patients with S. aureus cerebritis also had S. aureus endocarditis.

In Winkelman and Galloway's autopsy series, meningitis was most frequently associated with nosocomially acquired P. aeruginosa, a generally extremely rare cause of bacterial meningitis.[84] No significant relation was found

Table 14–4 CENTRAL NERVOUS SYSTEM COMPLICATIONS OF FATAL BURNS IN 143 PATIENTS

Complication	Patients, n (%)
Central nervous system infection	22 (15)
Hemorrhagic stroke	5 (3)
Ischemic stroke	15 (10)
Anoxic encephalopathy	18 (13)
Central pontine myelinolysis	11 (8)

Data from Winkelman and Galloway.[84]

with face or scalp burns. In half of the patients with Pseudomonas meningitis, cerebral infarcts were found that may potentially have been caused by local invasion of the organism in blood vessels. Cerebrospinal fluid confirmation of Pseudomonas involvement is important but hard to justify in patients with extensive burns, and treatment should probably be guided by confirmation from blood cultures and physical findings suggesting meningeal irritation. Treatment of Pseudomonas meningitis is complex and involves ceftazidime and parenterally administered anti-Pseudomonas penicillins or intrathecally administered aminoglycosides (see Chapter 5 for dose schedules).

The clinical diagnosis of Candida infection is difficult. Candida infections of the brain may result either in microabscesses (often too small to detect with current imaging methods) or in meningitis.

Peripheral Neuropathies

The incidence of peripheral neuropathy is derived from retrospective analysis. Common themes are close relation with severity of burn and frequent presence of mononeuritis multiplex. Prolonged use of vancomycin has been implicated in the largest reported series,[44] but although anecdotes have suggested a correlation,[41] it is very unlikely that antibiotics are a crucial factor in a patient population that whatever the critical illness will at some point be treated with antibiotics.

In a series of 800 patients, a mononeuritis multiplex was found in 11 of 19 patients with a neuropathy, probably explained by protein denaturation and clumping within vessels in extensive skin burns. Multiple compression neuropathies were considered unlikely, although conditions such as faulty position, incorrect splinting, and tight dressing were favorable. Surprisingly, a critical illness neuropathy was seldom seen despite a high incidence of sepsis.

SMOKE INHALATION

Severe burns may be associated with inhalation of toxic products of combustion, mostly carbon monoxide and cyanide. Facial burns should point to the possibility of smoke inhalation. Oxygenation may become compromised by direct inhalation damage as well, and the result may be fulminant acute respiratory distress syndrome.

Carbon Monoxide

Signs of carbon monoxide poisoning may not be immediately obvious in patients who have large burns and who are in hypovolemic shock. Concentrations of carbon monoxide in hemoglobin that are greater than 40% result in coma. In the lower range, these concentrations are poorly correlated with the level of consciousness.

Manifestations of carbon monoxide intoxication are variable.[8] The classic cherry red coloring sign is very infrequently seen;[8] many patients are more likely to be cyanotic and tachypneic at presentation. Headache, vomiting, and blurred vision are much more common. Severe papilledema with splinter hemorrhages may occur,[59] sometimes as a direct result of asphyxia.

Computed tomography (CT) scan may demonstrate the characteristic symmetrical lucencies in the globus pallidus and centrum semiovale,[48,52,78] but unilateral lesions are compatible with carbon monoxide intoxication. White matter hypodensities, often seen in comatose patients and patients with exposure of long duration, predict poor outcome. Globus pallidus lesions are generally less prognostic.[48,52] Treatment of acute carbon monoxide poisoning[55] is 100% oxygen and, if that is unsuccessful, hyperbaric oxygen.

Cyanide

Smoke inhalation victims may have significant blood levels of cyanide as a result of combustion of nitrogen-containing materials common in plastics and wood.[4,29,35,38] Both cyanide poisoning and carbon monoxide inhalation frequently occur in residential fires.[4]

Cyanide inhalation results in rapid development of ataxia, tonic-clonic seizures, unresponsive coma, and, very often, death at the scene. Diagnosis of cyanide inhalation is difficult. The detection of cyanide in blood is technically cumbersome and may take hours. High serum concentrations of lactate causing lactic acidosis are suggestive of cyanide poisoning in patients without burns.

Treatment of cyanide exposure is immediate administration of high-flow oxygen or hyperbaric oxygen when available.[31] Sodium thiosulfate produces a conversion in thiocyanate that is much less toxic and is excreted in urine. Amyl nitrite acts by converting hemoglobin to methemoglobin, which has a high affinity to cyanide. A dose of 12.5 g of sodium thiosulfate (Lilly cyanide antidote kit) is followed by amyl nitrite when life-threatening cardiac arrhythmias and seizures persist. Hydroxocobalamin is less toxic for the treatment of cyanide poisoning but is not yet approved.[38]

ELECTRICAL BURNS

The devastation of electrical burns is not immediately evident. Direct neurologic complications of deep conductive electrical injury are well documented, but a fall caused by sudden loss of consciousness may result in very significant head trauma or spine injury. Sustained tetanic contraction may also contribute to vertebral fractures similar to those in patients with status epilepticus[40] (see Chapter 2). The most common presentations of electrical burns are related to peripheral nerve damage, but the effects most likely depend on the voltage of the electric shock (Table 14–5).

Spinal Cord Damage

It has long been recognized that spinal cord damage can occur in patients with electrical burns.[37,39,42,53,58,73]

Table 14–5 NEUROLOGIC COMPLICATIONS OF ELECTRICAL BURNS IN 90 PATIENTS

Findings	Patients, n (%)
Acute peripheral neuropathy	21 (23)
Delayed peripheral neuropathy	11 (12)
Seizures	3 (3)
Transient hemiparesis	1 (1)
Delayed spinal cord injury	0 (0)

Data from Grube, et al.[27]

Direct electrical heating probably causes necrosis of the spinal cord. Autopsy findings are nonspecific, and demyelination of corticospinal tracts, lateral columns, and both fasciculi is usually found. In patients with delayed onset of spinal cord injury, thrombosis of the supplying arteries to the cord has been postulated as the mechanism.[33] The clinical picture may vary from only transient spinal cord signs to severe permanent quadriplegia.

In patients with transient electrical injuries, symptoms are generally mild, with only proximal leg weakness and extensor plantar responses that resolve within 24 hours. Other patients may have a more striking course, characterized by ascending paralysis, transverse myelitis, or clinical features similar to those of amyotrophic lateral sclerosis. Severe upper extremity wasting, spastic paraplegia, and minimal sensory involvement have been noted after electrical shocks with high voltage. Spinal cord injury varies in incidence and in one recent large series was surprisingly absent[27] (Table 14–6). Delayed onset of spinal cord injury—within days, months, or years after the injury—

results in permanent damage when injury is complete, but when spinal cord injury is limited, there is a chance of recovery. Three of five patients in the report by Varghese and associates[80] completely recovered when they initially had the ability to walk.

In general, significant recovery is not expected in patients with a complete spinal cord lesion after a symptom-free episode. Thoracic lesions appear more common, although there is no predilection for a specific location in the cord.

Peripheral Neuropathy

Polyneuropathy, mononeuropathy, and plexopathies have been described in association with major and minor electrical burns.[10,18,30] In Engrav and coworkers' series[19] and in Grube and coworkers' series,[27] acute peripheral nerve injury developed in 34% of patients, most frequently in the median and ulnar nerves. The mechanism of injury after electrical contact may be prominent muscle swelling causing nerve entrapment.[36,64] Many surgeons are inclined to immediately decompress the carpal tunnel and Guyon's canal, but the effectiveness of preventing permanent damage has not been demonstrated, and spontaneous improvement of ulnar nerve damage has been reported.

Central Nervous System Manifestations

Typically, electrical burns produce only sudden loss of consciousness followed by a confusional state.[11] Neurologic sequelae are rare, but homony-

Table 14–6 INCIDENCE OF SPINAL CORD INJURY AFTER ELECTRICAL BURNS IN A LARGE SERIES OF PATIENTS

Series (y)	Patients, n (%)	Total Patients (n)
DiVincente, et al., 1969[18]	2 (3)	65
Butler and Gant, 1977[10]	3 (2)	182
Varghese, et al., 1986[80]	5 (6)	85
Grube, et al., 1990[27]	0 (0)	90

mous hemianopia and hemiparesis from ischemic stroke have been described.[24]

Delayed coma was linked to thrombotic occlusion of the basilar artery in one case report.[28] High-voltage exposure or sudden impact from lightning produces cardiac arrest and, often, prolonged anoxia.[13] Very often, these victims are immediately unresponsive and remain in a persistent vegetative state if they survive the initial impact at all.

ACCIDENTAL HYPOTHERMIA

The neurologic findings in patients with accidental hypothermia suggest severe damage to the central nervous system and may include absence of brain stem reflexes. In all instances, therefore, neurologists should allow intensive care physicians to correct core temperature before brain damage is assessed.[22,54,56,62] The dictum "no one is dead until warm and dead" should be applied to every patient with accidental hypothermia.

Accidental hypothermia most frequently follows cold water immersion, winter outdoor exposure, and poisoning.[27] Primary hypothalamic disorders may result in spontaneous episodic hypothermia but remain extremely rare causes for hypothermia.

Most patients admitted to the intensive care unit have hypothermia after cold water or environmental exposure.[22] One of the largest series of hypothermia has been reported from San Francisco, where it can become deceptively cold (30°F) in the summer at night. Hypothermia may affect the relatively high proportion of homeless people in this city.

Clinical Features

The clinical changes produced by hypothermia are fairly typical, although a perfect match of neurologic and systemic signs with degree of hypothermia

does not exist. The level of consciousness is mostly decreased with core temperatures between 37°C and 32°C, although patients may still be alert at these temperatures. Nevertheless, during rapid cooling, confusion and combative behavior may prevail. Muscle tone may be slightly increased. Additional causes should be actively sought when at temperatures above 32°C, patients can only be aroused with vigorous stimuli. The frequent association of accidental hypothermia with alcohol abuse should point to Wernicke's encephalopathy, particularly if nystagmus or palsy of conjugate gaze is present. Coma, however, is very infrequent in Wernicke-Korsakoff syndrome. In Victor and associates' series of 229 patients, only 2 patients were in coma at presentation.[82] Rapid volume expansion with free water may also exacerbate signs of Wernicke's encephalopathy in patients with marginal thiamine stores. Therefore, high doses of thiamine (100 mg parenterally daily) should be administered to any alcoholic hypothermic patient, and improvement can be expected within hours. Another major pitfall is hypothyroid coma, which should be considered in patients who fail to rewarm. A large bolus of levothyroxine (500 μg) along with corticosteroid coverage is the first step in treatment.

Neurologic signs may begin to develop in patients with moderate hypothermia (core temperatures below 32°C) (Fig. 14–2), but the clinical presentation may still be limited to drowsiness and diminished judgment at these levels of hypothermia. Cardiac arrhythmias are more common and may show characteristic electrocardiographic features, such as "camel's hump" in the QRS complex, that can easily be recognized even by noncardiologists (Fig. 14–3). Depressed or absent brain stem reflexes appear in patients with severe hypothermia (less than 27°C), but, as noted previously, this cutoff point is not absolute. Some patients may have absent brain stem reflexes and apnea, closely mimicking brain death. Muscle tone,

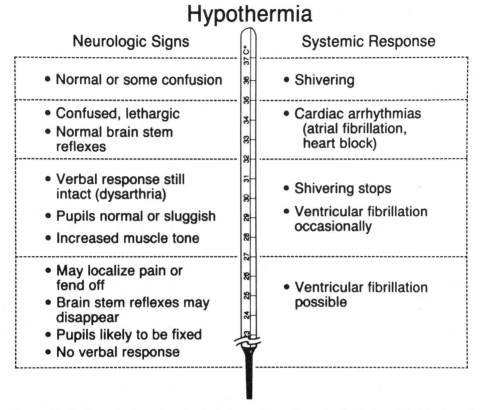

Figure 14−2. Neurologic and systemic factors of hypothermia. (Data from Fischbeck and Simon.[22])

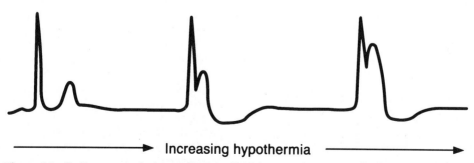

Increasing hypothermia

Figure 14−3. T wave on electrocardiogram. First tracing shows normal QRS complex. With increasing hypothermia, the QRS complex widens and an ST elevation is seen, with features of a "camel's hump." The hump increases with increasing hypothermia. The T wave appears at a temperature of 25°C.

however, is markedly increased rather than flaccid and may be misinterpreted as rigor mortis by novices. Electroencephalographic recordings in severe hypothermia may show many patterns, such as increased delta activity, triphasic waves, and, occasionally, isoelectricity.[63,72]

Treatment and Outcome

Most hypothermic patients are rewarmed by simple insulation with blankets.[20] This method results in a 7°C core temperature increase per hour. In coma from severe hypothermia that does not resolve after recovery, peritoneal lavage or cardiopulmonary bypass may be indicated.

Poor prognostic factors have been described but are impractical at the time of acute decision-making in the emergency room[14,15,71] (Table 14–7). Neurologic outcome can be remarkably good even after prolonged cardiac resuscitation,[76] core temperature of 20°C or lower, and absent brain stem reflexes. Any decision to discontinue resuscitation in a patient without brain stem reflexes who has severe hypothermia should be deferred until core temperature is above 32°C.

HEAT STROKE

A clear history and consistent recording of a rectal temperature above 40°C guide the diagnosis of heat stroke.[3,25,79] Well-known predisposing conditions are exertion in a hot environment and sudden heat waves in urban areas. Drugs that impair heat loss are often

Table 14–7 POOR PROGNOSTIC FACTORS OF HYPOTHERMIA

Increased potassium levels (>10 mmol/L)
Prehospital cardiac arrest
Low or absent blood pressure
Increased blood urea nitrogen
Severe underlying disease

Data from Schaller, et al.[71]

implicated, the most common of which are anticholinergic agents, phenothiazine derivatives, tricyclic antidepressants, amphetamine, and monoamine oxidase inhibitors.[70]

The incidence of heat stroke is unknown, mainly because many patients die early from cardiovascular compromise caused by high ambient temperatures. Heat stroke should be considered a medical emergency,[66] and early treatment is crucial to prevent neurologic complications.

Severe hyperthermia leads to multiorgan failure. Many patients are profoundly hypotensive from dehydration, and the direct effect of hyperthermia results in progressive hepatic failure, usually within a few days after the ictus. Bone marrow suppression leads to marked thrombocytopenia, but disseminated intravascular coagulation more likely produces a hypocoagulable state. Other typical findings are rhabdomyolysis with renal failure and severe electrolyte abnormalities (hypocalcemia, hyponatremia, hypophosphatemia), all of which may confound the neurologic assessment.

Clinical Features

Prodromes of heat stroke are acute confusional state and generalized weakness. A fair proportion of the patients may be psychotic, with vivid and often terrifying hallucinations. Headache and severely painful cramps in the truncal muscles may be present, often in association with hyponatremia from sweating. Patients may have hot and dry skin on the abdomen, but many already have had wet towels for cooling during transportation.

In heat stroke, progression into unresponsive coma is rapid but may take 1 to 2 days in some fatal cases.[23] Most patients have small pupils, profound rigidity, and spontaneous extensor responses.

In most patients with heat stroke and a fatal course, generalized tonic-clonic seizures occur at presentation. Any focal neurologic sign should point to a primary central nervous system disorder that may have directly contributed to hyperthermia, usually because the patient has been unable to prevent further deterioration by taking cover. Papilledema is found only in patients with massive cerebral edema. Except for some cortical effacement, CT scan findings are usually normal. Cerebrospinal fluid may show mild pleocytosis but is more often normal.

Treatment and Outcome

Treatment is supportive. Surface cooling should begin immediately after the airway is secured.[26,81] Shivering may be prevented by nondepolarizing muscle relaxants. Rehydration is crucial in the first hours. Although effective in many other causes of hyperthermia, dantrolene is not useful.[7]

Neurologic outcome is often poor, and patients who remain comatose after cooling die or have severe cognitive deficits (Table 14–8). Coma, stupor or seizures on presentation are not necessarily poor prognostic signs, however. In a series of 54 patients with heat stroke, only a minority, including 40% of the patients with Glasgow coma scale score of 3, had neurologic sequelae.[47] Nevertheless, death or neurologic morbidity is more likely in patients with extreme hyperthermia (greater than 42°C), although survivors have been reported.[74] Coma at presentation, coagulopathy, hypovolemic shock, high initial lactate levels, metabolic acidosis, association with predisposing medication, and electrolyte abnormalities indicate poor prognosis.

Cerebellar signs are frequent neurologic findings in survivors of heat stroke,[29] probably because hyperthermia may directly result in damage to Purkinje's cells. The cerebellar cortex is also exquisitely sensitive to anoxic-ischemic episodes. The pathologic changes in fatal cases—petechiae in the walls of the third and fourth ventricles and degenerative changes, most strikingly in the cerebellum, cerebral cortex, and basal ganglia—have been well described.[43,75] Many patients have slowed and scanning speech. Sitting in a chair while being weaned from the ventilator may unmask truncal instability and a tendency to fall to one side. The prospects of recovery are minimal.

NEAR-DROWNING

Patients entering the emergency room or intensive care unit after nearly drowning are unusually difficult to manage. Excellent survival can be expected in some aggressively resuscitated patients, but other patients remain in a persistent vegetative state. After resuscitation, general measures should focus on prevention of secondary brain damage from hypoxia and hypoglycemia, both common accompanying conditions in near-drowning victims.

Clinical Features

Neurologic examination of the nearly drowned patient may not produce reli-

Table 14–8 RECENT SERIES OF HEAT STROKE

	Patients (n)					
Series (y)	Total	In Stupor or Coma	With Seizures	Died	Disabled	Recovered
Tucker, et al., 1985[79]	34	26	2	6	3	25
Yaqub, et al., 1986[86]	30	15	2	3	2	25
Bouchama, et al., 1991[7]	52	20	6	1	4	47

able findings. Many patients with near-drowning are hypothermic from submersion in ice water associated with drug or alcohol intoxication. The patient may be severely hyponatremic from having swallowed large amounts of water, and this condition may be a potential cause of seizures. Near-drowning patients with flaccid, unresponsive limbs may be the most unfortunate, particularly if recovery halts in the first 48 hours. (Quadriplegia may also be caused by burst fractures of the cervical spine during submersion.)

Near-drowning is largely a diffuse hypoxic-ischemic insult (see Chapter 6). Cerebral edema is clinically insignificant but may be seen on CT scan as effacement of sulci and tailoring of ventricles. In general, differentiation of subtle cerebral edema on CT from normal findings in young patients can be extremely difficult.

Management and Outcome

Critical care management is focused on respiratory care.[21,49,50,57] In many patients, respiratory failure develops from acute respiratory distress syndrome or pulmonary infection that is caused by aspiration of contaminated water. These conditions may lead to sustained hypoxia in the first hours after resuscitation, but it is not clear whether neurologic outcome is less favorable when this happens.

Monitoring of intracranial pressure has been used, usually as part of an aggressive management approach, but successful control of intracranial pressure, if elevated at all, has not led to increased survival or recovery.[69]

Intracranial pressure monitoring in patients has demonstrated only occasional cerebral perfusion pressure decreases in the first 3 days after near-drowning. Initially increased intracranial pressure may predict poor outcome, but consistently normal pressure values have been found in patients who remained comatose.[16]

The general opinion is that use of in-

Table 14–9 POOR PROGNOSTIC FACTORS IN NEAR-DROWNING*

Submersion for more than 5 minutes
Metabolic acidosis of pH <7.1
Nonbreathing on admission to the emergency room
Fixed pupils
Glasgow coma scale score of <5

*Largely pediatric series.[60]

tracranial pressure monitoring in victims of near-drowning is of no value. This conclusion implies that aggressive measures that can lower intracranial pressure, such as osmotic diuretics, steroids, and barbiturates, are probably of no therapeutic use.

Outcome in near-drowning is difficult to predict, but the same rules of prognostication as those in postanoxic coma may apply (see Chapter 6 and Chapter 17) (Table 14–9). In this category of patients, a major confounding factor can be hypothermia. Outcome in hypothermic survivors is significantly better only when patients are immersed in ice water. Attempts to prolong the protective effect of hypothermia with high doses of barbiturates, however, have been unsuccessful and in addition may also aggravate neutropenia and lead to sepsis.[6]

CONCLUSIONS

The neurologic effects of environmental injuries involve three important rules.

First, the reliability of neurologic evaluation should be questioned in any patient with hypothermia, whether from outdoor exposure or from near-drowning. Every circumstance is different, and compounding factors, such as acute drug intoxication or an unexpected acute structural central nervous system lesion that has led to the injury, should be excluded. Core body temperatures should be around 32°C before a reliable assessment is attempted.

Second, care should be taken to prevent compression neuropathy in immobilized patients. Especially in burn patients, the incidence of peripheral neuropathy may be increased when appropriate measures are taken (for example, splinting, dressing changes).

Third, prognostication in these victims can be assessed. For most injured patients, prognostic factors have been identified that can ascertain the level of functioning in those who survive resuscitation.

REFERENCES

1. Andreasen, NJC, Hartford, CE, Knott, JR, and Canter, A: EEG changes associated with burn delirium. Dis Nerv Syst 38:27–31, 1977.
2. Antoon, AY, Volpe, JJ, and Crawford, JD: Burn encephalopathy in children. Pediatrics 50:609–616, 1972.
3. Austin, MG and Berry, JW: Observations on 100 cases of heatstroke. JAMA 161:1525–1529, 1956.
4. Baud, FJ, Barriot, P, Toffis, V, et al: Elevated blood cyanide concentrations in victims of smoke inhalation. N Engl J Med 325:1761–1766, 1991.
5. Bloedow, DC, Hansbrough, JF, Hardin, T, and Simons, M: Postburn serum drug binding and serum protein concentrations. J Clin Pharmacol 26:147–151, 1986.
6. Bohn, DJ, Biggar, WD, Smith, CR, et al: Influence of hypothermia, barbiturate therapy, and intracranial pressure monitoring on morbidity and mortality after near-drowning. Crit Care Med 14:529–534, 1986.
7. Bouchama, A, Cafege, A, Devol, EB, et al: Ineffectiveness of dantrolene sodium in the treatment of heatstroke. Crit Care Med 19:176–180, 1991.
8. Bour, H, Tutin, M, and Pasquier, P: The central nervous system and carbon monoxide poisoning. I. Clinical data with reference to 20 fatal cases. Prog Brain Res 24:1–30, 1967.
9. Bowdle, TA, Neal, GD, Levy, RH, and Heimbach, DM: Phenytoin pharmacokinetics in burned rats and plasma protein binding of phenytoin in burned patients. J Pharmacol Exp Ther 213:97–99, 1980.
10. Butler, ED and Gant, TD: Electrical injuries, with special reference to the upper extremities: A review of 182 cases. Am J Surg 134:95–101, 1977.
11. Christensen, JA, Sherman, RT, Balis, GA, and Wuamett, JD: Delayed neurologic injury secondary to high-voltage current, with recovery. J Trauma 20:166–168, 1980.
12. Cohen, BJ, Jordan, MH, Chapin, SD, et al: Pontine myelinolysis after correction of hyponatremia during burn resuscitation. J Burn Care Rehabil 12:153–156, 1991.
13. Critchley, M: Neurological effects of lightning and of electricity. Lancet i:68–72, 1934.
14. Danzl, DF, Hedges, JR, Pozos, RS, and Hypothermia Study Group: Hypothermia outcome score: Development and implications. Crit Care Med 17:227–231, 1989.
15. Danzl, DF, Pozos, RS, Auerbach, PS, et al: Multicenter hypothermia survey. Ann Emerg Med 16:1042–1055, 1987.
16. Dean, JM and McComb, JG: Intracranial pressure monitoring in severe pediatric near-drowning. Neurosurgery 9:627–630, 1981.
17. Demling, RH: Burns. N Engl J Med 313:1389–1398, 1985.
18. DiVincente, FC, Moncrief, JA, and Pruitt, BA Jr: Electrical injuries: A review of 65 cases. J Trauma 9:497–507, 1969.
19. Engrav, LH, Gottlieb, JR, Walkinshaw, MD, et al: Outcome and treatment of electrical injury with immediate median and ulnar nerve palsy at the wrist: A retrospective review and a survey of members of the American Burn Association. Ann Plast Surg 25:166–168, 1990.
20. Ferguson, J, Epstein, F, and van de Leuv, J: Accidental hypothermia. Emerg Med Clin North Am 1:619–637, Dec 1983.
21. Fields, AI: Near-drowning in the pediatric population. Crit Care Clin 8:113–129, Jan 1992.
22. Fischbeck, KH and Simon, RP: Neurological manifestations of accidental hy-

pothermia. Ann Neurol 10:384–387, 1981.

23. Freeman, W and Dumoff, SE: Cerebral syndrome following heat stroke. Arch Neurol Psychiatry 51:67–71, 1944.

24. Gans, M and Glaser, JS: Homonymous hemianopia following electrical injury. J Clin Neuroophthalmol 6:218–223, 1986.

25. Gauss, H and Meyer, KA: Heat stroke: Report of one hundred and fifty eight cases from Cook County Hospital, Chicago. Am J Med Sci 154:554–564, 1917.

26. Graham, BS, Lichtenstein, MJ, Hinson, JM, and Theil, GB: Nonexertional heatstroke: Physiologic management and cooling in 14 patients. Arch Intern Med 146:87–94, 1986.

27. Grube, BJ, Heimbach, DM, Engrav, LH, and Copass, MK: Neurologic consequences of electrical burns. J Trauma 30:254–258, 1990.

28. Haase, E and Luhan, JA: Protracted coma from delayed thrombosis of basilar artery following electrical injury. Arch Neurol 1:195–202, 1959.

29. Hall, AH and Rumack, BH: Clinical toxicology of cyanide. Ann Emerg Med 15:1067–1074, 1986.

30. Hanumadass, ML, Voora, SB, Kagan, RJ, and Matsuda, T: Acute electrical burns: A 10-year clinical experience. Burns Incl Therm Inj 12:427–431, 1986.

31. Hart, GB, Strauss, MB, Lennon, PA, and Whitcraft, DD III: Treatment of smoke inhalation by hyperbaric oxygen. J Emerg Med 3:211–215, 1985.

32. Haynes, BW Jr and Bright, R: Burn coma: A syndrome associated with severe burn wound infection. J Trauma 7:464–475, 1967.

33. Holbrook, LA, Beach, FXM, and Silver, JR: Delayed myelopathy: A rare complication of severe electrical burns. Br Med J 4:659–660, 1970.

34. Hughes, JR, Cayaffa, JJ, and Boswick, JA Jr: Seizures following burns of the skin. III. Electroencephalographic recordings. Dis Nerv Syst 36:443–447, 1975.

35. Jones, J, McMullen, MJ, and Dougherty, J: Toxic smoke inhalation: cyanide poisoning in fire victims. Am J Emerg Med 5:317–321, 1987.

36. Justis, DL, Law, EJ, and MacMillan, BG: Tibial compartment syndromes in burn patients: A report of four cases. Arch Surg 111:1004–1008, 1976.

37. Kanitkar, S and Roberts, AHN: Paraplegia in an electrical burn: A case report. Burns Incl Therm Inj 14:49–50, 1988.

38. Kulig, K: Cyanide antidotes and fire toxicology (editorial). N Engl J Med 325:1801–1802, 1991.

39. Langworthy, OR: Neurological abnormalities produced by electricity. J Nerv Ment Dis 84:13–26, 1936.

40. Layton, TR, McMurtry, JM, McClain, EJ, et al: Multiple spine fractures from electric injury. J Burn Care Rehabil 5:373–375, 1984.

41. Leibowitz, G, Golan, D, Jeshurun, D, and Brezis, M: Mononeuritis multiplex associated with prolonged vancomycin treatment (letter). BMJ 300:1344, 1990.

42. Levine, NS, Atkins, A, McKeel, DW Jr, et al: Spinal cord injury following electrical accidents: Case reports. J Trauma 15:459–463, 1975.

43. Malamud, N, Haymaker, W, and Custer, RP: Heat stroke: A clinico-pathologic study of 125 fatal cases. Mil Surg 99:397–449, 1946.

44. Marquez, S, Turley, JJE, and Peters, WJ: Neuropathy in burn patients. Brain 116:471–483, 1993.

45. Martyn, J: Clinical pharmacology and drug therapy in the burned patient. Anesthesiology 65:67–75, 1986.

46. Martyn, JAJ: Acute Management of the Burned Patient. WB Saunders, Philadelphia, 1990.

47. Mehta, AC and Baker, RN: Persistent neurological deficits in heat stroke. Neurology 20:336–340, 1970.

48. Miura, T, Mitomo, M, Kawai, R, and Harada, K: CT of the brain in acute carbon monoxide intoxication: Characteristic features and prognosis. AJNR Am J Neuroradiol 6:739–742, 1985.

49. Modell, JH: Drowning. N Engl J Med 328:253–256, 1993.

50. Modell, JH, Graves, SA, and Ketover, A: Clinical course of 91 consecutive near-

drowning victims. Chest 70:231–238, 1976.

51. Mohnot, D, Snead, OC III, and Benton, JW Jr: Burn encephalopathy in children. Ann Neurol 12:42–47, 1981.

52. Nardizzi, LR: Computerized tomographic correlate of carbon monoxide poisoning. Arch Neurol 36:38–39, 1979.

53. Naville, F and de Morsier, G: Symptômes neurologiques consécutifs aux électrocutions industrielles. Rev Neurol (Paris) 1:337–355, 1932.

54. Niazi, SA and Lewis, FJ: Profound hypothermia in man: Report of a case. Ann Surg 147:264–266, 1958.

55. Norkool, DM and Kirkpatrick, JN: Treatment of acute carbon monoxide poisoning with hyperbaric oxygen: A review of 115 cases. Ann Emerg Med 14:1168–1171, 1985.

56. Nozaki, R, Ishibashi, K, Adachi, N, et al: Accidental profound hypothermia (letter). N Engl J Med 315:1680, 1986.

57. Orlowski, JP: Drowning, near-drowning, and ice-water submersions. Pediatr Clin North Am 34:75–92, Feb 1987.

58. Panse, F: Electrical lesions of the nervous system. In Vinken, PJ and Bruyn, GW (eds): Handbook of Clinical Neurology. Vol 7: Diseases of Nerves. North-Holland Publishing, Amsterdam, 1970, pp 344–387.

59. Pye, IF and Blandford, RL: Papilledema associated with respiratory failure. Postgrad Med 53:704–709, 1977.

60. Quan, L, Wentz, KR, Gore, EJ, and Copass, MK: Outcome and predictors of outcome in pediatric submersion victims receiving prehospital care in King County, Washington. Pediatrics 86:586–593, 1990.

61. Resch, CS and Sullivan, WG: Unexplained blindness after a major burn. Burns Incl Therm Inj 14:225–227, 1988.

62. Reuler, JB: Hypothermia: Pathophysiology, clinical settings, and management. Ann Intern Med 89:519–527, 1978.

63. Reutens, DC, Dunne, JW, and Gubbay, SS: Triphasic waves in accidental hypothermia. Electroencephalogr Clin Neurophysiol 76:370–372, 1990.

64. Rosenberg, DB: Neurologic sequelae of minor electric burns. Arch Phys Med Rehabil 70:914–915, 1989.

65. Rosenbloom, C and Kravath, R: Neurological disturbances following minor burns. Lancet ii:1423, 1969.

66. Salem, SN: Neurological complications of heat-stroke in Kuwait. Ann Trop Med Parasitol 60:393–400, 1966.

67. Salz, JJ and Donin, JF: Blindness after burns. Can J Ophthalmol 7:243–246, 1972.

68. Sanders, R: Neurological disturbances and minor burns. Lancet ii:1133, 1969.

69. Sarnaik, AP, Preston, G, Lieh-Lai, M, and Eisenbrey, AB: Intracranial pressure and cerebral perfusion pressure in near-drowning. Crit Care Med 13:224–227, 1985.

70. Sarnquist, F and Larson, CP: Drug-induced heat stroke. Anesthesiology 39:348–350, 1973.

71. Schaller, M-D, Fischer, AP, and Perret, CH: Hyperkalemia: A prognostic factor during acute severe hypothermia. JAMA 264:1842–1845, 1990.

72. Scott, JW, McQueen, D, and Callahagn, JC: The effect of lowered body temperature on the EEG (abstr). Electroencephalogr Clin Neurophysiol 5:465, 1953.

73. Silversides, J: The neurological sequelae of electrical injury. Can Med Assoc J 91:195–204, 1964.

74. Slovis, CM, Anderson, GF, and Casolaro, A: Survival in a heat stroke victim with a core temperature in excess of 46.5 C. Ann Emerg Med 11:269–271, 1982.

75. Snider, RS, Thomas, W, and Snider, SR: Focal brain hyperthermia. I. The cerebellar cortex. Experientia 34:479–481, 1978.

76. Southwick, FS and Dalglish, PH Jr: Recovery after prolonged asystolic cardiac arrest in profound hypothermia: A case report and literature review. JAMA 243:1250–1253, 1980.

77. Stanford, GK, and Pine, RH: Postburn delirium associated with use of intravenous lorazepam. J Burn Care Rehabil 9:160–161, 1988.

78. Taylor, R and Holgate, RC: Carbon monoxide poisoning: Asymmetric and uni-

lateral changes on CT. AJNR Am J Neuroradiol 9:975–977, 1988.

79. Tucker, LE, Stanford, J, Graves, B, et al: Classical heatstroke: Clinical and laboratory assessment. South Med J 78:20–25, 1985.

80. Varghese, G, Mani, MM, and Redford, JB: Spinal cord injuries following electrical accidents. Paraplegia 24:159–166, 1986.

81. Vicario, SJ, Okabajue, R, and Haltom, T: Rapid cooling in classic heatstroke: Effect on mortality rates. Am J Emerg Med 4:394–398, 1986.

82. Victor, M, Adams, RD, and Collins, GH: The Wernicke-Korsakoff Syndrome and Related Neurologic Disorders Due to Alcoholism and Malnutrition, ed 2. FA Davis, Philadelphia, 1989.

83. Williams, IM: Neuro-ophthalmic deterioration after burns. Proc Aust Assoc Neurol 11:49–56, 1974.

84. Winkelman, MD and Galloway, PG: Central nervous system complications of thermal burns: A postmortem study of 139 patients. Medicine (Baltimore) 71:271–283, 1992.

85. Xiao, J, Xu, H, and Kong, FY: Bilateral visual loss after severe burns in a child. Burns 17:423–424, 1991.

86. Yaqub, BA, Al-Harthi, SS, Al-Orainey, IO, et al: Heatstroke at the Mekkah pilgrimage: Clinical characteristics and course of 30 patients. Q J Med 59:523–530, 1986.

Chapter 15

NEUROLOGIC COMPLICATIONS OF MULTISYSTEM TRAUMA

Patients with multiple injuries are often admitted to designated surgical or trauma units, mostly because many have hemodynamic deterioration after emergency admission or become hypoxic from direct chest or airway trauma. In this hectic environment, cranial computed tomography (CT) scan does not have immediate priority over surgical stabilization of the patient. Failure to recognize head or neck injury may have devastating consequences. Decreased level of consciousness that initially appears as a direct result of hypoxemia, hypercarbia, or shock should be reassessed after stabilization. The threshold for additional imaging should be low, particularly if the level of responsiveness does not improve within reasonable time.[138]

Appropriate triage to hospitals with neurointensive care or neurosurgical facilities should follow after major trauma. Adequate oxygenation, rapid correction of hypotension, and treatment of increased intracranial pressure are all hallmarks of emergency management, with the ultimate goal to prevent secondary brain damage in a patient with a recently injured and vulnerable brain. These concerns are not trivial. Transfer from the emergency room to the intensive care unit increases the likelihood of secondary insult from hypoxia, hypotension, or surges of increased intracranial pressure.[8] In many clinical situations, both the neurologist and the neurosurgeon become closely involved in patient care.

The major focus of this chapter is the discussion of priorities of evaluation and management guidelines in patients with intracranial and spinal injuries. Specific neurosurgical and orthopedic interventions are not addressed; these subspecialties have their own texts.

NEURORADIOLOGIC FINDINGS IN HEAD INJURY

Any patient with multiple trauma or a history of significant head injury should undergo baseline head CT scanning with additional bone-setting views. First, CT scanning may detect abnormalities that may determine management in the first hours.[138] Second, certain radiologic findings[164] may signal a potential for rapid neurologic deterioration[105] in, for example, patients with small extradural hematomas, bilateral frontal contusions, or a unilateral temporal lobe mass.

Third, an initial CT scan may help in prognostication. Multiple intracranial hematomas with diffuse cerebral swelling almost certainly indicate that a dismal outcome is likely. Predictive factors for intracerebral hematomas have been identified that may guide trauma surgeons in consulting the neurologist and the need for emergency CT scanning. These predictors are age (with a notable increase in incidence after the fourth decade), injury from fall, low Glasgow coma scale score on admission, pupillary inequality, and skull fracture. Factors that do not predict intracerebral hematomas are unilateral or bilateral fixed pupils, injury caused by mechanisms other than fall, trauma to multiple organs, and alcohol intoxication.[162]

The traumatic lesions that can be demonstrated on CT can be divided into diffuse axonal injury with edema, intracerebral hematoma, or a combination (Fig. 15 – 1), but the CT scan can be initially normal in 50% of the patients admitted comatose to an emergency room. Although magnetic resonance imaging (MRI) has repeatedly been reported to have, as expected, higher sensitivity than conventional CT, it may not become the first diagnostic test in patients with acute multiple injuries despite improvement in acquisition time.[70,71,76,84,160,171,181] Although prospective MRI studies demonstrate a higher incidence of intra-axial lesions and parenchymal lesions not seen on initial CT, CT scan remains superior in demonstration of hemorrhagic lesions in the first days of trauma.[157]

Diffuse Brain Injury

The main features of diffuse axonal brain injury are multiple small hemorrhagic shear lesions and cerebral edema associated with loss of visibility of the mesencephalic cisterns. Recently, a new classification system of CT scanning in diffuse head injury was proposed; the most pertinent features are summarized in Table 15 – 1.[110] These categories may predict outcome (see Chapter 17) and may also predict increased intracranial pressure, but data are not yet available.

Frequently found on CT scan in patients with diffuse closed head injury are small tissue-tear hemorrhages accompanied by a halo of edema.[17,102] They are commonly seen at the frontal cortex and white matter interface, basal ganglia, thalamus, and internal capsule (see Fig. 15 – 1). Subarachnoid or intraventricular blood is found in half the patients with shear lesions.[170] Shear le-

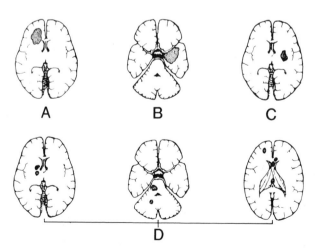

Figure 15 – 1. Spectrum of computed tomography scan intraparenchymal hemorrhages in closed head injury. *A*, Frontal hemorrhagic contusion. *B*, Temporal lobe hemorrhagic contusion. *C*, Basal ganglia hemorrhage. *D*, Typical locations of shear lesions (corpus callosum, midbrain, frontal cortex interface).

Table 15–1 COMPUTED TOMOGRAPHY (CT) CLASSIFICATION OF DIFFUSE BRAIN INJURY

Category	Definition
I	No visible intracranial disease on CT scan
II	Cisterns present Midline shift of 0 to 5 mm or lesion density, or both No high- or mixed-density lesion >25 mL May include bone fragments and foreign bodies
III	Cisterns compressed or absent Midline shift of 0 to 5 mm No high- or mixed-density lesion >25 mL
IV	Midline shift >5 mm No high- or mixed-density lesion >25 mL

Modified from Marshall, et al.[110]

sions from trauma are infrequently associated with cerebral edema and increased intracranial pressure. Shearing injuries in multiple sites do not necessarily imply a poor outcome (see Chapter 17), but high-intensity lesions in both the corpus callosum and the interpeduncular midbrain have been singled out as markers of poor outcome.[102] Shearing abnormalities of corpus callosum are often associated with small lesions in the thalamus, splenium, or septum pellucidum, consistent with a fronto-occipital course of acceleration.

Isolated shearing injury in the midbrain caused by sudden displacement in the sagittal plane from a frontal or occipital impact ruptures the perforating arteries to the midbrain.[159] If shearing injury is not present in other locations, good neurologic outcome can be expected.[115] It is important to differentiate these punctate midbrain lesions from acute traumatic midbrain hemorrhages, which carry a more dismal outcome. Acute traumatic midbrain hemorrhages may occur as a primary event, causing damage that occupies the ventral rim of the aqueduct to the interpeduncular fossa and extends inferiorly to the pontomesencephalic junction.[139]

Traumatic Intracerebral Hematomas

Initial CT scanning should identify mixed-density lesions or intracerebral hematomas in most patients with major head injury. Delayed traumatic intracerebral hematomas (spät-apoplexie) may occur after an initial normal CT scan but are extremely rare. Sudden deterioration from large intracerebral hematomas has been noted in patients with initial CT scans that showed a depressed skull fracture and small midline subdural hematoma.[52] Delayed intracerebral hematomas mostly occur in patients with initial neurologic impairment, but maximal Glasgow coma scale scores occur in up to 20% of patients who harbor intracerebral hematomas.

In a series of 656 patients, 9 with delayed intracerebral hematoma were identified 8 hours to 13 days after the impact,[47] but in another series with serial CT scans, the vast majority of delayed intracerebral hematomas were identified within 2 days.[73]

Most traumatic parenchymal lesions are located in the frontal and temporal lobes. Bilateral frontal contusions are associated with a significant risk of further deterioration from massive edema and brain stem compression in the anteroposterior direction[158] (Fig. 15–2). Patients with temporal lobe hematomas or hematomas in temporoparietal locations also are more at risk for clinical deterioration.[6] In patients with frontal or temporal lobe locations, any subtle change in neurologic findings should warrant placement of an intracranial pressure monitor.

Another potentially dangerous location is the posterior fossa.[61,145] A traumatic hematoma in this small, contained compartment may produce a rapid and at times abrupt clinical deterioration. Both intracerebellar and extradural hematomas may cause clinical deterioration, but an extradural infratentorial hematoma is most likely from bleeding from the transverse sinus and without appreciable fourth ven-

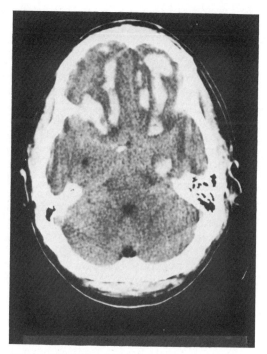

Figure 15–2. Bilateral frontal lobe contusions.

tricle compression can be managed conservatively.

Basal ganglia hemorrhages and hemorrhage in the corpus callosum[152] are traumatic hemorrhages that have been associated with shearing of midsized cerebral blood vessels (Fig. 15–3).

Basal ganglia hemorrhages are rare (3% in two large series) and indicate diffuse axonal and tissue shear injury.[38,91,99,108] Traumatic basal ganglia hemorrhage may be differentiated from spontaneous basal ganglia hemorrhage by its preferred location in the lenticulate nucleus and external capsule and its frequent association with corpus callosum lesions and other small white matter shear lesions that are sometimes evident only on MRI. Outcome in traumatic basal ganglia hemorrhage, therefore, is related more to the presence of additional lesions.[38,91,99,108] Traumatic intraventricular hematomas[66,87] are often seen in association with parenchymal lesions, but subependymal tears may cause the primary location to be in ventricles. Outcome is variable.

Emergency ventricular shunting is not effective.

GENERAL PRINCIPLES OF MANAGEMENT

Patients with multitrauma often receive large volumes of fluids. Uncontrolled fluid resuscitation may lead to massive fluid intakes and may theoretically exacerbate cerebral edema. Little is known about the ideal fluid balance in patients with severe head injuries. These patients, similar to those with subarachnoid hemorrhage, may be at risk for hypovolemia, but whether hypovolemia contributes to further ischemic damage is not known.[169] Vasospasm[32] and delayed cerebral ischemia have been demonstrated in severe head injury, but the role of volume depletion is not clear.[118]

Patients with head injury should be kept normovolemic (central venous pressure of 8 to 10 mm Hg; pulmonary wedge pressure of 12 to 14 mm Hg), and free water should be restricted.

Blood pressure is very often increased as part of an adrenergic stress response with outpouring of catecholamines.[153] Guidelines for appropriate blood pressure levels are not available, because no study has addressed the effect of antihypertensive agents on cerebral perfusion pressure and outcome in severe head injury. Sedation is probably more effective than treatment with antihypertensive medication. For patients with persistent hypertension with clinical signs of left ventricular failure or pulmonary edema (rales, third heart sound, or pulse deficit), a bolus of labetalol (20 mg intravenously; maximum of 300 mg) is mandated, with the intent to produce a 25% decrease in mean arterial pressure below baseline. In many patients, intracranial pressure monitoring is needed to maintain sufficient cerebral perfusion pressure (cerebral perfusion pressure equals mean arterial pressure minus intracranial pressure) (for specific antihypertensive treatment, see Chapter 8). It is important to

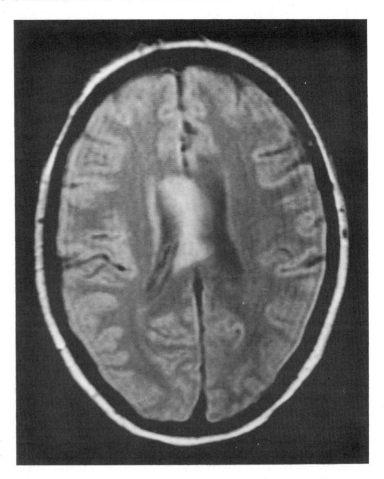

Figure 15–3. Traumatic corpus callosum hematoma on magnetic resonance imaging.

avoid hypovolemia, and hypotension can be expected when antihypertensive agents are used in this situation. Use of anticonvulsants is controversial, but phenytoin in a high therapeutic dosage range decreases the incidence of post-traumatic seizures during the first week.[163] Anticonvulsant therapy can be discontinued if no seizures have occurred during the first 2 weeks of hospital admission. Glucocorticoids in conventional doses or megadoses have been unsuccessful in improving outcome and in one study resulted in greater mortality.[43]

Nutrition in head-injured patients is not easily managed. The demand is high, many patients are hypercatabolic, gastric emptying is disturbed, and enteral feeding is cumbersome.[36,178,179] In addition, full-strength, full-rate feedings are often tolerated only after 1 week. In patients with prolonged intolerance, a feeding tube should be placed in the jejunum.[124] Most dietitians will begin administration of low-residual, high-caloric commercial enriched mixtures that are delivered continuously by a volumetric feeding pump. If this therapy is unsuccessful, total parenteral nutrition is indicated, because starvation decreases alertness and subsequently increases the risk of aspiration and decreases the ability to fend off infections.

Skull and basal skull fractures pose difficult management problems. Conservative treatment of closed skull fractures[22,165] is standard care for many neurosurgeons. Compound skull fractures generally undergo exploration, debridement, and dura mater repair. The risk of epilepsy is increased, approaching 60% when post-traumatic amnesia lasts more than 24 hours and a dural tear is present. In this case, anticonvulsants should be strongly considered.[88]

Cerebrospinal fluid fistulas are estimated to occur in 5% to 10% of basal skull fractures. Rhinorrhea is most likely to occur immediately after the impact and can be proved by glucose determination or detection of beta$_2$ and tau fractions in the cerebrospinal fluid.[123,177] The risk of bacterial meningitis from cerebrospinal fluid fistulas is low, and antibiotic prophylaxis is not indicated. If rhinorrhea persists, surgical repair is indicated.

MANAGEMENT OF INCREASED INTRACRANIAL PRESSURE

Increased intracranial pressure, defined as pressure higher than 15 mm Hg on several occasions, cannot be estimated by determination of the Glasgow coma scale score alone.

Guidelines for placement of intracranial pressure monitoring devices are summarized in Table 15–2, but the indications may differ in various institutions. In any patient without purposeful movements, particularly when CT scan shows absence of ambient cisterns, intraventricular or subarachnoid blood,

Table 15–2 GUIDELINES FOR INTRACRANIAL PRESSURE (ICP) MONITORING IN PATIENTS WITH MULTISYSTEM TRAUMA, INCLUDING HEAD INJURY

- No purposeful movements
- Need for prolonged sedation and neuromuscular paralysis
- Computed tomography scan abnormalities indicating increased ICP:
  Bifrontal and temporal lobe contusion
  Intraventricular and subarachnoid hemorrhage
  Absence of ambient cisterns or narrowing of third ventricle

or an intracerebral hematoma, placement of a monitoring device should be strongly considered. Other trauma centers use Glasgow coma sum scores of 8 or less as a cutoff point to decide whether an intracranial device should be placed.

Fiberoptic systems in which the probe is placed directly into the white matter are currently used[42,107] (Fig. 15–4). In contrast to other new intracranial pressure devices, this technology has been validated. Infectious complications and intracerebral hematoma at the site of placement are extremely rare. An important drift in intracranial pressure readings can be expected only after 5 days of placement, but intracranial pressure monitoring is often no longer indicated at that time.

Treatment of increased intracranial pressure includes recognition of common triggers.

Combative behavior and patient intolerance of mechanical ventilation can be counteracted by sedation, preferably with short-acting sedatives in low doses (e.g., midazolam or propofol) or narcotics. Fear of not detecting an important clinical neurologic deterioration should not prevent taking this measure to mute potential catastrophic surges in intracranial pressure. In patients with extreme agitation and profuse sweating, neuromuscular blockade and narcotics are needed occasionally to maximize oxygen delivery. Positive end-expiratory pressure mode is often necessary to ensure adequate oxygenation in patients with additional lung trauma. Positive end-expiratory pressure of less than 10 cm H$_2$O does not significantly raise intracranial pressure, perhaps because decreased lung compliance in these patients with acute lung concussion or flail chests prevents transmural conductance of airway pressure to the right atrium.[40] Endotracheal suctioning may cause important increases in intracranial pressure. These marked increases cannot be ameliorated by simple hyperoxygenation.[143] Patients with marked increases in intracranial pressure after endotracheal suctioning

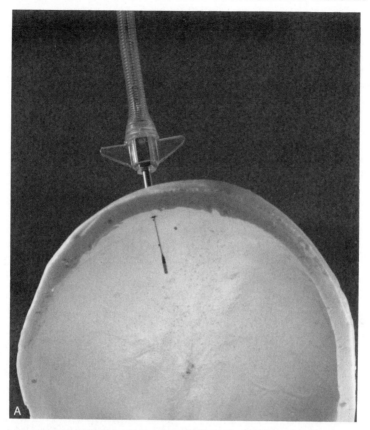

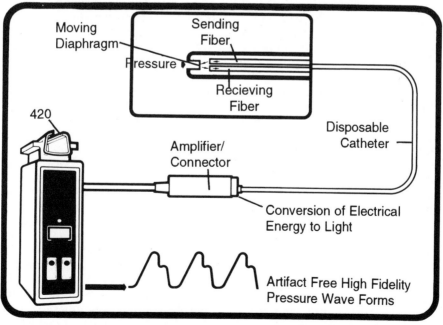

Figure 15–4. *A*, Intracranial monitoring device in demonstration model. *B*, Diagram of complete fiberoptic parenchymal intracranial pressure monitoring system (Camino Laboratories).

should receive lidocaine, 1 mg/kg, or thiopental, 0.5 to 1 mg/kg, intravenously to blunt this response. In addition, the number of suction passes should be limited to one.[142,143]

Patients with head injury should have elevation of the head to 30° in neutral position, although in some patients intracranial pressure may not change or may paradoxically increase.[140] For this reason, it is prudent to determine which position optimizes cerebral perfusion pressure in an individual patient rather than to use head elevation indiscriminately. Recent studies have suggested that hydrostatic displacement of the cerebrospinal fluid from the cranial cavity to the spinal space and facilitation of venous outflow are the most likely mechanisms for decrease of intracranial pressure after head elevation.[57] After cervical spine injury is excluded, a rigid collar should be removed because it may also contribute to venous congestion.[41]

The preferred treatment for control of increased intracranial pressure is hyperventilation with a goal of PCO_2 in the low 30s.[19,107] Experimental data suggest, however, that the effect on cerebrospinal fluid pH and vessel diameter is brief and is attenuated after 6 hours. When hyperventilation is the only mode of treatment (e.g., in patients with severe renal failure), addition of tromethamine (THAM) (0.3 M at a rate of 1 mL/kg per hour) is indicated.[174] A recent randomized study with tromethamine found that fluctuations in intracranial pressure could be controlled, but outcome in head injury was not significantly improved.[174] Prolonged hyperventilation in head injury should be avoided, and recent evidence suggests a higher incidence of poor outcome.[120]

Treatment with osmotic agents remains the cornerstone of intracranial pressure reduction,[19,107,156] aiming at serum osmolality of 310 to 320 mOsm/L. This can be readily achieved with mannitol in a starting dose of 0.25 to 2 g/kg. Plasma osmolality of more than 325 mOsm/L will result in renal failure. Reduction of intracranial pressure can

be expected 20 minutes after a bolus, and the first-pass effect may last 6 hours. A difference of less than 10 mOsm/kg between measured and calculated osmolality, determined as follows:

$$2[Na^+] + \frac{[glucose]}{18}$$

$$+ \frac{[blood\ urea\ nitrogen]}{2.8}$$

should indicate the need for an additional bolus of mannitol. A rebound effect of mannitol is seldom encountered. In one study, a rebound was demonstrated in only 12% of 65 patients and did not occur more often in patients treated with higher doses or faster infusion rates.[122]

Lack of response to treatment with mannitol, 2g/kg, and no new CT scan findings other than diffuse abnormalities or cerebral edema may be followed by a more aggressive (but also potentially harmful) treatment. Furosemide with albumin to prevent hypovolemia can be reasonably tried first[136] in combination with mannitol, but this regimen is fraught with complications and only at times successful. Hypertonic saline 3% is as successful as mannitol (50 mL in 10 minutes).[175] Barbiturates can be considered next, but only 50% of patients with refractory increased intracranial pressure responded to high-dose barbiturate therapy (loading dose of pentobarbital, 10 to 20 mg/kg; maintenance dose, 1 to 3 mg/kg per hour). No clinical study with barbiturates in head injury has demonstrated improved outcome. Moreover, it is not clear whether treatment with pentobarbital increases the number of patients with severe disability and vegetative state whose course otherwise would have been rapid deterioration to brain death.

Barbiturate treatment has significant complications. Hypotension occurred in 50% of 38 patients with severe trauma.[148] Other frequent complications were hypokalemia, hepatic and renal dysfunction, and sepsis. Barbiturates may depress lung mucociliary clearance[62] and therefore may account for an increased risk of pulmonary infections.[137,149] Nonetheless, one may feel compelled to use aggressive treatment with barbiturates as the last resort in young patients with head injury. Propofol infusion has recently been used as an alternative means of sedation in patients with head injury,[56,83] with additional reduction of intracranial pressure. A recent study, however, seriously questioned the role of propofol (2 mg/kg by intravenous bolus followed by infusion of 150 $\mu g \cdot kg^{-1} \cdot min^{-1}$) after demonstrating a reduction in intracranial pressure but also cerebral perfusion pressure from hypotension.[56,129] We do not routinely use propofol for this reason and use it only if intracranial pressure and cerebral perfusion pressure can be monitored or, as alluded to previously, for sedation.

MANAGEMENT OF TRAUMATIC INTRACRANIAL HEMATOMAS

After stabilization of airway, circulation, and fractures, head CT scanning is a logical next step in patients with severe trauma, although some physicians may assess the need for CT scanning on the basis of whether a skull fracture is present, the level of responsiveness, and the type of trauma. A major treatment dilemma occurs when a small extradural hematoma without appreciable shift is found. Options for trauma unit management of intracranial hematomas are presented in this section.

Epidural Hematoma

Of the total population of head injury patients admitted to emergency rooms, 3% to 5% have epidural hematoma. Mortality is extremely variable in large series, ranging from 20% to 55%. It is intuitively obvious that mortality from epidural hematoma is related to the Glasgow coma scale score before evacuation. Two thirds of patients with an epidural hematoma and Glasgow motor score of 3 or less die or remain in a vegetative state.[150] Good outcome can be expected in patients who have withdrawal to pain before evacuation is attempted. Prognosis for good recovery is worse in patients with an associated intracerebral lesion, although immediate mortality is not greatly influenced.

The clinical presentation of epidural hematoma is typically dramatic, with a rapid lapse into coma. Often, the ipsilateral pupil dilates and becomes fixed, and this reaction soon follows in the opposite pupil. Asymmetry in motor response may be noted but does not localize the hematoma.

It has been argued whether an exploratory burr hole should be drilled before a CT scan is performed. Andrews and associates[7] reported, in a large series, that 86% of extradural hematomas could be localized by an ipsilateral burr hole. A contralateral epidural or subdural hematoma was found in 2 of 56 explorations. In 33 patients, "complete" burr hole exploration (bilateral temporal, frontal, and parietal burr holes) produced negative findings. Both poor outcome and the 44% negative rate at exploration in these patients make this heroic procedure difficult to justify. In most patients, there should be enough time for a "limited" CT scan, but immediate surgical exploration at the site of pupil enlargement or skull fracture may be considered in patients with rapid loss of brain stem reflexes in the emergency room.

Acute bilateral epidural hematomas are infrequent,[9] representing approximately 15% of all epidural hematomas. Mortality is high, usually because major trauma is needed to produce bilateral epidural hematomas, but a 1991 report found that with bilateral frontal epidural hematoma the chance of good recovery was relatively high (60%).[46] Posterior fossa epidural hematomas are rare, seldom associated with concomitant supratentorial contusion, and outcome is excellent after immediate surgical intervention. In several reported series from Italy, mortality was relatively low (12% to 18%).[106,132,134]

An important controversial issue is the management of small epidural hematomas that do not produce appreciable clinical signs. Knuckey and associates[95] attempted to prospectively manage a series of 22 patients with small epidural hematomas seen within several hours after trauma. All were initially managed conservatively. Patients with associated skull fractures that traversed the arteria meningea media or major dural vessels, such as the transverse sinus, had a 55% chance of delayed expansion requiring surgical intervention. Approximately 60% of these patients did not have clinical deterioration in the course of conservative management. Another important and consistent warning radiologic sign is a radiolucent region within the denser clot, probably a sign of active bleeding.[80,95] Other, more obvious warning signs are depressed level of consciousness, volume of hematoma, and midline shift.[80] Delayed epidural hemorrhage has been noted in patients hypotensive from multiple trauma whose condition deteriorated after correction of hypotension[11,26,48,77,100,121,155] (Fig. 15–5). Conservative management of asymptomatic epidural hematomas may be appropriate except when CT scans show a volume of more than 30 mL, thickness of more than 15 mm, and a midline shift beyond 5 mm. Enlargement may occur with or without clinical deterioration.[34] In this subcategory, early evacuation probably is needed.

Subdural Hematoma

Venous hemorrhage from bridging veins ruptured by trauma is associated

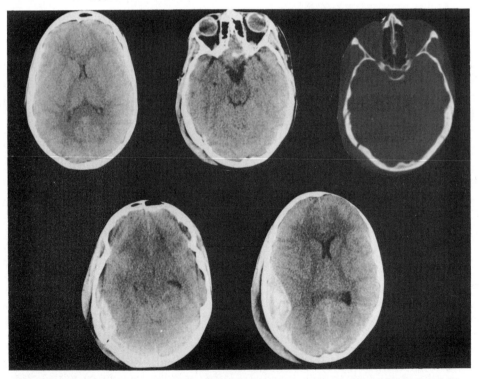

Figure 15–5. A series of computed tomography scans in a patient with multiple facial injuries shows small epidural hematoma and associated skull fracture. Repeated scan verified marked increase in volume that was detected by suddenly dilated fixed pupils during surgical repair of facial lacerations. Outcome was excellent after evacuation.

with high mortality, particularly in the elderly.[89,127,135] A large study of acute subdural hematomas found that old age (defined as older than 65 years) quadrupled the mortality rate.[85] None of these elderly patients with Glasgow coma scale scores of less than 13 had a functional outcome after surgical evacuation. A more recent study[172] of 101 patients with acute subdural hematomas noted a mortality of 66% and 19% functional recovery. Poor predictors for outcome were age older than 65 years, admission Glasgow coma scale score of 3 or 4, and postoperative intracranial pressure greater than 45 mm Hg.

Patients with an acute subdural hematoma generally present with Glasgow coma scale scores of less than 7.[172] In 7% of patients, an associated cerebral contusion is found, and poor outcome is presumably related to diffuse head injury rather than to brain shift alone.[31]

Computed tomography scanning may occasionally show isodense subdural hematoma in the acute phase and is frequently associated with anemia (hemoglobin less than 10 g/dL) or disseminated intravascular coagulation.[21]

Interhemispheric location of subdural hematomas has also been described on CT scan, and conservative treatment can be considered in patients who do not have symptoms or who have maximal Glasgow coma scale scores.[44,166] Delayed subdural hematomas are less common than epidural hematomas[20,105,128] and may also occur after removal of a contralateral epidural hematoma from release of its tamponade effect.[58,113,176]

The initial management of traumatic acute subdural hematoma may remain conservative if the thickness of the hematoma is similar to the skull bone thickness and no midline shift is noted.[131] Low Glasgow coma scale scores in these patients with small subdural hematomas should be attributed to additional post-traumatic lesions or systemic factors. Therefore, it is prudent to wait and act only in case of enlargement associated with clinical deterioration. Recent data suggest that rapid operative removal does not affect outcome.

Intraparenchymal Hematoma

Large contusions on CT scan are prone to cause deterioration and are best handled by neurosurgical evacuation.[75] Frontal and temporal hematomas should be removed, with additional lobe resection when located in the nondominant hemisphere. Hematomas in the deep white matter are treated medically in many large trauma centers. The management of a patient with a small intracerebral hematoma and minimal neurologic deficit is conservative, but as mentioned previously, intracranial pressure monitoring should be used in frontal and temporal lobe localizations, and then sustained elevation of intracranial pressure may prompt evacuation.[27]

TRAUMA OF SPINE AND SPINAL CORD

A potential consequence of major trauma is injury to the spine and spinal cord, usually subtle and at times unaccompanied by pertinent clinical findings.

Management of spinal trauma demands proper judgment and extensive experience. This section is a practical summary of spine and spinal cord injury and initial management. Remaining problems and decisions can be found in excellent textbooks[53,116] and should be left to the discretion of the consulting neurosurgeon and orthopedic surgeon.

Most patients should be evaluated with anteroposterior, lateral, oblique, and open-mouth odontoid radiographic views. A lateral cervical spine film to "clear C-spine" is not sufficient, and 25% of cervical spine injuries can be overlooked.[141]

Plain cervical spine films should be scrutinized for soft-tissue abnormalities, abnormalities in alignment, abnormality in disc space height, and

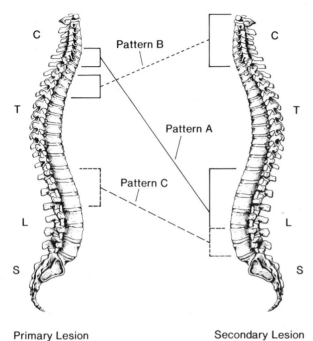

Primary Lesion   Secondary Lesion

Figure 15–6. Multilevel fractures: *Pattern A*, C-5 through C-7 associated with T-11 through L-5; *Pattern B*, T-2 through T-4 associated with C-1 through C-7; and *Pattern C*, T-11 through L-2 associated with L-4 and L-5. (Modified from Errico, et al.[53])

fractures. Multiple spine fractures may occur, and three multilevel patterns have been recognized[130] (Fig. 15–6). Questionable radiologic findings should prompt further imaging with CT, but many institutions already simultaneously image head and cervical spine in patients with multisystem trauma. Important cervical spine fractures, however, may be over-

Table 15–3 CHECKLIST FOR THE DIAGNOSIS OF CLINICAL INSTABILITY IN THE MIDDLE AND LOWER CERVICAL SPINE

Element	Point Value
Anterior elements destroyed or unable to function	2
Posterior elements destroyed or unable to function	2
Positive stretch test	2
Radiographic criteria	4
A. Flexion/extension radiographs	
1. Sagittal plane translation > 3.5 mm or 20% (2 points)	
2. Sagittal plane rotation > 20° (2 points)	
or	
B. Resting radiographs	
1. Sagittal plane displacement > 3.5 mm or 20% (2 points)	
2. Relative sagittal plane angulation > 11° (2 points)	
Abnormal disc narrowing	1
Developmentally narrow spinal canal (sagittal diameter < 13 mm)	1
Spinal cord damage	2
Nerve root damage	1
Dangerous loading anticipated	1
Total of 5 or more points = unstable	

Adapted from White, AA III and Panjabi, MM: Clinical Biomechanics of the Spine, ed 2. JB Lippincott, Philadelphia, 1990, p 314.

looked with 4- to 10-mm slices, and occasionally a segment is not displayed on CT scan. Nevertheless, CT scanning has the major advantages of a lack of superimpositions and the potential for reconstruction. MRI,[126] because of its ability to image in multiple planes, should be considered the best method to date to demonstrate spinal cord damage.

Cervical Spine Injuries

Cervical spine injuries can be classified by mechanism of injury, which may guide choice of treatment.[3,37,53,59,82] Many trauma centers use White and Panjabi's classification for instability (Table 15–3). The most common cervical spine injuries are outlined in Figure 15–7.

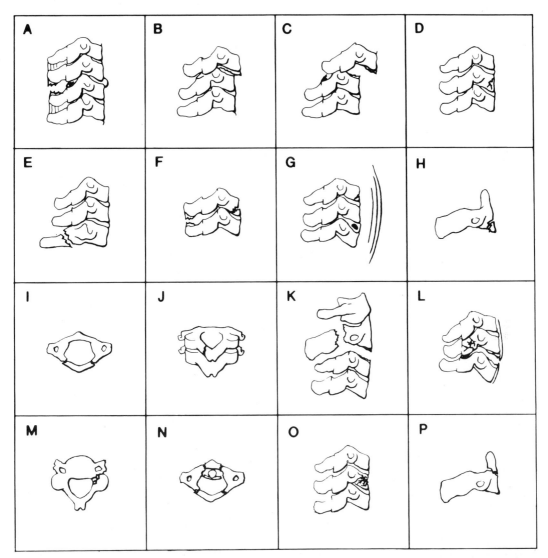

Figure 15–7. Cervical fractures. *A*, Hyperflexion sprain (stable but may become unstable; see text). *B*, Unilateral facet dislocation (unstable). *C*, Bilateral facet dislocation (unstable). *D*, Anterior wedge compression fracture (stable). *E*, Clay shoveler's fracture (stable). *F*, Teardrop fracture-dislocation (unstable). *G*, Hyperextension strain (stable). *H*, Teardrop fracture of axis (stable). *I*, Posterior arch fracture of atlas (stable). *J*, Laminar fracture (stable). *K*, Hangman's fracture (unstable). *L*, Hyperextension fracture-dislocation (unstable). *M*, Pillar fracture (stable). *N*, Jefferson C-1 fracture (unstable). *O*, Burst fracture of cervical body (stable). *P*, Odontoid fracture (unstable).

HYPERFLEXION INJURIES

Hyperflexion forces result in rupture of the posterior ligamentous complex, sometimes including the posterior portion of the annulus fibrosis. Rupture causes additional traumatic disc prolapse and compression fractures of the vertebral body.

Acute Anterior Subluxation (Hyperflexion Sprain) (Fig. 15–7A). Many patients will experience excruciating neck pain that limits neck flexion and extension. Neurologic findings are rarely demonstrated at the time of examination and seldom appear at later stages. Among the many posterior ligaments that can be torn with this type of injury are the supraspinous and interspinous ligaments, capsules of the interfacetal joints, and the posterior longitudinal ligament. When torn, they produce the characteristic radiographic findings of hyperkyphotic angulation, anterior glide of vertebra with some forward subluxation of the superior facets, and, often more evident, widening of the interspinous spaces.

This type of injury is potentially unstable, because significant angulation and subluxation may occur, necessitating follow-up flexion and extension views. Most patients are initially treated with a Philadelphia collar.

Unilateral Facet Dislocation (Fig. 15–7B). Common at C4-7 levels, this cervical spine injury is unstable. Nerve root injury may occur at the time of injury or during reduction. Radiologic features are anterior displacement of the superior vertebral body, usually within 50% of the anterior-posterior width of the vertebral body below the displaced segment. The retropharyngeal space is characteristically enlarged.

When the anterior displacement reaches 60% of the width of the underlying vertebral body, both facet joints are generally subluxed or dislocated. Impaction fractures of the interfacetal joint or articular mass may be an associated radiologic feature. Operative fixation is indicated.

Bilateral Facet Dislocation (Fig. 15–7C). A free-floating vertebral body, seen on the lateral view, predominantly involves the C5-6 and C6-7 levels and indicates complete disruption of all soft tissue structures. This type of cervical injury is unstable, and spinal cord damage is common. Open reduction is indicated when traction results in worsening of neurologic symptoms or is unable to reduce the dislocation. MRI or myelographic CT is indicated before open reduction to rule out an associated disc herniation. If a disc herniation is identified, the extruded fragment must be removed anteriorly before posterior reduction is done. Failure to follow this protocol may lead to cord compression from the extruded fragment during reduction, with potentially devastating neurologic sequelae.[51]

Anterior Wedge Compression Fracture (Fig. 15–7D). Wedge fractures of the C-5 or C-6 vertebral body are often associated with transient facet separation or other cervical injuries. This type of injury should be differentiated from a burst fracture of the vertebral body, which has a vertical fracture line and is caused by axial force rather than sudden flexion. Neurologic findings are usually absent. If there is no evidence of facet subluxation, this injury is stable and needs only radiologic follow-up to detect delayed instability.

Clay Shoveler's Fracture (Fig. 15–7E). A typical hyperflexion injury occurs in approximately 15% of all patients with cervical spine injury. This spinous process avulsion fracture is frequently seen in the C-7, T-1, or T-2 region on lateral projection films. The avulsed fragment may be small and dislocated, at times mimicking nuchal ligament calcification. Neurologic findings are absent, and this condition, if isolated, is generally stable, but radiologic follow-up with flexion and extension radiographs is necessary to detect instability.

Teardrop Fracture-Dislocation (Fig. 15–7F). Complete disruption of all ligaments and the vertebral disc at the level of injury produces a highly unstable injury and is sometimes detected on films only by a small triangular fragment in the anteroinferior corner. Other radiologic findings are posterior kyphotic angulation, retropulsion of the posterior portion of the vertebral body, and bilateral dislocated facet joints. Displacement of the vertebral body into the spinal canal frequently causes spinal cord injury, most commonly anterior spinal cord syndrome. Operative removal of disc material or bone fragments during operative stabilization unfortunately may not improve the overall poor outcome.

HYPEREXTENSION INJURIES

Retroflexion or hyperextension injuries may produce only ligamentous or muscular injuries. In the elderly population with cervical spondylosis, these injuries produce spinal cord syndromes.

Hyperextension Strain (Fig. 15–7G). The most important hallmark is conspicuous lack of radiologic features in a patient with otherwise severe cord injury. Subtle findings are prevertebral swelling, small horizontally oriented avulsion chips from the anteroinferior margin of the vertebral body, gas phenomena or vacuum defect, and widening of a disc space. The clinical findings are striking, consisting of either a complete cord lesion or a central cord syndrome.[119] Both pincer action and vertical tearing of nervous tissue produce hemorrhage in the central cord. The typical clinical features of a central cord syndrome are arm and hand weakness more prominent than leg weakness and preservation of the sacral segments and perianal sensation.[119] Bladder and bowel function as well as some upper arm function may return, but spasticity of the legs usually remains in some degree.

Teardrop Fracture of Axis (Fig. 15–7H). In patients with severe osteoporosis or advanced cervical spondylosis, a large triangular fragment may chip from the body of the axis and can be recognized radiologically by larger vertical height than transverse width and by prevertebral soft tissue swelling. This fracture should be differentiated from a teardrop fracture in a flexion injury. This fracture is stable in flexion and is not associated with spinal cord damage.

Posterior Arch Fracture of Atlas (Fig. 15–7I). Absence of bilateral displacement of lateral masses of C-1 relative to C-2 on the open mouth odontoid view and absence of anterior arch fracture differentiate this fracture from the Jefferson burst fracture. (The fracture line is posterior to lateral masses and the transverse atlantal ligament.) The fracture is stable and is uncommonly associated with neurologic symptoms. However, one should carefully look for associated hyperextension fractures and type II odontoid fractures.

Laminar Fractures (Fig. 15–7J). Hyperextension injuries are most common in elderly persons with spondylosis. Neurologic abnormalities can be expected only when laminar fragments are displaced into the spinal canal. CT scan may be more sensitive than plain films for diagnosis. This injury is stable because the anterior column and facet joints are intact.

Traumatic Spondylolisthesis of C-2 (Hangman's Fracture) (Fig. 15–7K). This uncommon cervical spine injury (7% of all cervical injuries) is caused by abrupt deceleration and is frequently accompanied by severe closed head injury, facial trauma, and lung contusion. Traumatic spondylolisthesis seldom produces neurologic signs. In a series of 181 patients, 8 (4%) had some neurologic findings but 6 of the 8 completely recovered.[63]

The degree and type of displacement of the anterior fragment are important. Type I fractures are isolated hairline fractures of the axis ring with minimal displacement. The disc space between C-2 and C-3 is normal, and the injury at this stage is stable. In type II fractures, the disc space C2-3 is abnormal, and the body of C-2 is displaced. The body of C-2 usually shows some anterior angulation. Type III fractures are characterized by definite displacement and flexion of the body of C-2 and bilateral interfacetal dislocation of C-2 and C-3.

Both types II and III fractures are considered unstable and are frequently treated with closed reduction with traction before halo vest placement. Type III fractures often require operative intervention. This flexion-distraction injury pattern is unstable in traction, and stretch of the spinal cord may occur. Direct application of a halo vest without traction is the appropriate form of management of this injury.[103]

Hyperextension Fracture-Dislocation (Fig. 15–7L). Anterior displacement of the vertebral body (usually at the C4–7 level), horizontal rotation of the fractured articular pillar, and anterior displacement of the pillar into the intervertebral foramen are typical radiologic findings. Either the facet is severely comminuted or the inferior facet of the superior vertebra is driven upward. The condition is unstable, largely because the facet joints are disrupted.

Pillar Fracture (Fig. 15–7M). Simultaneous hyperextension and bending to one side may cause vertical fractures of the articular mass that may extend into the transverse process of the pedicle or posteriorly into the lamina. Pillar views or CT scanning is necessary to demonstrate this fracture, which occasionally produces an acute radiculopathy.

VERTICAL COMPRESSION

Typically, heavy weights dropped on top of the skull or, more commonly, hitting of the skull on the bottom of a swimming pool causes vertical compression fractures.

Jefferson C-1 Fracture (Fig. 15–7N). This uncommon fracture complex consists of two fractures on each side involving the anterior and posterior sides of the arch of C-1. Prevertebral soft tissue swelling may be prominent, and with disruption of the transverse ligament, one of the lateral masses may spread more than 7 mm.

Widening of the lateral atlantodental interval is another feature of disruption of the transverse ligament (more than 3 mm). The involvement of the transverse ligament determines instability of the injury.

In a review of 15 patients from the Northwestern University Acute Spine Center, 4 had spinal cord injury.[116] Management is generally conservative, but posterior C1-2 fusion (after healing of the C-1 fracture) is an option in unstable injuries with disruption of the transverse ligament.

Burst Fracture of the Cervical Body (Fig. 15–7O). All ligamentous structures are intact; therefore, the bony lesion is stable, but spinal cord injury is common because disc material and fragments are forced into the spinal canal. Surgical removal and bone grafting are frequently done when canal intrusion is significant.

MISCELLANEOUS CERVICAL SPINE INJURIES

The mechanisms underlying these injuries are not understood. Most likely, multiple vector forces contribute.

Odontoid Fractures (Fig. 15–7P). Odontoid fractures can be classified into three types.[5,65,81] Type I is an avulsion of the tip, type II (the most common) is a fracture through the neck of the odontoid, and type III is a fracture extending into the body of C-2.

Most patients have only neck stiffness, pain, or torticollis, which may occur weeks after injury. Surgical fixation is often required in type II fractures. Other types heal successfully with conservative treatment.

A common pitfall is os odontoideum in type II fractures. Radiologic differences are difficult to interpret, but in os odontoideum, the ossicle is rounded and widely separated from the base of the odontoid.

Thoracolumbar Spine Injuries

Many algorithms have been proposed for management of thoracolumbar fractures.[1] In many of them, CT, myelographic, or MRI demonstration of cord compression with more than 50% narrowing of the bone canal is an indication for decompression and fusion.

COMPRESSION FLEXION FRACTURE (FIG. 15–8A)

Neurologic findings can be expected in patients with fractures that cause narrowing of the spinal canal. The neurologic signs and symptoms may also progressively worsen over time, and then usually within 2 days after the onset of trauma. The chance of cord damage, however, remains relatively small, approximately 10%. (This type of fracture should be differentiated from a burst fracture, which is invariably caused by axial damage and has an up to 60% chance of cord injury; in general, if the canal is narrowed, it is most likely a burst fracture.)

Operative treatment is indicated only in the most severe compression fractures.

DISTRACTIVE FLEXION FRACTURE (FIG. 15–8B)

This fracture is well known because of its association with lap seatbelt injury. The impact often causes rupture of a hollow viscus, such as the duodenum. Radiologically, a wide disruption through the body, spinous process, and disc is seen, at times associated with

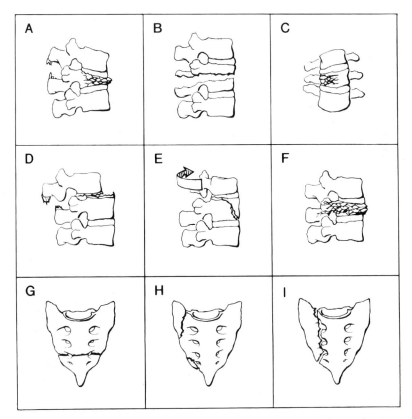

Figure 15–8. Thoracolumbar and sacral fractures. *A*, Compression flexion fracture. *B*, Distractive flexion fracture. *C*, Lateral flexion fracture. *D*, Fracture-dislocation. *E*, Rotation dislocation. *F*, Burst fracture. *G*, Transverse sacral fracture. *H* and *I*, Vertical sacral fractures.

fracture of the spinous process, so-called chance fracture. Most injuries are ligamentous and do not involve the bone. Bony injuries often heal with bracing, whereas ligamentous injuries generally require surgery.

LATERAL FLEXION FRACTURE (FIG. 15–8C)

An acute lateral bending of the spine causes shortening of the vertebral body. Neurologic involvement is rare.

FRACTURE-DISLOCATIONS (FIG. 15–8D)

A high incidence of spinal cord injury can be expected if fractures are located in the thoracic area. Transection is less common in the lumbar area because the spinal canal is wider.

ROTATION DISLOCATION (FIG. 15–8E)

Tension and compression may cause a very unstable fracture of the thoraco-lumbar spine severe enough to produce complete transection of the spinal cord. Operative stabilization is mandatory.

BURST FRACTURE (FIG. 15–8F)

Many of these types of fractures are located between T-10 and L-2,[12] and the vertical impact frequently causes lower extremity fractures, particularly of the knee and calcaneus. Whether the approach should be conservative or operative is controversial. The proponents of surgical stabilization[96,168] have reasoned that post-traumatic kyphosis and progressive neurologic deterioration may occur with the conservative approach. Nevertheless, even with compression of the spinal canal, neurologic deterioration does not necessarily occur.

MISCELLANEOUS THORACOLUMBAR INJURIES

Rare fractures of the thoracic and lumbar spine are distractive extension and lumbosacral dislocation, both with infrequent neurologic damage.

Isolated chip fractures of the transverse processes or spinous processes may be found but do not produce any nerve damage, except that T1-2 transverse fractures may damage the brachial plexus.

Sacral Fractures

Sacral fractures are almost invariably associated with pelvic fractures.[28,29] The mechanism of neurologic injury may involve direct bony compression of nerve roots at the level of the foramina entry, stretching and avulsion of plexus lumbosacral roots, or a cauda equina lesion. The incidence of neurologic involvement depends on the type of sacral fracture.[35,50,125,144]

TRANSVERSE SACRAL FRACTURES (FIG. 15–8G)

Most transverse sacral fractures are at the level of the os coccyx, so that neurologic function remains intact. Higher level fractures are unstable, and their proximity to the foramina produces nerve root damage in most patients.

VERTICAL SACRAL FRACTURES (FIG. 15–8H AND 15–8I)

Denis and associates[45] divided sacral fractures into three zones. Zone I fractures are avulsion fractures of the sacrotuberous ligament or alar fractures, both with a low incidence of nerve root or bladder function damage. Zone II involves a fracture line through the foramina. In one series, L-5 involvement was most frequent, resulting in footdrop. Bladder involvement occurred in 4 of 23 patients.[45] Fractures into the central canal (zone III) may spare nerve roots in 50% of the patients, but bowel, bladder, and sexual dysfunction is common. Operative decompression may result in significant improvement in ambulation and bladder function.

ACUTE SPINAL CORD INJURY

Fractures and dislocations of the spine may contuse the spinal cord,[14-16,167] but direct forces may injure the cord over several segments as well. Complete transection of the cord is rare. Patients who enter the trauma intensive care unit may have maximal deficits from spinal shock rather than permanent immediate complete damage. Likewise, pharmacologic treatment of acute spinal cord injury assumes that additional biochemical damage is causing secondary injury that can potentially be arrested or ameliorated. The pathophysiology of secondary spinal cord injury is not elucidated, but many investigators in this field have postulated that lipid peroxidation leads to neuronal damage through release of free radicals and excitatory amino acids and that the post-traumatic microvascular injury results from vasoconstriction, platelet aggregation, and edema. Animal experiments have supported the existence of complex cascades of tissue injuries, and the reader is referred to scholarly reviews on this subject.[79,161] Early randomized trials have already resulted in promising agents for treatment, such as methylprednisolone and GM-1 ganglioside.[23,24,68,180]

Spinal cord injury is very dramatic in presentation and does not necessarily have to remain unrecognized in emergency trauma units. High-level cervical spinal cord injury (above the C-3 level) instantaneously paralyzes the respiratory muscles. The generation of sufficient tidal volumes is impossible because diaphragmatic expansion and abdominal muscle function are lost.[98,109] In patients with cervical cord injury above C-3, paradoxical inward movement of the rib cage and excessive use of neck muscles can be observed, but most patients are already intubated and mechanically ventilated. (Guidelines for intubation, with use of fiberoptic bronchoscopy, in presumed cervical spine injury have been described.[49,93])

More commonly, however, respiratory function in patients with multisystem trauma is compromised because fractured ribs or hemothorax is present. Neurogenic pulmonary edema may occur in acute spinal cord injury,[25,30,92,133,173] but cardiac or lung contusion may be a more common mechanism. In lower cervical spinal cord injury, respiration is characterized by postural dependence of breathing, and vital capacity increases in the supine position secondary to the pressure effect of the abdominal contents. Abdominal binders are needed for mobilization. Neurologic involvement between the C-1 and T-6 segments results in sympathetic loss, hypotension, hypothermia, and bradycardia from unopposed vagal function. Hypotension may theoretically increase secondary spinal cord injury[111] and should be aggressively treated with anti-Trendelenburg positioning, fluid administration, dopamine, or phenylephrine.[2,97] Nevertheless, differentiation from hypovolemic shock is virtually impossible in the acute stage. In spinal shock, peritoneal signs and symptoms may be absent. Therefore, in many trauma centers, when hypotension is present an abdominal tap, echocardiogram, or abdominal CT scan is done in patients with multitrauma.

Bradyarrhythmias, when refractory to atropine or beta-adrenergic agonist, may need cardiac pacing, but this situation seldom occurs.[54]

In the flaccid paralysis of spinal shock, fecal and urinary retention occurs, but it may disappear in some patients after months. In an atonic bladder, an indwelling catheter should be immediately placed.[39] A nasogastric tube should also be placed, because gastric atony may result in a considerable risk for aspiration. Neurologic assessment of the level of cord damage should be done immediately. Several key points in motor and sensory examination may assist in localization (Fig. 15–9).

Medical treatment of spinal cord injury has been advanced by the recent results of the National Acute Spinal

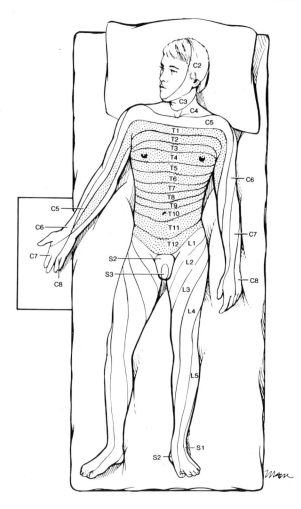

Figure 15-9. Distribution of sensory segments.

Cord Injury Study (NASCIS), which showed that recovery was significantly greater in patients treated with methylprednisolone within 8 hours after cord damage (intravenous bolus of 30 mg/kg followed by infusion with 5.4 mg/kg per hour for 23 hours).[23,24] GM-1 gangliosides are effective as well but are not yet routinely used.[68]

POST-TRAUMATIC NEUROPATHIES ASSOCIATED WITH FRACTURES

Isolated nerve injuries and plexopathies are uncommon in patients with multitrauma and require the expertise of neurosurgeons and orthopedic surgeons. Clinical decision-making often focuses on whether to explore the injured area or wait for spontaneous recovery.

Brachial Plexopathies

Traumatic brachial plexus palsy is frequently seen in young patients after motorcycle accidents.[67] In the initial assessment of brachial plexus injuries, careful evaluation of the magnitude of nerve damage is important, because secondary deterioration may be associated with the development of a false aneurysm or an arteriovenous fistula in an axillary artery that needs immediate surgical intervention.

Closed brachial plexus injuries may be approached by differentiating patients who have a proximal injury from those who have a postganglionic injury.

Proximal brachial plexus injury is manifested by Horner's syndrome (C-8 to T-1), winging of the scapula, and paralysis of the rhomboids. Diaphragmatic paralysis is occasionally present. Electromyographic and sensory nerve studies are usually performed 6 to 8 weeks after the initial insult and may differentiate a preganglionic from a postganglionic lesion. Normal sensory conduction from the anesthetic median or radial nerve area of the hand strongly suggests a preganglionic injury at the C6-7 level. Somatosensory studies may also be helpful. Subsequently, myelography, CT myelography, or MRI[74] is done to exclude rootlet avulsion in case plexus repair is considered. (In most patients, 3 months must have elapsed without spontaneous improvement.)

Similarly, in postganglionic injuries of the brachial plexus, operative repair is considered if no clinical or electromyographic improvement is found after 3 months. Detailed discussion of nerve repair techniques can be found in textbooks and review articles.[4,94,101]

Lumbosacral Plexus Injury

Far less common than traumatic brachial plexus lesions, lumbosacral plexus injury can result from compression or stretching of the plexus in sacral and pelvic fractures.[154] External iliac artery injury occasionally accompanies the nerve damage.[18] MRI may be useful in establishing lumbosacral nerve root avulsion,[64] which precludes operative correction. Outcome of traumatic lumbosacral plexus injury is unpredictable but often poor.

Miscellaneous Isolated Neuropathies Associated with Fractures

Fractures of the ulna have been associated with complete paralysis of the anterior interosseous nerve, a motor branch of the median nerve. A characteristic feature is weakness of the flexor pollicis longus or flexor digitorum profundus and pronator quadratus without any sensory deficit. Patients may notice abnormal pinching, which can easily be demonstrated when they are asked to make a circle with thumb and index finger. Complete recovery may take months.[117]

Acute median nerve damage may also occur in wrist fractures[10] (for example, Colles' fractures) or may be exacerbated after immobilization of wrist fractures in marked flexion.[69] Entrapment of the ulnar nerve at the elbow region may occur in supracondylar humeral fractures.[114] Neurolysis with anterior transposition has resulted in satisfactory outcomes, but a comparison with conservative management is not available.[13]

Radial nerve paralysis associated with fractures of the humerus has been frequently reported, usually with fractures of the distal part of the humerus. Excellent recovery was reported in a series of 62 patients, 95% of whom regained normal radial nerve function.[151] Clinical recovery occurred within 1 month in one third of the patients, and the remainder improved within 6 months.

Other peripheral nerve injuries are axillary nerve damage (anterior dislocation of the shoulder) and damage to the sciatic nerve (dislocation of the acetabulum of the pelvis), both with potential for complete recovery.

FAT EMBOLISM SYNDROME

Embolization of fat and fatty acids from bone marrow of long bones that have been fractured probably occurs in most patients with multitrauma, but a typical clinical fat embolism syndrome develops in only a minority (3% to 4%).[104] In general, 12 to 75 hours after the initial traumatic impact, the patient's condition deteriorates in parallel with laboratory changes.

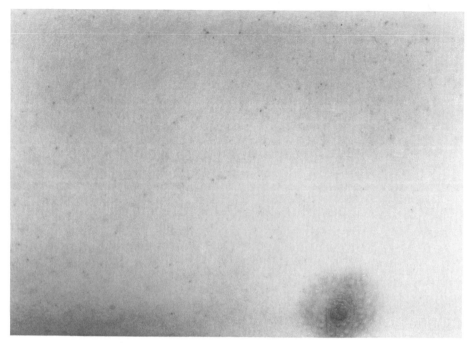

Figure 15–10. Petechiae on chest in fat embolism syndrome.

Sudden tachypnea and tachycardia, fever, and development of a large A-a gradient are the first clinical indicators of the lodging of fat globules in the pulmonary vasculature. A pleural friction rub may be heard, but this sign is almost always absent. A pathognomonic sign, present in 50% of patients, is a petechial rash appearing suddenly on the chest (Fig. 15–10), axillary folds, and, occasionally, conjunctiva. Cotton-wool spots, petechial hemorrhages, and intravascular fat globules may be seen in the fundi but only in patients with widespread skin petechiae and thrombocytopenia.

Central nervous involvement is most often manifested by an acute confusional state,[55,60,72,77,78,86,104] but focal signs and generalized tonic-clonic seizures may be temporarily seen. Laboratory findings that support the diagnosis are urinary fat bodies identified by Sudan red staining. The diagnostic criteria for fat embolism syndrome are summarized in Table 15–4. The clinical diagnosis becomes fairly certain when at least one major and four minor criteria are present. Recently, bronchoalveolar lavage was shown to rapidly confirm the diagnosis, and this may become the preferred diagnostic test in patients with unexplained neurologic deterioration after multitrauma and fractures.[33]

In patients without pulmonary symptoms, cerebral fat embolization can at times be explained by a patent foramen ovale. In other patients, however, the pathway of fat globules is presumably similar to that of air emboli small enough to pass through the lungs. Neuropathologic studies in patients with central nervous system involvement have repeatedly demonstrated fat droplets in both white and gray matter and multiple microinfarcts. Petechiae are often found in the centrum semiovale, brain stem, and cerebellum.[90]

Imaging studies of the brain are often nondiagnostic, but multiple hypodensities in the frontal white matter[147] have been noted on CT scan. A massive pontine hemorrhagic infarct has been re-

Table 15−4 CLINICAL CRITERIA FOR FAT EMBOLISM SYNDROME

Major	*Minor*
• Axillary or subconjunctival petechiae • $PaO_2 < 60$ mm Hg, $FIO_2 \leq 0.4$ • Central nervous system symptoms • Pulmonary edema, acute respiratory distress syndrome	• Tachycardia > 110/min • Temperature > 38.5°C • Retinal emboli • Fat in urine • Fat in sputum • Decreased hematocrit and platelets, increased erythrocyte sedimentation rate

Modified from Gurd, AR: Fat embolism syndrome: An aid to diagnosis. J Bone Joint Surg Br 52:732–737, 1970.

ported in one patient with nontraumatic fat embolism.[112] Multiple scattered spotty white matter lesions resembling demyelination have been documented on T2-weighted MRI, with complete resolution in one patient.[146]

Fat embolism syndrome can be rapidly fatal, but in most patients clinical signs resolve within 24 hours. Treatment should be focused on immediate stabilization of the fracture. Early repair of the fracture decreases the risk of fat embolization.

CONCLUSIONS

Management of patients with multitrauma starts in the field and in the emergency department. The risks of secondary brain damage in these patients are well documented, even in designated trauma centers. The most challenging patient is the one who "talks and deteriorates" after normal findings on the initial CT scan. Important causes are subdural or epidural hematoma, fat embolization, and delayed hemorrhagic frontal or temporal lobe contusion. In patients with limited subdural or epidural hematoma, placement of a fiberoptic monitor may detect increasing intracranial pressure if emergency surgery for reasons other than head injury is contemplated (for example, abdominal exploration, orthopedic surgery). Ideally, patients with multitrauma and head injury should also be cared for by neurointensive care specialists and neurosurgeons, who can appreciate delicate changes in neurologic condition and changes in imaging studies of the brain and spine.

REFERENCES

1. Aebi, M, Mohler, J, Zäch, G, and Morscher, E: Analysis of 75 operated thoracolumbar fractures and fracture dislocations with and without neurological deficit. Arch Orthop Trauma Surg 105:100–112, 1986.
2. Alexander, S and Kerr, FWL: Blood pressure responses in acute compression of the spinal cord. J Neurosurg 21:485–491, 1964.
3. Allen, BL Jr, Ferguson, RL, Lehmann, TR, and O'Brien, RP: A mechanistic classification of closed, indirect fractures and dislocations of the lower cervical spine. Spine 7:1–27, 1982.
4. Alnot, JY: Traumatic brachial plexus palsy in the adult: Retro- and infraclavicular lesions. Clin Orthop 237:9–16, 1988.
5. Anderson, LD and D'Alonzo, RT: Fractures of the odontoid process of the axis. J Bone Joint Surg [Am] 56:1663–1674, 1974.
6. Andrews, BT, Chiles, BW, Olsen, WL, and Pitts, LH: The effect of intracerebral hematoma location on the risk of brain-stem compression and on clinical outcome. J Neurosurg 69:518–522, 1988.
7. Andrews, BT, Pitts, LH, Lovely, MP, and Bartkowski, H: Is computed tomographic scanning necessary in patients with tentorial herniation? Results of immediate surgical exploration without computed tomography in

100 patients. Neurosurgery 19:408–414, 1986.

8. Andrews, PJD, Piper, IR, Dearden, NM, and Miller, JD: Secondary insults during intrahospital transport of head-injured patients. Lancet 335:327–330, 1990.

9. Arienta, C, Baiguini, M, Granata, G, and Villani, R: Acute bilateral epidural hematomas: Report of two cases and review of the literature. J Neurosurg Sci 30:139–142, 1986.

10. Aro, H, Koivunen, T, Katevuo, K, et al: Late compression neuropathies after Colles' fractures. Clin Orthop 233:217–225, 1988.

11. Ashkenazi, E, Constantini, S, Pomeranz, S, et al: Delayed epidural hematoma without neurologic deficit. J Trauma 30:613–615, 1990.

12. Atlas, SW, Regenbogen, V, Rogers, LF, and Kim, KS: The radiographic characterization of burst fractures of the spine. AJR Am J Roentgenol 147:575–582, 1986.

13. Barrios, C, Ganoza, C, de Pablos, J, and Cañadell, J: Posttraumatic ulnar neuropathy versus non-traumatic cubital tunnel syndrome: Clinical features and response to surgery. Acta Neurochir 110:44–48, 1991.

14. Bedbrook, GM: Treatment of thoracolumbar dislocation and fractures with paraplegia. Clin Orthop 112:27–43, 1975.

15. Bedbrook, GM: Spinal injuries with tetraplegia and paraplegia. J Bone Joint Surg Br 61:267–284, 1979.

16. Bedbrook, GM and Clark, WB: Thoracic spine injuries with spinal cord damage. J R Coll Surg Edinb 26:264–271, 1981.

17. Bešenski, N, Jadro-Šantel, D, and Grčević, N: Patterns of lesions of corpus callosum in inner cerebral trauma visualized by computed tomography. Neuroradiology 34:126–130, 1992.

18. Birchard, JD, Pichora, DR, and Brown, PM: External iliac artery and lumbosacral plexus injury secondary to an open book fracture of the pelvis: Report of a case. J Trauma 30:906–908, 1990.

19. Borel, C, Hanley, D, Diringer, MN, and Rogers, MC: Intensive management of severe head injury. Chest 98:180–189, 1990.

20. Borovich, B, Braun, J, Guilburd, JN, et al: Delayed onset of traumatic extradural hematoma. J Neurosurg 63:30–34, 1985.

21. Boyko, OB, Cooper, DF, and Grossman, CB: Contrast-enhanced CT of acute isodense subdural hematoma. AJNR Am J Neuroradiol 12:341–343, 1991.

22. Braakman, R: Depressed skull fracture: Data, treatment, and follow-up in 225 consecutive cases. J Neurol Neurosurg Psychiatry 35:395–402, 1972.

23. Bracken, MB, Shepard, MJ, Collins, WF, et al: A randomized, controlled trial of methylprednisolone or naloxone in the treatment of acute spinal cord injury. N Engl J Med 322:1405–1411, 1990.

24. Bracken, MB, Shepard, MJ, Collins, WF Jr, et al: Methylprednisolone or naloxone treatment after acute spinal cord injury: 1-year follow-up data. J Neurosurg 76:23–31, 1992.

25. Brisman, R, Kovach, RM, Johnson, DO, et al: Pulmonary edema in acute transection of the spinal cord. Surg Gynecol Obstet 139:363–366, 1974.

26. Bucci, MN, Phillips, TW, and McGillicuddy, JE: Delayed epidural hemorrhage in hypotensive multiple trauma patients. Neurosurgery 19:65–68, 1986.

27. Bullock, R, Golek, J, and Blake, G: Traumatic intracerebral hematoma—which patients should undergo surgical evacuation? CT scan features and ICP monitoring as a basis for decision making. Surg Neurol 32:181–187, 1989.

28. Byrnes, DP, Russo, GL, Ducker, TB, and Cowley, RA: Sacrum fractures and neurological damage: Report of two cases. J Neurosurg 47:459–462, 1977.

29. Carl, A, Delman, A, and Engler, G: Displaced transverse sacral fractures: A case report, review of the literature, and the CT scan as an aid in management. Clin Orthop 194:195–198, 1985.

30. Carter, RE: Respiratory aspects of spi-

nal cord injury management. Paraplegia 25:262–266, 1987.

31. Cervantes, LA: Concurrent delayed temporal and posterior fossa epidural hematomas: Case report. J Neurosurg 59:351–353, 1983.

32. Chan, K-H, Dearden, NM, and Miller, JD: The significance of posttraumatic increase in cerebral blood flow velocity: A transcranial Doppler ultrasound study. Neurosurgery 30:697–700, 1992.

33. Chastre, J, Fagon, J-Y, Soler, P, et al: Bronchoalveolar lavage for rapid diagnosis of the fat embolism syndrome in trauma patients. Ann Intern Med 113:583–588, 1990.

34. Chen, T-Y, Wong, C-W, Chang, C-N, et al: The expectant treatment of "asymptomatic" supratentorial epidural hematomas. Neurosurgery 32:176–179, 1993.

35. Chiaruttini, M: Transverse sacral fracture with transient neurologic complication. Ann Emerg Med 16:111–113, 1987.

36. Clifton, GL, Robertson, CS, Grossman, RG, et al: The metabolic response to severe head injury. J Neurosurg 60:687–696, 1984.

37. Cloward, RB: Acute cervical spine injuries. Clin Symp 32:1–32, 1980.

38. Colquhoun, IR and Rawlinson, J: The significance of haematomas of the basal ganglia in closed head injury. Clin Radiol 40:619–621, 1989.

39. Comarr, AE: Neurourology of spinal cord-injured patients. Semin Urol 10:74–82, 1992.

40. Cooper, KR, Boswell, PA, and Choi, SC: Safe use of PEEP in patients with severe head injury. J Neurosurg 63:552–555, 1985.

41. Craig, GR and Nielsen, MS: Rigid cervical collars and intracranial pressure. Intensive Care Med 17:504–505, 1991.

42. Crutchfield, JS, Narayan, RK, Robertson, CS, and Michael, LH: Evaluation of a fiberoptic intracranial pressure monitor. J Neurosurg 72:482–487, 1990.

43. Dearden, NM, Gibson, JS, McDowall, DG, et al: Effect of high-dose dexamethasone on outcome from severe head injury. J Neurosurg 64:81–88, 1986.

44. Delfini, R, Santoro, A, Innocenzi, G, et al: Interhemispheric subdural hematoma (ISH): Case report. J Neurosurg Sci 35:217–220, 1991.

45. Denis, F, Davis, S, and Comfort, T: Sacral fractures: An important problem; retrospective analysis of 236 cases. Clin Orthop 227:67–81, 1988.

46. Dharker, SR and Bhargava, N: Bilateral epidural haematoma. Acta Neurochir (Wien) 110:29–32, 1991.

47. Diaz, FG, Yock, DH Jr, Larson, D, and Rockswold, GL: Early diagnosis of delayed posttraumatic intracerebral hematomas. J Neurosurg 50:217–223, 1979.

48. Di Rocco, A, Ellis, SJ, and Landes, C: Delayed epidural hematoma. Neuroradiology 33:253–254, 1991.

49. Doolan, LA and O'Brien, JF: Safe intubation in cervical spine injury. Anaesth Intensive Care 13:319–324, 1985.

50. Dowling, T, Epstein, JA, and Epstein, NE: S1-S2 sacral fracture involving neural elements of the cauda equina: A case report and review of the literature. Spine 10:851–853, 1985.

51. Eismont, FJ, Arena, MJ, and Green, BA: Extrusion of an intervertebral disc associated with traumatic subluxation or dislocation of cervical facets. J Bone Joint Surg [Am] 73:1555–1560, 1991.

52. Elsner, H, Rigamonti, D, Corradino, G, et al: Delayed traumatic intracerebral hematomas: "Spät-Apoplexie": Report of two cases. J Neurosurg 72:813–815, 1990.

53. Errico, TJ, Bauer, RD, and Waugh, T (eds): Spinal Trauma. JB Lippincott, Philadelphia, 1991.

54. Evans, DE, Kobrine, AI, and Rizzoli, HV: Cardiac arrhythmias accompanying acute compression of the spinal cord. J Neurosurg 52:52–59, 1980.

55. Fabian, TC, Hoots, AV, Stanford, DS, et al: Fat embolism syndrome: Prospective evaluation in 92 fracture patients. Crit Care Med 18:42–46, 1990.

56. Farling, PA, Johnston, JR, and Coppel, DL: Propofol infusion for sedation of patients with head injury intensive

care: A preliminary report. Anaesthesia 44:222–226, 1989.

57. Feldman, Z, Kanter, MJ, Robertson, CS, et al: Effect of head elevation on intracranial pressure, cerebral perfusion pressure, and cerebral blood flow in head-injured patients. J Neurosurg 76:207–211, 1992.

58. Feuerman, T, Wackym, PA, Gade, GF, et al: Intraoperative development of contralateral epidural hematoma during evacuation of traumatic extraaxial hematoma. Neurosurgery 23:480–484, 1988.

59. Fielding, JW: Injuries to the upper cervical spine. Instr Course Lect 36:483–494, 1987.

60. Findlay, JM and DeMajo, W: Cerebral fat embolism. Can Med Assoc J 131:755–757, 1984.

61. Firsching, R, Frowein, RA, and Thun, F: Intracerebellar haematoma: Eleven traumatic and nontraumatic cases and a review of the literature. Neurochirurgia (Stuttg) 30:182–185, 1987.

62. Forbes, AR and Gamsu, G: Depression of lung mucociliary clearance by thiopental and halothane. Anesth Analg 58:387–389, 1979.

63. Francis, WR, Fielding, JW, Hawkins, RJ, et al: Traumatic spondylolisthesis of the axis. J Bone Joint Surg [Br] 63:313–318, 1981.

64. Freedy, RM, Miller, KD Jr, Eick, JJ, and Granke, DS: Traumatic lumbosacral nerve root avulsion: Evaluation by MR imaging. J Comput Assist Tomogr 13:1052–1057, 1989.

65. Fuji, E, Kobayashi, K, and Hirabayashi, K: Treatment in fractures of the odontoid process. Spine 13:604–609, 1988.

66. Fujitsu, K, Kuwabara, T, Muramoto, M, et al: Traumatic intraventricular hemorrhage: Report of twenty-six cases and consideration of the pathogenic mechanism. Neurosurgery 23:423–430, 1988.

67. Gebarski, KS, Glazer, GM, and Gebarski, SS: Brachial plexus: Anatomic, radiologic, and pathologic correlation using computed tomography. J Comput Assist Tomogr 6:1058–1063, 1982.

68. Geisler, FH, Dorsey, FC, and Coleman, WP: Recovery of motor function after spinal cord injury: A randomized, placebo-controlled trial with GM-1 ganglioside. N Engl J Med 324:1829–1838, 1991.

69. Gelberman, RH, Szabo, RM, and Mortensen, WW: Carpal tunnel pressures and wrist position in patients with Colles' fractures. J Trauma 24:747–749, 1984.

70. Gentry, LR, Godersky, JC, and Thompson, B: MR imaging of head trauma: Review of the distribution and radiopathologic features of traumatic lesions. AJR Am J Roentgenol 150:663–672, 1988.

71. Gentry, LR, Godersky, JC, Thompson, B, and Dunn, VD: Prospective comparative study of intermediate-field MR and CT in the evaluation of closed head trauma. AJR Am J Roentgenol 150:673–682, 1988.

72. Gossling, HR and Pellegrini, VD Jr: Fat embolism syndrome: A review of the pathophysiology and physiological basis of treatment. Clin Orthop 165:68–82, 1982.

73. Gudeman, SK, Kishore, PRS, Miller, JD, et al: The genesis and significance of delayed traumatic intracerebral hematoma. Neurosurgery 5:309–312, 1979.

74. Gupta, RK, Mehta, VS, Banerji, AK, and Jain, RK: MR evaluation of brachial plexus injuries. Neuroradiology 31:377–381, 1989.

75. Gutman, MB, Moulton, RJ, Sullivan, I, et al: Risk factors predicting operable intracranial hematomas in head injury. J Neurosurg 77:9–14, 1992.

76. Hadley, DM, Teasdale, GM, Jenkins, A, et al: Magnetic resonance imaging in acute head injury. Clin Radiol 39:131–139, 1988.

77. Hagley, SR: The fulminant fat embolism syndrome. Anaesth Intensive Care 11:167–170, 1983.

78. Hagley, SR, Lee, FC, and Blumbergs, PC: Fat embolism syndrome with total hip replacement. Med J Aust 145:541–543, 1986.

79. Hall, ED: The neuroprotective pharmacology of methylprednisolone. J Neurosurg 76:13–22, 1992.

80. Hamilton, M and Wallace, C: Nonoper-

ative management of acute epidural hematoma diagnosed by CT: The neuroradiologist's role. AJNR Am J Neuroradiol 13:853–859, 1992.

81. Hanssen, AD and Cabanela, ME: Fractures of the dens in adult patients. J Trauma 27:928–934, 1987.

82. Harris, JH Jr and Edeiken-Monroe, B: Radiology of Acute Cervical Spine Trauma. Williams & Wilkins, Baltimore, 1987.

83. Herregods, L, Verbeke, J, Rolly, G, and Colardyn, F: Effect of propofol on elevated intracranial pressure. Preliminary results. Anaesthesia 43 Suppl: 107–109, 1988.

84. Hesselink, JR, Dowd, CF, Healy, ME, et al: MR imaging of brain contusions: A comparative study with CT. AJR Am J Roentgenol 150:1133–1142, 1988.

85. Howard, MA III, Gross, AS, Dacey, RG Jr, and Winn HR: Acute subdural hematomas: An age-dependent clinical entity. J Neurosurg 71:858–863, 1989.

86. Jacobson, DM, Terrence, CF, and Reinmuth, OM: The neurologic manifestations of fat embolism. Neurology 36:847–851, 1986.

87. Jayakumar, PN, Kolluri, VRS, Basavakumar, DG, et al: Prognosis in traumatic intraventricular haemorrhage. Acta Neurochir (Wien) 106:48–51, 1990.

88. Jennett, B, Miller, JD, and Braakman, R: Epilepsy after nonmissile depressed skull fracture. J Neurosurg 41:208–216, 1974.

89. Jones, NR, Blumbergs, PC, and North, JB: Acute subdural haematomas: Aetiology, pathology and outcome. Aust N Z J Surg 56:907–913, 1986.

90. Kamenar, E and Burger, PC: Cerebral fat embolism: A neuropathological study of a microembolic state. Stroke 11:477–484, 1980.

91. Katz, DI, Alexander, MP, Seliger, GM, and Bellas, DN: Traumatic basal ganglia hemorrhage: Clinicopathologic features and outcome. Neurology 39:897–904, 1989.

92. Kiker, JD, Woodside, JR, and Jelinek, GE: Neurogenic pulmonary edema associated with autonomic dysreflexia. J Urol 128:1038–1039, 1982.

93. King, H-K, Wang, L-F, Khan, AK, and Wooten, DJ: Translaryngeal guided intubation for difficult intubation. Crit Care Med 15:869–871, 1987.

94. Kline, DG and Judice, DJ: Operative management of selected brachial plexus lesions. J Neurosurg 58:631–649, 1983.

95. Knuckey, NW, Gelbard, S, and Epstein, MH: The management of "asymptomatic" epidural hematomas: A prospective study. J Neurosurg 70:392–396, 1989.

96. Krompinger, WJ, Fredrickson, BE, Mino, DE, and Yuan, HA. Conservative treatment of fractures of the thoracic and lumbar spine. Orthop Clin North Am 17:161–170, Jan. 1986.

97. Lambert, DH, Deane, RS, and Mazuzan, JE Jr: Anesthesia and the control of blood pressure in patients with spinal cord injury. Anesth Analg 61:344–348, 1982.

98. Ledsome, JR and Sharp, JM: Pulmonary function in acute cervical cord injury. Am Rev Respir Dis 124:41–44, 1981.

99. Lee, J-P and Wang, AD-J: Post-traumatic basal ganglia hemorrhage: analysis of 52 patients with emphasis on the final outcome. J Trauma 31:376–380, 1991.

100. Lee, ST and Lui, TN: Delayed intracranial haemorrhage in patients with multiple trauma and shock-related hypotension. Acta Neurochir (Wien) 113:121–124, 1991.

101. Leffert, RD: Brachial-plexus injuries. N Engl J Med 291:1059–1067, 1974.

102. Levi, L, Guilburd, JN, Lemberger, A, et al: Diffuse axonal injury: Analysis of 100 patients with radiological signs. Neurosurgery 27:429–432, 1990.

103. Levine, AM and Edwards, CC: The management of traumatic spondylolisthesis of the axis. J Bone Joint Surg Am 67:217–226, 1985.

104. Levy, D: The fat embolism syndrome: A review. Clin Orthop 261:281–286, 1990.

105. Lobato, RD, Rivas, JJ, Gomez, PA, et al: Head-injured patients who talk and deteriorate into coma: Analysis of 211 cases studied with computerized to-

mography. J Neurosurg 75:256–261, 1991.

106. Lui, T-N, Lee, S-T, Chang, C-N, and Cheng, W-C: Epidural hematomas in the posterior cranial fossa. J Trauma 34:211–215, 1993.

107. Lyons, MK and Meyer, FB: Cerebrospinal fluid physiology and the management of increased intracranial pressure. Mayo Clin Proc 65:684–707, 1990.

108. MacPherson, P, Teasdale, E, Dhaker, S, et al: The significance of traumatic haematoma in the region of the basal ganglia. J Neurol Neurosurg Psychiatry 49:29–34, 1986.

109. Mansel, JK and Norman, JR: Respiratory complications and management of spinal cord injuries. Chest 97:1446–1452, 1990.

110. Marshall, LF, Bowers Marshall, S, Klauber, MR, et al: A new classification of head injury based on computerized tomography. J Neurosurg 75 Suppl:S14–S20, 1991.

111. Marshall, LF, Knowlton, S, Garfin, SR, et al: Deterioration following spinal cord injury: A multicenter study. J Neurosurg 66:400–404, 1987.

112. McCarthy, M and Norenberg, MD: Pontine hemorrhagic infarction in nontraumatic fat embolism. Neurology 38:1645–1647, 1988.

113. Meguro, K, Kobayashi, E, and Maki, Y: Acute brain swelling during evacuation of subdural hematoma caused by delayed contralateral extradural hematoma: Report of two cases. Neurosurgery 20:326–328, 1987.

114. Meya, U and Hacke, W: Anterior interosseous nerve syndrome following supracondylar lesions of the median nerve: Clinical findings and electrophysiological investigations. J Neurol 229:91–96, 1983.

115. Meyer, CA, Mirvis, SE, Wolf, AL, et al: Acute traumatic midbrain hemorrhage: Experimental and clinical observations with CT. Radiology 179:813–818, 1991.

116. Meyer, PR Jr (ed): Surgery of Spine Trauma. Churchill Livingstone, New York, 1989.

117. Mirovsky, Y, Hendel, D, and Halperin, N: Anterior interosseous nerve palsy following closed fracture of the proximal ulna: A case report and review of the literature. Arch Orthop Trauma Surg 107:61–64, 1988.

118. Mirvis, SE, Wolf, AL, Numaguchi, Y, et al: Posttraumatic cerebral infarction diagnosed by CT: Prevalence, origin, and outcome. AJR Am J Roentgenol 154:1293–1298, 1990.

119. Morse, SD: Acute central cervical spinal cord syndrome. Ann Emerg Med 11:436–439, 1982.

120. Muizelaar, JP, Marmarou, A, Ward, JD, et al: Adverse effects of prolonged hyperventilation in patients with severe head injury: A randomized clinical trial. J Neurosurg 75:731–739, 1991.

121. Nelson, AT, Kishore, PRS, and Lee, SH: Development of delayed epidural hematoma. AJNR Am J Neuroradiol 3:583–585, 1982.

122. Node, Y and Nakazawa, S: Clinical study of mannitol and glycerol on raised intracranial pressure and on their rebound phenomenon. Adv Neurol 52:359–363, 1990.

123. Oberascher, G: Cerebrospinal fluid otorrhea—new trends in diagnosis. Am J Otol 9:102–108, 1988.

124. Ott, L, Young, B, Phillips, R, et al: Altered gastric emptying in the head-injured patient: Relationship to feeding intolerance. J Neurosurg 74:738–742, 1991.

125. Patterson, FP and Morton, KS: Neurologic complications of fractures and dislocations of the pelvis. Surg Gynecol Obstet 112:702–706, 1961.

126. Perovitch, M, Perl, S, and Wang, H: Current advances in magnetic resonance imaging (MRI) in spinal cord trauma: Review article. Paraplegia 30:305–316, 1992.

127. Phonprasert, C, Suwanwela, C, Hongsaprabhas, C, et al: Extradural hematoma: Analysis of 138 cases. J Trauma 20:679–683, 1980.

128. Piepmeier, JM and Wagner, FC Jr: Delayed post-traumatic extracerebral hematomas. J Trauma 22:455–459, 1982.

129. Pinaud, M, Lelausque, J-N, Chetan-

neau, A, et al: Effects of propofol on cerebral hemodynamics and metabolism in patients with brain trauma. Anesthesiology 73:404–409, 1990.

130. Powell, JN, Waddell, JP, Tucker, WS, and Transfeldt, EE: Multiple-level noncontiguous spinal fractures. J Trauma 29:1146–1150, 1989.

131. Pozzati, E and Tognetti, F: Spontaneous healing of acute extradural hematomas: Study of twenty-two cases. Neurosurgery 18:696–700, 1986.

132. Pozzati, E, Tognetti, F, Cavallo, M, and Acciarri, N: Extradural hematomas of the posterior cranial fossa: Observations on a series of 32 consecutive cases treated after the introduction of computed tomography scanning. Surg Neurol 32:300–303, 1989.

133. Reines, HD and Harris, RC: Pulmonary complications of acute spinal cord injuries. Neurosurgery 21:193–196, 1987.

134. Rivano, C, Borzone, M, Altomonte, M, and Capuzzo, T: Traumatic posterior fossa extradural hematomas. Neurochirurgia 35:43–47, 1992.

135. Rivas, JJ, Lobato, RD, Sarabia, R, et al: Extradural hematoma: Analysis of factors influencing the courses of 161 patients. Neurosurgery 23:44–51, 1988.

136. Roberts, PA, Pollay, M, Engles, C, et al: Effect on intracranial pressure of furosemide combined with varying doses and administration rates of mannitol. J Neurosurg 66:440–446, 1987.

137. Rockoff, MA, Marshall, LF, and Shapiro, HM: High-dose barbiturate therapy in humans: A clinical review of 60 patients. Ann Neurol 6:194–199, 1979.

138. Rockswold, GL, Leonard, PR, and Nagib, MG: Analysis of management in thirty-three closed head injury patients who "talked and deteriorated." Neurosurgery 21:51–55, 1987.

139. Ropper, AH and Miller, DC: Acute traumatic midbrain hemorrhage. Ann Neurol 18:80–86, 1985.

140. Ropper, AH, O'Rourke, D, and Kennedy, SK: Head position, intracranial pressure, and compliance. Neurology 32:1288–1291, 1982.

141. Ross, SE, Schwab, CW, David, ET, et al: Clearing the cervical spine: Initial radiologic evaluation. J Trauma 27:1055–1060, 1987.

142. Rudy, EB, Baun, M, Stone, K, and Turner, B: The relationship between endotracheal suctioning and changes in intracranial pressure: A review of the literature. Heart Lung 15:488–494, 1986.

143. Rudy, EB, Turner, BS, Baun, M, et al: Endotracheal suctioning in adults with head injury. Heart Lung 20:667–674, 1991.

144. Sabiston, CP and Wing, PC: Sacral fractures: Classification and neurologic implications. J Trauma 26:1113–1115, 1986.

145. St. John, JN and French, BN: Traumatic hematomas of the posterior fossa: A clinicopathological spectrum. Surg Neurol 25:457–466, 1986.

146. Saito, A, Meguro, K, Matsumura, A, et al: Magnetic resonance imaging of a fat embolism of the brain: Case report. Neurosurgery 26:882–885, 1990.

147. Sakamoto, T, Sawada, Y, Yukioka, T, et al: Computed tomography for diagnosis and assessment of cerebral fat embolism. Neuroradiology 24:283–285, 1983.

148. Sato, M, Tanaka, S, Suzuki, K, et al: Complications associated with barbiturate therapy. Resuscitation 17:233–241, 1989.

149. Schalén, W, Messeter, K, and Nordström, C-H: Complications and side effects during thiopentone therapy in patients with severe head injuries. Acta Anaesthesiol Scand 36:369–377, 1992.

150. Seelig, JM, Marshall, LF, Toutant, SM, et al: Traumatic acute epidural hematoma: Unrecognized high lethality in comatose patients. Neurosurgery 15:617–619, 1984.

151. Shah, JJ and Bhatti, NA: Radial nerve paralysis associated with fractures of the humerus: A review of 62 cases. Clin Orthop 172:171–176, 1983.

152. Shigemori, M, Kojyo, N, Yuge, T, et al: Massive traumatic haematoma of the corpus callosum. Acta Neurochir (Wien) 81:36–39, 1986.

153. Shiozaki, T, Taneda, M, Kishikawa, M, et al: Transient and repetitive rises in blood pressure synchronized with plasma catecholamine increases after head injury: Report of two cases. J Neurosurg 78:501–504, 1993.

154. Sidhu, JS and Dhillon, MK: Lumbosacral plexus avulsion with pelvic fractures. Injury 22:156–158, 1991.

155. Smith, HK and Miller, JD: The danger of an ultra-early computed tomographic scan in a patient with an evolving acute epidural hematoma. Neurosurgery 29:258–260, 1991.

156. Smith, HP, Kelly, DL Jr, McWhorter, JM, et al: Comparison of mannitol regimens in patients with severe head injury undergoing intracranial monitoring. J Neurosurg 65:820–824, 1986.

157. Snow, RB, Zimmerman, RD, Gandy, SE, and Deck, MDF: Comparison of magnetic resonance imaging and computed tomography in the evaluation of head injury. Neurosurgery 18:45–52, 1986.

158. Statham, PF, Johnston, RA, and MacPherson, P: Delayed deterioration in patients with traumatic frontal contusions. J Neurol Neurosurg Psychiatry 52:351–354, 1989.

159. Takenaka, N, Mine, T, Suga, S, et al: Interpeduncular high-density spot in severe shearing injury. Surg Neurol 34:30–38, 1990.

160. Tanaka, T, Sakai, T, Uemura, K, et al: MR imaging as predictor of delayed posttraumatic cerebral hemorrhage. J Neurosurg 69:203–209, 1988.

161. Tator, CH and Fehlings, MG: Review of the secondary injury theory of acute spinal cord trauma with emphasis on vascular mechanisms. J Neurosurg 75:15–26, 1991.

162. Teasdale, GM, Murray, G, Anderson, E, et al: Risks of acute traumatic intracranial haematoma in children and adults: Implications for managing head injuries. BMJ 300:363–367, 1990.

163. Temkin, NR, Dikmen, SS, Wilensky, AJ, et al: A randomized, double-blind study of phenytoin for the prevention of post-traumatic seizures. N Engl J Med 323:497–502, 1990.

164. Thornbury, JR, Masters, SJ, and Campbell, JA: Imaging recommendations for head trauma: A new comprehensive strategy. AJR Am J Roentgenol 149:781–783, 1987.

165. Van Den Heever, CM and van der Merwe, DJ: Management of depressed skull fractures: Selective conservative management of nonmissile injuries. J Neurosurg 71:186–190, 1989.

166. Vaz, R, Duarte, F, Oliveira, J, et al: Traumatic interhemispheric subdural haematomas. Acta Neurochir (Wien) 111:128–131, 1991.

167. Waters, RL, Adkins, RH, and Yakura, JS: Definition of complete spinal cord injury. Paraplegia 29:573–581, 1991.

168. Weinstein, JN, Collalto, P, and Lehmann, TR: Thoracolumbar "burst" fractures treated conservatively: A long-term follow-up. Spine 13:33–38, 1988.

169. Wijdicks, EFM, Vermeulen, M, ten Haaf, JA, et al: Volume depletion and natriuresis in patients with a ruptured intracranial aneurysm. Ann Neurol 18:211–216, 1985.

170. Wilberger, JE, Rothfus, WE, Tabas, J, et al: Acute tissue tear hemorrhages of the brain: Computed tomography and clinicopathological correlations. Neurosurgery 27:208–213, 1990.

171. Wilberger, JE Jr, Deeb, Z, and Rothfus, W: Magnetic resonance imaging in cases of severe head injury. Neurosurgery 20:571–576, 1987.

172. Wilberger, JE Jr, Harris, M, and Diamond, DL: Acute subdural hematoma: Morbidity, mortality, and operative timing. J Neurosurg 74:212–218, 1991.

173. Winslow, EBJ, Lesch, M, Talano, JV, and Meyer, PR Jr: Spinal cord injuries associated with cardiopulmonary complications. Spine 11:809–812, 1986.

174. Wolf, AL, Levi, L, Marmarou, A, et al: Effect of THAM upon outcome in severe head injury: A randomized prospective clinical trial. J Neurosurg 78:54–59, 1993.

175. Worthley, LIG, Cooper, DJ, and Jones, N: Treatment of resistant intracranial hypertension with hypertonic saline:

Report of two cases. J Neurosurg 68:478–481, 1988.

176. Yagüe, LG, Rodríguez-Sánchez, J, Polaina, M, et al: Contralateral extradural hematoma following craniotomy for traumatic intracranial lesion: Case report. J Neurosurg Sci 35:107–109, 1991.

177. Yokoyama, K, Hasegawa, M, Shiba, KS, et al: Diagnosis of CSF rhinorrhea: Detection of tau-transferrin in nasal discharge. Otolaryngol Head Neck Surg 98:328–332, 1988.

178. Young, AB, Ott, LG, Beard, D, et al: The acute-phase response of the brain-injured patient. J Neurosurg 69:375–380, 1988.

179. Young, B, Ott, L, Twyman, D, et al: The effect of nutritional support on outcome from severe head injury. J Neurosurg 67:668–676, 1987.

180. Young, W: Medical treatments of acute spinal cord injury (editorial). J Neurol Neurosurg Psychiatry 55:635–639, 1992.

181. Zimmerman, RA, Bilaniuk, LT, Hackney, DB, et al: Head injury: Early results of comparing CT and high-field MR. AJR Am J Roentgenol 147:1215–1222, 1986.

Chapter 16

NEUROLOGIC COMPLICATIONS OF ORGAN TRANSPLAN-TATION

Organ transplantations are done widely, and many institutions have meticulously organized transplantation programs. Immediately after the operative procedure, patients are admitted to surgical intensive care units (ICUs) or to units specially equipped for transplant recipients. Neurologists should expect to be frequently consulted in the perioperative period. Neurologic complications are confined largely to use of immunosuppressive drugs or to infectious complications in immunocompromised patients. Other neurologic complications, particularly peripheral nerve damage, are related to the operative procedure. Although significant risks are imposed on transplant recipients, neurologic complications may be unrelated to transplantation. Adair and associates,[1] for example, made the important observation that most cerebrovascular events in their large series of cardiac transplantations were not directly attributable to transplantation.

Currently, the kidney, liver, heart, lung, and bone marrow are successfully transplanted, with comparatively low morbidity and mortality, and most patients rate their quality of life as good or excellent after transplantation.[86]

GENERAL CONSIDERATIONS IN TRANSPLANTATION

Transplantation programs may have subtle differences in procedures and postoperative care, but most critical care aspects are uniform. A brief overview of the first postoperative weeks may help in understanding the circumstances in which neurologic complications occur.

Renal Transplantation

The recipient of a renal graft is least likely to have a prolonged intensive care stay. Most patients do well, are already extubated a few hours after surgery, and have graft function without major clinical intervention. Occasionally, cadaver kidneys may take hours to resume production of urine. Uremia may occur suddenly, most frequently from acute tubular necrosis, acute accelerated rejection, or renal vein thrombosis, but these conditions are rare. The patients characteristically lapse into rapidly progressive drowsiness, stupor, and seizures in the immediate postoperative course (see Chapter 8). In this situation, filtration can be temporarily maintained through dialysis before second transplantation.

Renal transplant recipients may have significant cardiovascular disease and, therefore, are prone to postoperative ischemic cardiac disease. Many patients may need invasive monitoring with pulmonary artery catheters to optimize renal perfusion. Because end-stage renal disease often results from long-standing diabetes mellitus, other immediate medical problems are marked hyperglycemia — and certainly corticosteroids increase the risk — and gastrointestinal hemorrhage that may result in hypovolemic shock (in many patients, a combined kidney-pancreas procedure is done).

Heart and Lung Transplantation

The hemodynamic function of the graft in the first postoperative days determines care in the ICU. One may theoretically expect a large increase in cardiac output and relative hypertension when a poorly functioning heart has been replaced by an adequate muscle pump. In clinical practice, however, a tendency to become hypotensive is the rule. The transplanted heart has been subjected to many insults during procurement, and massive sympathetic outpouring before the diagnosis of brain death may result in contraction necrosis. (Many harvesting programs, however, require echocardiography to assess ejection fraction and wall motion abnormalities.) Additionally, the denervated heart cannot adjust easily to marked changes in filling pressure, and cardiac output is frequently maintained with inotropic agents. However, use of cyclosporine and increasing doses of inotropic agents may cause overcompensation to hypertension, which is generally well controlled with nitroprusside. Furthermore, cerebral perfusion is seriously threatened by frequent episodes of bradycardia that can at times be resolved only with demand-type pacemakers. Rejection of the transplanted heart may be manifested by fever and hypotension. In other patients, the clinical manifestations include extreme fatigue, drowsiness, and dyspnea. (Many patients cannot sustain elevation of the head and limbs from the bed.) Less severe rejection, however, can be asymptomatic, only to be demonstrated on endomyocardial biopsy.

The number of lung transplantations is increasing, but the critical care experience is still limited. Early complications include cytomegalovirus pneumonitis and obstructive bronchiolitis, which may lead to loss of the graft. Many of the neurologic manifestations in lung transplantations in the early postoperative course, therefore, are related to severe hypoxemia caused by airway obstruction. Occasionally, transient brachial plexopathy occurs from forceful splitting of the rib cage during thoracotomy.

Liver Transplantation

The fundamentals of postoperative care in liver recipients include management of coagulopathy, pulmonary care, and management of blood pressure and fluids.[101,102] The production of clotting factors (for example, factor V) is one of the indicators of graft function, but severe coagulopathy may persist in the first postoperative days. Infusion of fresh frozen plasma and platelets is often needed. In the first postoperative days, fluid loss from third space sequestration and protein loss from drains are common, but fluid status may rapidly switch into hypervolemia associated with hypertension. Intravascular volume overload may result in hyponatremia, and rapid correction may cause seizures or central pontine demyelination. Central pontine myelinolysis has been associated with marked shifts in sodium levels and osmolality.

The postoperative period in liver transplantation is frequently dominated by nosocomial infections that cause death from sepsis. Selective gut decontamination and antifungal prophylaxis may limit the risk of infection, but the multiplicity of lines, catheters, and drains also predisposes to infection and emphasizes the need for strict sterile techniques.

Bone Marrow Transplantation

Use of bone marrow transplantation, effective in diseases of the lymphohematopoietic system, is increasing. In the pretransplantation period, neurologic side effects, including seizures, transverse myelitis, leukoencephalopathy, meningitis, and isolated cranial nerve palsies, can occur from high doses of multiple chemotherapeutic agents.[19] The specific toxicities of chemotherapy and radiotherapy regimens are outside the scope of this chapter. Details can be found in reviews.[31,55]

After bone marrow infusion, pancytopenia is expected for 2 to 5 weeks before a significant response is mounted. During this critical period, overwhelming gram-negative sepsis, severe bleeding from thrombocytopenia, and disseminated intravascular coagulation are the most feared complications.[19]

A potentially devastating complication (although mild in some cases) is graft-versus-host disease.[105] Graft-versus-host disease is diagnosed by skin biopsy, but many other organs can be involved in various degrees.

NEUROLOGIC MANIFESTATIONS OF IMMUNOSUPPRESSIVE AGENTS

Most transplantation programs have adopted triple drug therapy (cyclosporine, azathioprine, prednisone), but with the recent introduction of new and possibly less toxic immunosuppressive agents, protocols are continuously adjusted. The neurologic side effects of immunosuppressive agents have been well described, although for most of the agents used, the pathophysiologic mechanism is a mystery. The neurologic manifestations of the immunosuppressive agents can be nonspecific, including seizures and diminished alertness, but more typical adverse effects have been reported.

Neurologic manifestations have not been reported with antithymocyte globulin and azathioprine use.

Cyclosporine

As part of triple or quadruple therapy (additional antilymphocyte globulin or OKT3), cyclosporine has greatly advanced the efficacy of organ transplantation. Cyclosporine mainly inhibits T-lymphocyte maturation, but reduction of interleukin-2 production in helper T cells is equally important.[28]

The systemic side effects of cyclosporine are usually reversible. These are nephrotoxicity from its vasoconstrictive effect and severe hypertension either alone or in combination with nephrotoxicity. Neurotoxicity associated with cyclosporine most often develops within the first 2 weeks after transplantation.[14,29,33,61,67,83,91]

Cyclosporine neurotoxicity has been linked to several clinical syndromes with striking radiologic abnormalities. The pathogenesis, frequently in conjunction with hypocholesterolemia or hypertension, is mysterious. Hypertensive encephalopathy, which has many features of cyclosporine toxicity in its presentation (see Chapter 8), has been dismissed as a potential mechanism because malignant hypertension (e.g., mean arterial pressure greater than 130 mm Hg) and papilledema do not occur. Predisposing factors that have received considerable attention are aluminum overload and high doses of corticosteroids, but the possibility of interactions with commonly used drugs should be considered as well (Table 16–1).

Table 16-1 DRUGS THAT INCREASE THE CHANCE OF CYCLOSPORINE TOXICITY

Erythromycin
Itraconazole
Ketoconazole
Diltiazem
Nicardipine
Verapamil
Metoclopramide
Cimetidine
Ranitidine

Two major theories of cyclosporine toxicity have been proposed, but both are largely speculative. Cyclosporine may have a direct damaging effect on the vascular endothelium, which may cause vasoconstriction from increased plasma endothelium levels[113] or from an altered balance of prostacyclin and thromboxane.[104] Transcranial Doppler studies in these patients may demonstrate evidence of severe vasospasm, but data are not yet available. Another attractive, but unproven, hypothesis[27] suggests that cyclosporine neurotoxicity is caused by intracellular transport by means of the low-density lipoprotein receptor. These receptors may be sensitized and increased in patients with low cholesterol levels and may also bind low-density lipoprotein particles with increased concentrations of cyclosporine. This theory assumes a disturbed blood-brain barrier and low cholesterol levels; both have been inconsistently demonstrated in series with neurotoxicity. A large proportion of cyclosporine is bound to low-density lipoprotein fractions, and recently cyclosporine neurotoxicity was described after intralipid infusion, which lowers the low-density lipoprotein fraction and increases the free fraction of cyclosporine.[30]

Neurologic manifestations of cyclosporine toxicity are infrequent, and the clinical features, although distinct, are derived from a small number of patients.[74,103,113] Mild side effects of cyclosporine almost always are manifested by fine finger tremor, sometimes associated with paresthesias, and resolve after the dose of cyclosporine is reduced. Headaches have been regularly reported and are often refractory to common analgesics. Propranolol (20 mg every 6 to 8 hours) has been very effective in most patients, who otherwise may need narcotics for pain control.[48] Other typically dose-related side effects are confusional states with delusions, hallucinations, and depression, but increasing lack of interest and lethargy are often the first indicators of cyclosporine toxicity.

As early as the first postoperative day, patients may become inactive, and mild aphasia with paraphasic errors may appear and progressively worsen within hours. Visual hallucinations,[103] often with bright colors, may occur intermittently. Some patients may have cortical blindness[43,88,122] with corresponding bilateral parieto-occipital hypodensities and increased T2 signal on imaging studies that may resolve after tapering of the dose.[113] In many patients with cortical blindness, months may be required for visual acuity to return to normal.[62,89] Blindness appears to be linked to demyelination and petechial hemorrhage in autopsy studies. In other patients, bizarre behavior with echolalia may occur.

When toxicity is unrecognized, patients may lapse into coma or have cerebellar or spinal cord symptoms. Severe spasticity with brisk reflexes and Babinski's response is invariably found and resolves after withdrawal of cyclosporine. Recently, oculogyric crises, grimacing, and tongue protrusion as part of severe orofacial dyskinesia were reported in three patients, two of whom recovered completely.[13] In one patient, central pontine myelinolysis was subsequently found on magnetic resonance imaging (MRI), and incomplete recovery was related to extrapontine locations in the basal ganglia.

Many reports have demonstrated virtually complete resolution of neurologic symptoms and MRI findings after administration was discontinued. Neurologic symptoms did not recur after rechallenge with lower doses of cyclosporine.[33]

Magnetic resonance imaging is most sensitive in demonstrating cyclosporine neurotoxicity. Typically, abnormalities are restricted to white matter areas or the occipital lobes and are often identical to MRI findings in hypertensive encephalopathy[113] (see Chapter 8) (Fig. 16–1). However, cyclosporine toxicity may occur without these MRI abnormalities and must remain a strong contender when changes in level of consciousness or behavior are found. Discontinuation of cyclosporine is often entertained first, and when renal failure is present in addition, recovery from cyclosporine toxicity may require days. Treatment of cyclosporine neurotoxicity also may include low-dose haloperidol.

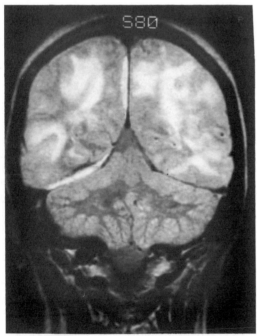

Figure 16–1. Magnetic resonance imaging scan in a patient with cyclosporine toxicity. Note also rim of subdural blood on the tentorium. (Courtesy of Dr. P. de Groen, Department of Gastroenterology, Mayo Clinic, Rochester, MN.)

OKT3

OKT3 has recently been introduced as rescue treatment for failing grafts in patients unresponsive to high doses of corticosteroids or antilymphocyte globulin but may also serve as a primary agent. This agent consists of a monoclonal IgG antibody against the T3 receptor of T lymphocytes and blocks recognition of classes I and II major histocompatibility complex antigens.

Its adverse effects are considerable but, as with many other immunosuppressive agents, self-limiting. Usually, within 1 hour after the first or any subsequent dose, patients have nonspecific signs, such as fever, chills, vomiting, diarrhea, wheezing, and dyspnea, but many patients may also have myalgias, rigors, and headache.[107]

The neurotoxicity of OKT3 is limited to aseptic meningitis and a toxic encephalopathy that seems more severe than that from cyclosporine.

OKT3 aseptic meningitis may resemble any of the bacterial or fungal meningitides in immunosuppressed patients. Its true incidence is not known, and in many patients cerebrospinal fluid (CSF) pleocytosis may remain undetected.[38,87] However, in patients who had CSF examination in association with nonspecific clinical signs such as fever, meningism, and headache, the cell count was increased. The spinal fluid formula with polymorphic or mononuclear cells appeared to coincide with the degree of fever.[2,65] Many patients do not have obvious neck stiffness, and aseptic meningitis has been found immediately after the first dose, with complete resolution within 2 days despite continuation of therapy. In 1991, Adair and associates[2] noted onset of meningitis 5 to 16 days after completion of daily administration of OKT3.

A dramatic toxic encephalopathy may emerge in OKT3 administration, yet almost nothing is known about its true incidence. Several patients with wild psychotic episodes, hallucinations, multifocal myoclonus, asterixis, and seizures have been reported.[18,107] Out-of-body experience, preoccupation with death, aggressive response to hallucinated objects, and auditory hallucinations occurred before the patients became drowsy or lapsed into unresponsive coma 24 to 75 hours after initiation of OKT3 therapy.[64]

A recent report of OKT3 encephalopathy highlighted cerebral edema diagnosed on computed tomography (CT) and high CSF opening pressures.[108] Complete resolution was noted after 3 days.[21] Chan and associates[20] found that patients receiving renal transplants who had OKT3 encephalopathy had been premedicated with indomethacin, which is known to cause an aseptic meningoencephalitis (see Chapter 5, Table 5–3).

At the Mayo Clinic in Rochester, Minnesota, OKT3 is used for primary treatment in cardiac transplantation. The OKT3 encephalopathy described previously has not yet been observed, most likely because particular attention is paid to not exceeding the dose. Only 3 of 67 patients with cardiac transplants receiving OKT3 who were seen at the Mayo Clinic had aseptic meningitis (Dr. C. G. A. McGregor, personal communication). However, headache alone was generally more common but easily treated with acetaminophen. Lumbar punctures are usually not performed on patients without fever or meningismus; therefore, mild aseptic meningitis cannot be completely ruled out.

FK 506

A new, promising, and less toxic immunosuppressive agent may replace cyclosporine.[5,110] FK 506 suppresses T-lymphocyte activation and inhibits the synthesis of cytokines. Experience is limited, although results of the first trials are very favorable in liver transplantation. Hypertension is 50% less than that with cyclosporine, but nephrotoxicity and glucose intolerance remain the principal undesirable effects.[5,110]

Neurotoxicity of FK 506 has also been reported and correlated with neuropathologic findings. In a preliminary study, the incidences of central nervous system (CNS) infection, central pontine myelinolysis, and intracranial hemorrhages were similar to those with cyclosporine.[62]

Many of the neurotoxic effects of FK 506, including its clinical presentation and a white matter abnormality on CT scan, are similar to those of cyclosporine.[37,42] In one report, however, bilateral thalamic hypodensities not known in cyclosporine toxicity were found.[42] Many patients have hand tremors. Some severe tremor results in difficulty writing and inability to sign checks.[121] Tremor is not associated with trough plasma or serum levels and appears to be an all-or-nothing phenomenon (Fig. 16–2). Nevertheless, neurotoxicity often appears during the intravenous phase of drug administration; lowering the dose resolves the problem. In a recent study, FK 506 neurotoxicity was dramatically reduced in maintenance doses of 0.075 mg/kg twice a day. Tremor may become less troublesome but never completely disappears. Painful dysesthesias in the hands and feet sometimes occur without objective neurologic findings of small fiber neuropathy. Speech apraxia or mutism occasionally occurs. MRI may show white matter abnormalities or may remain normal.[84] Characteristically in these patients, auditory comprehension of language is intact, but simple oral non-

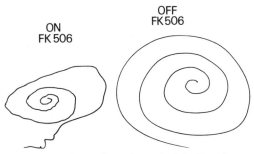

Figure 16–2. Archimedes spiral in liver transplantation patient with "therapeutic" levels of FK 506 (*left*) and after discontinuation (*right*). Note marked improvement in skilled movement.

Table 16–2 NEUROTOXICITY OF FK 506 IN 44 CONSECUTIVE PATIENTS WITH ORTHOTOPIC LIVER TRANSPLANTATION

Clinical Characteristics	Patients (n)
Tremors	10
Tingling hands and feet	3
Mood swings and psychosis	3
Apraxia of speech	3
Seizures	2

Data from Wijdicks, et al.[121]

speech motor acts (e.g., whistling) cannot be performed. The defect may resolve completely, but stuttering speech may remain for months.[121] Other significant reported signs are florid nightmares, bizarre behavior, severe mood swings, inappropriate crying, and acoustic hallucinations (Table 16–2). Although blood and plasma levels of FK 506 are usually similar in patients with and without neurotoxicity, peak plasma levels may have a better correlation. Deciding whether neurotoxicity of FK 506 can explain the clinical symptoms should not depend on FK 506 plasma trough levels. In all patients, despite FK 506 levels in the estimated normal range, dose reduction results in striking clinical improvement.[121]

NEUROLOGIC COMPLICATIONS IN TRANSPLANTATION

Within the range of transplantation-related complications, neurologic manifestations are comparatively minor. Among the patients with neurologic complications, neurologists must confront difficult issues, the most pressing of which is whether the usually excellent outcome of solid organ transplantation is compromised.

Central Nervous System Infections

Immunocompromised patients have an enhanced susceptibility to systemic infection but rarely within the 1-month duration of immunosuppression. Well-known nosocomial infections, such as those caused by gram-negative organisms, *Staphylococcus*, and *Candida albicans*, are as frequent in transplant patients as in any other critically ill patients and are related to contamination of central intravenous catheters and surgical wound sepsis.

Very early CNS infections are virtually never seen except for those caused by *Aspergillus* species, and opportunistic infections occur mostly in patients who are still critically ill after 1 month. Nonetheless, the threshold for additional imaging or CSF studies should be low.

This section is divided into brief discussions of the most relevant CNS infections in the post-transplantation period (Table 16–3). Anecdotal reports of rare parasital or fungal CNS infections, which may occur only in highly endemic areas, are not relevant to most patients and will not be discussed in this text.

PARASITIC INFECTIONS

Many parasite species may gain access to the CNS. Some are endemic, and others have a widespread geographic prevalence. *Toxoplasma gondii* remains the most common agent in the immunosuppressed population, but strongyloidiasis and cysticercosis have been reported in renal transplantation.[35] Histoplasmosis endemic in Alabama, Indianapolis, and Texas has been reported in HIV infection only.[56] It may be present as a single mass on CT scan and may mimic lymphoma.

Toxoplasma gondii. One of the most serious parasitic infections in compromised hosts is caused by *Toxoplasma gondii*.[23,40,63,118] Several instances of acute toxoplasma encephalitis have been reported, mostly in patients with renal[23] or bone marrow[63] transplantation. Recently, a neuropathologic survey noted toxoplasma encephalitis in two patients who had a heart-lung transplantation.

**Table 16–3 CENTRAL NERVOUS SYSTEM
INFECTIONS IN TRANSPLANTATION**

Microorganism	Transplanted Organ*	Days After Transplantation
Listeria	Heart, kidney, bone marrow	≥70
Nocardia	Liver, kidney, heart	≥84
Toxoplasma	Kidney, bone marrow, heart and lung	≥9
Cysticercus	Kidney	≥150
Strongyloides	Kidney	≥150
Cryptococcus	Liver, kidney	≥180
Aspergillus	Bone marrow, liver, heart	≥12
Adenovirus	Bone marrow	≥360
Varicella	Kidney	≥360

*May occur in any type of transplantation, but associations with listed grafts are those reported in the literature.

Diagnosis of CNS toxoplasma may be difficult during life. Clinical symptoms can be minimal or absent despite multiple mass lesions on CT scan. Headache, low-grade fever, and confusion may be the only findings, but focal signs may occur, and then patients have mild hemiparesis or cerebellar signs. Surprisingly, toxoplasmic abscesses are often located in the basal ganglia without always producing movement disorders. Acute, fatal toxoplasma encephalitis is often seen, and patients may also die from infestation in the myocardium that leads to refractory cardiac arrhythmias. Chorioretinitis is infrequently seen, and funduscopy cannot assist in the diagnosis. Before the CT scan era, the diagnosis of CNS toxoplasma was very rarely confirmed, because toxoplasma tachyzoites almost never appear in the CSF. The CSF typically shows a nonspecific but profound mononuclear pleocytosis with a pronounced increase in protein concentration and a normal glucose value. Serologic tests in immunocompromised patients are not helpful, but toxoplasmosis occurs more often in seropositive patients. In a recent study, 23 of 25 bone marrow transplant recipients with disseminated toxoplasmosis had unchanged IgG titers, and specific IgM antibodies were detected in only 2 patients.[34]

Computed tomography scan findings are fairly typical. Ring-enhancing necrotic abscesses (Fig. 16–3A) are multiple but can be single on CT scan, with a predilection for the basal ganglia and cerebellum. (MRI usually demonstrates lesions that are missed by CT scan.) In acute fulminant toxoplasmosis, CT scan is negative or may demonstrate multiple abscesses and edema or multiple rounded hemorrhages[118] (Fig. 16–3B).

Treatment is very effective, and apart from clinical improvement, CNS lesions may markedly decrease in size or even vanish within 10 to 14 days. Drug treatment consists of a 100-mg loading dose of pyrimethamine followed by 50-mg daily doses together with sulfadiazine, 2 to 6 g daily, and folinic acid, 10 mg.

VIRAL INFECTIONS

In a critical phase after transplantation, systemic viral infections may emerge. A systemic viremia is often present in patients with CNS involvement. Some viral infections in immunocompromised patients can cause fulminant and lethal disseminated infections. The most plausible mechanism is reactivation or infection introduced by the graft itself.

Adenovirus. Adenovirus infection is frequent after bone marrow transplantation,[25] and invasive infection has been reported in 20% of patients. Many patients have severe liver failure, gross

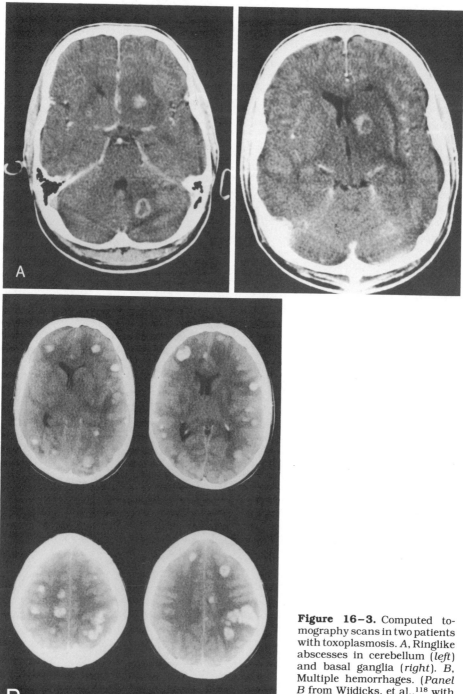

Figure 16-3. Computed tomography scans in two patients with toxoplasmosis. *A*, Ringlike abscesses in cerebellum (*left*) and basal ganglia (*right*). *B*, Multiple hemorrhages. (*Panel B* from Wijdicks, et al.,[118] with permission of the Annals of Neurology.)

hematuria, and pneumonia. Adenovirus can be cultured from specimens.

An acute meningoencephalitis characterized by nonspecific findings such as headache, drowsiness, and seizures and by ultrastructurally proven intranuclear viral aggregates has been reported. There is no effective treatment when this fulminant, uniformly fatal complication occurs.[25]

Varicella Zoster Virus. Reactivation of latent infection of sensory ganglion neurons with varicella zoster virus may occur in renal transplant recipients. Many patients have a cutaneous dissemination. The neurologic manifestations include meningoencephalitis, acute transverse myelitis, and, in some patients, involvement of only a single cranial nerve. Detailed neuropathologic studies in transplant recipients have not been reported.

Cytomegalovirus. Cytomegalovirus is perhaps the most common viral infection after organ transplantation, but a cytomegalovirus encephalitis is seldom diagnosed during life. Ganciclovir may be effective not only in eradication of the virus but also in prevention. Its use is advocated in many transplantation protocols, particularly among recipients of bone marrow. Unfortunately, strains of cytomegalovirus resistant to conventional treatment with ganciclovir have been reported. It has been suggested that in selected patients, ganciclovir should be combined with intrathecally delivered beta-interferon.[11]

The incidence of cytomegalovirus infection of the brain may have been underestimated. Microglial nodules in cerebral and cerebellar cortex have been reported in recipients of renal, liver, and bone marrow transplants and confirmed with in situ hybridization.

The clinical presentation of cytomegalovirus encephalitis is nonspecific and may include severe refractory headache with profound vomiting, behavior changes, slowly developing memory deficits, and seizures. In a recent large series of neurologic complications of bone marrow transplantation, six patients had neuropathologic evidence of cytomegalovirus infection and, in retrospect, signs of encephalopathy that could not be linked to acute metabolic abnormalities.[76]

Convincing cases of cytomegalovirus encephalitis after organ transplantation diagnosed during life are seldom reported. In situ hybridization and polymerase chain reaction were diagnostically useful in one patient with a renal transplant.[11] Cytomegalovirus may also cause Guillain-Barré syndrome or acute transverse myelitis. In these patients the diagnosis of disseminated cytomegalovirus infection was confirmed by positive cultures of buffy coat and bronchoalveolar lavage fluid and a marked (16 fold) rise in IgG antibody titer. Paraparesis and urinary retention completely resolved.[100]

Epstein-Barr Virus. Epstein-Barr virus is involved not only in the development of lymphoma from B-cell proliferation but also in causing a fatal mononucleosis in liver transplant recipients.[82] Clinical manifestations are similar to those of infectious mononucleosis, with characteristic generalized lymphadenopathy, but occasionally jaundice, headache, and nuchal rigidity are found. It may occur with overwhelming lymphomatous invasion of the CNS, always as part of a systemic dissemination that causes multiple granulomas in many other organs.

FUNGAL INFECTIONS

Cryptococcus neoformans and *Aspergillus* are most frequently involved in transplant recipients who have fungal meningitis or brain abscesses.[112] In addition, many anecdotal reports are on record of fungal infections in patients who were immunosuppressed and visited or lived in endemic areas. Coccidioidomycosis is endemic in the southwestern United States, Mexico, and parts of South America, and an increased incidence of infections has been reported in Native Americans, African-Americans, and Filipinos.[36]

Coccidioidal meningitis has been reported in heart transplant recipients and is rapidly fatal. CNS histoplasmosis has a worldwide distribution but is rare in transplant recipients; it may result in subacute or chronic meningitis.[56] Only the most common fungal infections in transplant recipients are discussed in this text.

Cryptococcus neoformans. Cryptococcosis frequently is manifested as a primary pulmonary infection followed by hematogenous dissemination and is associated with a poor prognosis in transplant recipients.[57,117]

The most typical manifestation of *Cryptococcus* infestation is a meningitis. Clinical symptoms are very often absent or subtle. Persistent headache may be the only symptom that points to cryptococcal meningitis. Focal neurologic signs, neck stiffness, and papilledema may be absent unless mass lesions emerge. CSF examination can be normal except for high opening pressures. In 95% of patients, the diagnosis can be confirmed by CSF culture, positive India ink preparation, and serologic detection of cryptococcal antigen titers of 1 : 32 or more.

Computed tomography scan may demonstrate parenchymal cryptococcoma and hydrocephalus, but findings can be completely normal in patients with cryptococcal cerebritis. A study of patients with intracranial cryptococcal infection showed normal CT scan findings in 43%, diffuse atrophy in 34%, mass lesions in 11%, hydrocephalus in 9%, and diffuse cerebral edema in only one patient.[80] MRI may help in recognition by demonstration of deleted Virchow-Robin spaces or miliary enhancing nodules, or both, not seen by conventional CT scanning.[109]

Standard treatment for *Cryptococcus neoformans* meningitis or abscesses is amphotericin B intravenously in high doses (1 to 1.5 mg/kg daily) for 4 to 6 weeks. Flucytosine may be added and can significantly lower the dose of amphotericin (0.3 mg/kg), and in patients who received treatment, less nephrotoxicity, fewer relapses, and more rapid eradication have been claimed. Recent evidence that recurrence of cryptococcal meningitis results from persistence of the initial strain should influence the decision to use more aggressive combination therapies.[99] As a last resort, fluconazole and itraconazole have been successfully used.[17,32]

Aspergillus fumigatus. *Aspergillus* infection in transplant recipients may go largely unnoticed, and, unfortunately, CNS inoculation is seldom diagnosed before death. In 1990, Boon and associates[16] emphasized a relatively high incidence (9 of 44 autopsied brains) in liver transplant recipients. In only two patients with CNS aspergillosis, the diagnosis was made shortly before death.

Aspergillus tends to cause meningoencephalitis, but brain abscesses may develop.[79,111] Hemorrhagic necrosis resulting in intracerebral hematoma is frequently a feature of *Aspergillus* infestation.[111] Therefore, sudden intracerebral hematomas after liver transplantation in patients with severe coagulopathy can result from aspergillosis. *Aspergillus* infection with intracerebral hematoma has also been described in heart-lung and bone marrow transplantation, and outcome is invariably poor.

The neuropathologic findings in a series of 22 patients from Pittsburgh were reviewed in 1993.[111] Seizures were observed in 41% of the patients. Rapidly progressive decrease in level of consciousness was associated with grand mal seizures in approximately half of the patients. Meningeal signs were uncommon. At the Mayo Clinic, CNS aspergillosis occurred in 4 of 430 liver transplantations. All instances were fatal. One patient had a solitary abscess at presentation with evidence of hemorrhage on MRI, as described previously by others.[22,24] Systemic aspergillosis became more evident later with pulmonary involvement. Recurrent seizures and, finally, multiorgan failure preceded death. Another patient presented

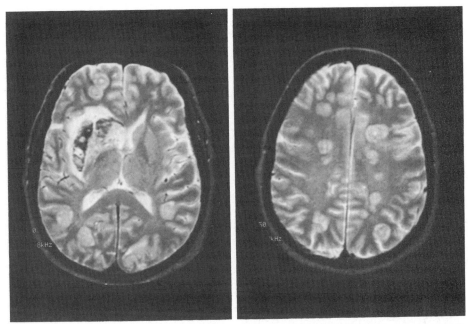

Figure 16-4. Magnetic resonance imaging scans of *Aspergillus* abscess in a patient with liver transplantation. Multiple abscesses with large (fatal) basal ganglia hemorrhage are shown.

with multiple abscesses and a large basal ganglia hemorrhage (Fig. 16-4).

Aspergillus infection can manifest as a spinal cord syndrome from an epidural abscess.[75] Similarly, progression is rapidly fatal. Possibly, increased awareness of this devastating fungal infection may increase survival if treatment with high doses of amphotericin B (up to 1.5 mg/kg per day) is initiated early, but mortality with CNS aspergillosis remains 100%. The most critical interval appears to be the first 2 months. Of particular interest in the Pittsburgh series was the frequent combination of infection with intense antirejection therapy and retransplantation.[79]

BACTERIAL INFECTIONS

Mundane bacterial infection in the ICU can be expected in the days after transplantation, but hosts with immunocompromised systems are particularly susceptible to *Listeria monocytogenes* and *Nocardia asteroides*.

Listeria monocytogenes. Systemic listeriosis is a well-recognized clinical entity in transplant recipients. In a 1992 report, most renal transplant recipients were infected within 1 month after transplantation.[95] Most patients were treated with additional monoclonal antibodies and high doses of steroids to counteract acute rejection. The most frequent clinical presentation of listeriosis is acute meningitis with fever and headache. Again, nuchal rigidity is usually difficult to appreciate in immunosuppressed patients and is absent in almost 75% of the cases.[95] Bacteremia is often present, and blood cultures may already show the offending organism before CSF results are available. The outcome in immunosuppressed patients after adequate treatment with penicillin G, ampicillin, or piperacillin is generally good, but mortality remains 30%.

Patients with *Listeria* meningitis may experience recurrence, and any patient who had one episode during rejection should have prophylactic antibiotic treatment in times of increasing doses of immunosuppressive agents.[59]

Listeria may cause brain abscesses, frequently accompanied by focal signs, and when this happens, mortality doubles. Multiple abscesses like those in toxoplasmosis are infrequent, although the preferred location in basal ganglia is similar.[26,115] In one report, *Listeria* abscess occurred 6 months after renal transplantation, in other reports, years later.[26] Stereotactic neurosurgical intervention is usually necessary to isolate the organism. Continuing or fractionated drainage of the abscess is not mandatory, because it may resolve after systemic antibiotic therapy. Additional complications, such as hydrocephalus, cerebral edema, and cerebral infarction, may develop in patients with *Listeria* meningitis.[12] An autopsy study in an elderly patient who had renal transplantation documented an occlusion of the middle cerebral artery from septic emboli.[72]

Nocardia. Patients with ringlike and hemorrhagic parenchymal lesions may have nocardial abscess, especially if they have bilateral pleural effusions, pulmonary nodules, or pulmonary abscesses. It has also been suggested that skin lesions predict disseminated disease and cerebral lesions.[69,81]

Nocardial infection is treated with high doses of sulfonamides or cyclosporine, tetracycline, and chloramphenicol. Conservative treatment of brain abscesses can be successful with a combination of amikacin, ciprofloxacin, and amoxicillin with clavulanic acid.[81]

In summary, one should probably perform a biopsy on a new-onset mass lesion in a transplant recipient. For patients with locations suspicious for toxoplasma, a trial of drug treatment is preferred. A differential diagnosis of mass lesions in immunosuppressed transplant recipients is presented in Table 16–4.

Table 16–4 DIFFERENTIAL DIAGNOSIS OF MASS LESIONS IN TRANSPLANT PATIENTS

Nocardia asteroides
Toxoplasma gondii
Cryptococcus neoformans
Listeria monocytogenes
Mycobacteria
Lymphoma
Progressive multifocal leukoencephalopathy

Cerebrovascular Complications

Successful grafting can be offset by a devastating stroke[1,7] (Table 16–5). Causes of stroke vary, but the perioperative circumstances may play a crucial role.[4,94]

Table 16–5 CEREBROVASCULAR COMPLICATIONS AFTER TRANSPLANTATION

Series	Year	Total Patients (n)	TX	Patients (n)			
				ICH	SDH	SAH	IS
Andrews, et al.[7]	1990	90	Heart	2	0	0	3
Estol, et al.[39]	1991	1357	Liver	3*	2	3	5
Adair, et al.[1]	1992	275	Heart	1	0	0	3
Adams, et al.[4]	1986	467	Kidney	3	1	1†	2
Mayo series, unpublished	1994	505	Liver	9	2	0	3

*Five patients had ICH-SDH and ICH-SAH combinations.
†No evidence of polycystic kidney disease.
ICH = intracerebral hematoma; IS = ischemic stroke; SAH = subarachnoid hemorrhage; SDH = subdural hematoma; TX = transplanted organ.

In heart transplants, ischemic stroke is frequently related to effects of cardiac bypass, retained thrombi within the graft, or catheterization of the right side of the heart for endomyocardial biopsy (see Chapter 3). Adair and colleagues,[1] however, correctly noted that a history of stroke and preoperative carotid stenosis of more than 50% significantly increase the risk for ischemic stroke. Hemorrhagic stroke in cardiac transplant recipients may be related to associated coagulopathy from thrombocytopenia. Intracerebral hemorrhages, often in multiple intracranial compartments, are more common in liver transplantation and have been associated with severe coagulopathy.[104] Many cases in the literature, however, have also been linked to *Aspergillus* inoculation.[3,7,8,39,66,116]

In the Mayo liver transplantation program, 10 patients were seen with intracerebral hemorrhages (4%). Eight patients had intracerebral hemorrhages, and two had subdural hematomas. In one patient with a relatively small hematoma, a *Candida*-associated mycotic aneurysm was found (Fig. 16–5A). In one patient, hemorrhage was associated with systemic aspergillosis. When these patients were compared with a control series of patients without intracerebral hemorrhage and liver transplantation, no statistically significant differences were found in the incidence of coagulopathy, extracranial bleeding sites, or cyclosporine toxicity, but bacteremia or fungemia was statistically more common, suggesting that intracerebral hematoma may have an origin in overwhelming infection. The cause of spontaneous intracerebral hemorrhage in patients after transplantation remains unknown.[119] In the cytopenic stage of bone marrow transplantation, intracranial hemorrhages may occur and are often fatal. In a series of 105 bone marrow transplantations, subarachnoid hemorrhage occurred in 13% of the patients, subdural hematoma in 10%, and intraparenchymal hematoma in 5%.[70] Ischemic strokes have been poorly characterized in this population but may occur with nonbacterial thrombotic endocarditis as a consequence of a hypercoagulable state; chemotherapy may additionally contribute[54] when it is used in the conditioning pretransplantation regimen (Fig. 16–5).

Seizure Disorders

In the transplant recipient, seizures are often the first indication that the immunosuppressive agent has reached toxic levels.[10,29] New-onset seizures may have multiple causes, including drug withdrawal, drug toxicity, and severe acute metabolic derangements (see Chapter 2). The highly selected population of transplant recipients is at risk for seizures. The most commonly reported circumstances are outlined in Table 16–6.[47,124]

The incidence of seizures frequently is high in liver transplant recipients, and cyclosporine-induced hypomagnesemia has been implicated.[58] However, in liver transplant recipients, focal or generalized tonic-clonic seizures or epileptiform activity on electroencephalograms (interictal spike and sharp waves, triphasic waves) usually indicates severe ischemic-anoxic damage or subdural or subarachnoid hemorrhage.[124] It is difficult to be certain that cyclosporine use is causing the seizures. The many other potential triggers for seizures in the first weeks after transplantation make the association with cyclosporine, unless a toxic level is demonstrated, fortuitous. Complex partial status epilepticus, with rapid reversal after intravenously administered benzodiazepines, has been reported in association with therapeutic levels of cyclosporine as well.[9]

De Novo Central Nervous System Malignant Lesions

The incidence of post-transplantation malignant lesions involving the CNS is low. Most CNS tumors are B-cell

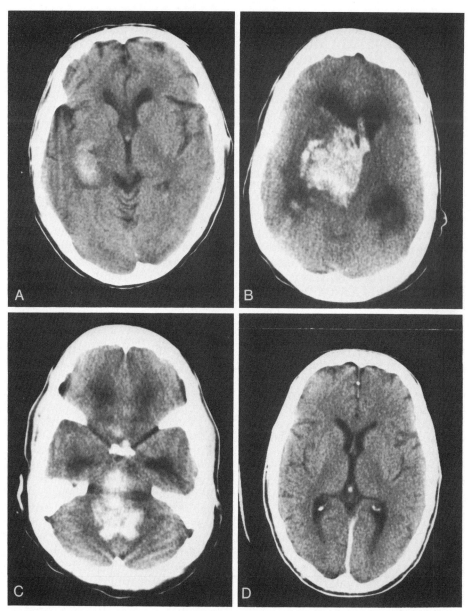

Figure 16–5. Types of intracranial hemorrhages in liver transplantation.[119] *A*, Small intracerebral hematoma associated with mycotic aneurysm demonstrated at autopsy. *B* and *C*, Massive putamen hemorrhage with intraventricular extension and acute hydrocephalus. No cause was found. *D*, Small subdural rim of blood. No cause was found except a flurry of seizures from cyclosporine toxicity.

lymphomas, but glioblastoma multiforme with a rapidly fatal course has developed, usually years after transplantation. Astrocytomas have been reported in bone marrow transplantation and heart transplantation, but in either case other predisposing factors, such as

prophylactic cranial irradiation[90] or genetic propensity,[120] were present (Fig. 16–6).

Penn[77,78] noticed in his transplant tumor registry that the incidence of lymphomas has increased and that lymphomas have occurred earlier. Lym-

**Table 16–6 POTENTIAL CAUSES OF EARLY
NEW-ONSET SEIZURES IN TRANSPLANT RECIPIENTS**

Type of Transplant	Incidence (%)	Metabolic	Structural
Liver	10–20	Hypocalcemia, hyponatremia, hypomagnesemia, hyperglycemia Cyclosporine, FK 506 toxicity	Ischemic-anoxic encephalopathy, subdural hematoma, intracerebral hemorrhage, subarachnoid hemorrhage, extrapontine myelinolysis, fungal or bacterial abscess
Renal	1–5	Acute uremia, hyponatremia	Intracranial hemorrhage, fungal or bacterial abscess
Cardiac	10–15	Cyclosporine toxicity	Ischemic stroke, air emboli, *Toxoplasma* or *Aspergillus* abscess
Bone marrow	5–10	Drug-related*	Cortical venous thrombosis, intracerebral hemorrhage

*Drugs used before bone marrow transplantation, such as busulfan in high doses.[44]

phoma of the brain occurs in 7% of transplant recipients. Most post-transplantation lymphomas are monoclonal B-cell lymphomas, but multiclonal lymphomas (from different progenitor cells) or T-cell lymphomas have been reported.[45,49] The addition of both OKT3 and cyclosporine or the use of any intensive immunosuppressive therapy to counteract rejection of the graft has been tentatively linked to higher incidences of lymphoma. On the other hand, risk of post-transplantation lymphoma is not higher in patients who re-

quired a second transplantation. The interval to the onset of lymphoma has become relatively short: an average of 3 to 6 months after transplantation. In a 1990 series,[106] a systemic lymphoproliferative disorder developed in several patients 1 month after cardiac transplantation. Its presentation was characterized largely by organ failure or sepsis without CNS localization.

Epstein-Barr virus infection has been linked to B-cell lymphoma because the genome DNA of the virus could be demonstrated in the tumor in some pa-

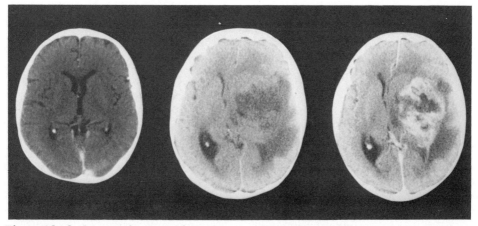

Figure 16–6. Computed tomography scans in a patient with neurofibromatosis in whom astrocytoma developed 1 year after heart transplantation (*left*, pretransplantation scan). (From Wijdicks, et al,[120] with permission of Neurology.)

tients.[51,52] Nevertheless, serologic evidence of active Epstein-Barr virus infection is absent in 10% to 20% of patients with B-cell lymphoma after transplantation. In T-cell lymphoma, human T-cell lymphotrophic virus 1 may have a role, but data are contradictory.

The clinical manifestations of CNS lymphoma may include brain and spinal cord involvement. Systemic localization is absent in most patients. CT scan shows a solitary mass lesion,[53] which can be similar to those in progressive multifocal leukoencephalopathy, a condition usually seen years after initial transplantation[41,50] (review of this condition is outside the scope of this chapter). Multiple localizations, sometimes with diffuse subependymal nodules, can occur, and MRI increases their yield.

The presenting symptoms are often behavior changes with visual hallucinations and hemiparesis. Headache is noted by one third of the patients and points to meningeal involvement. The lack of focal signs and preponderance of personality changes in patients with intracranial lymphoma may delay detection.

Aggressive treatment with radiation may result in complete resolution of the lesion on CT scan and of the neurologic findings in both types of lymphomas, but the prospect of long-term survival is low.

NEUROLOGIC COMPLICATIONS OF GRAFT-VERSUS-HOST DISEASE

Viable immunocompetent donor bone marrow cells may react to target organs, such as skin, liver, and the gastrointestinal tract. Acute graft-versus-host disease (GVHD) is usually apparent 20 to 100 days after bone marrow inoculation. Survival is determined by infectious complications. The incidence of GVHD, which may reach 70%, increases with age. A chronic form of GVHD may occur as early as 3 months after bone marrow transplantation. Chronic GVHD strongly resembles vasculitis syndromes, such as systemic lupus erythematosus and scleroderma and sicca syndrome. The principal neurologic complications are polymyositis and myasthenia gravis.[73,76] Peripheral nerve abnormalities are rarely described, except for herpes zoster, neuralgia, Guillain-Barré syndrome,[71] and, in one patient, mononeuritis multiplex involving the peroneal and cutaneous femoral lateral nerves.[73,76,123]

Polymyositis

Polymyositis may appear 2 to 54 months after allogeneic bone marrow transplantation.[6,41,85,92,96,114] Only one patient with autologous bone marrow transplantation for recurrent Hodgkin's disease is known.[92]

Clinical presentation is similar to that in any other patient with polymyositis, although early contractures are common and most likely associated with marked skin changes. Many patients complain of stiffness with movement and pain in proximal shoulder muscles. These symptoms are often followed by marked weakness and wasting of neck flexors and shoulder girdle muscles. Many patients have a low-grade fever. Serum creatine phosphokinase levels are increased but are within normal range in patients with only minimal weakness and nontender muscles. Muscle biopsies invariably demonstrate necrotic fibers with endomysial lymphocytes and phagocytosis without immunoglobulin deposits or blood vessel abnormalities.

Outcome is good if the patient survives the devastating consequences of chronic GVHD. Excellent return of muscle function has been reported after treatment with prednisone (1 to 3 mg/kg of body weight), prednisone with antithymocyte globulin (7 mg of IgG/kg), or azathioprine (100 mg daily).

Myasthenia Gravis

Nine patients with myasthenia gravis have been reported.[15,46,93,97] Six of the nine patients had bone marrow transplantation for aplastic anemia. All features known in typical myasthenia gravis have been described. However, most patients with myasthenia gravis as part of GVHD were comparatively young (range, 9 to 26 years; mean, 18.4 years). It has been speculated that patients with HLA-B7 and HLA-DR2 antigens are at risk.[68] Ptosis may begin unilaterally but becomes bilateral in all patients. Bulbar involvement may occur, and diaphragmatic failure requiring support by mechanical ventilation develops in some patients.

Acetylcholine receptor antibody concentrations are increased.[60,93,98] All but one study found that IgG acetylcholine receptor antibody levels were increased 2 to 13 months after bone marrow transplantation in 20% of patients who otherwise did not have clinical myasthenia gravis. In a more recent study,[60] 41% of the patients had anti-acetylcholine antibodies. The clinical impression of myasthenia gravis is usually confirmed by edrophonium chloride (Tensilon) test (positive in all reported patients with myasthenia gravis associated with bone marrow transplantation) and conventional or single-fiber electromyography. Prednisone and azathioprine are successful in treatment, but tapering of the dose may lead to exacerbation, and long-term maintenance therapy is crucial.

CONCLUSIONS

When neurologic symptoms occur after organ transplantation, several patterns emerge. The transplantation literature is rife with neurologic manifestations of the major immunosuppressive agents: cyclosporine, OKT3, and the recently discovered FK 506. The likelihood of toxicity from cyclosporine or FK 506 is great in patients with postoperative behavioral changes and seizures, although plasma or blood concentrations may be in the normal range. Limited data suggest that liver transplantation in patients with preoperative hepatic encephalopathy is associated with a considerably higher risk of toxicity, but toxic effects also occur in heart, lung, and renal transplantation.

Other underlying causes of postoperative waxing and waning levels of consciousness worthy of pursuit are nonconvulsive status epilepticus and central pontine myelinolysis after liver transplantation. Opportunistic CNS infections and lymphoma may occur in the postoperative months. There is a low probability of cerebrovascular complications at any time after organ transplantation. Intracranial hemorrhages may be associated with fungal infections, particularly those caused by *Aspergillus*.

An intracranial mass may be manifested by new-onset seizures or focal signs. Malignant lymphoma, nocardia, toxoplasma, and progressive multifocal leukoencephalopathy are possible causes. Brain biopsy may yield a final diagnosis.

REFERENCES

1. Adair, JC, Call, GK, O'Connell, JB, and Baringer, JR: Cerebrovascular syndromes following cardiac transplantation. Neurology 42:819–823, 1992.
2. Adair, JC, Woodley, SL, O'Connell, JB, et al: Aseptic meningitis following cardiac transplantation: Clinical characteristics and relationship to immunosuppressive regimen. Neurology 41 (2 Part 1):249–252, 1991.
3. Adams, DH, Ponsford, S, Gunson, B, et al: Neurological complications following liver transplantation. Lancet i:949–951, 1987.
4. Adams, HP Jr, Dawson, G, Coffman, TJ, and Corry, RJ: Stroke in renal transplant recipients. Arch Neurol 43:113–115, 1986.
5. Alessiani, M, Cillo, U, Fung, JJ, et al:

Adverse effects of FK 506 overdosage after liver transplantation. Transplant Proc 25:628–634, 1993.

6. Anderson, BA, Young, PV, Kean, WF, et al: Polymyositis in chronic graft vs host disease: A case report. Arch Neurol 39:188–190, 1982.

7. Andrews, BT, Hershon, JJ, Calanchini, P, et al: Neurologic complications of cardiac transplantation. West J Med 153:146–148, 1990.

8. Ang, LC, Gillett, JM, and Kaufmann, JCE: Neuropathology of heart transplantation. Can J Neurol Sci 16:291–298, 1989.

9. Appleton, RE, Farrell, K, Teal, P, et al: Complex partial status epilepticus associated with cyclosporin A therapy. J Neurol Neurosurg Psychiatry 52:1068–1071, 1989.

10. Baliga, R and Etheredge, EE: Cyclosporine-associated convulsions in a child after renal transplantation. Transplantation 51:1126–1128, 1991.

11. Bamborschke, S, Wullen, T, Huber, M, et al: Early diagnosis and successful treatment of acute cytomegalovirus encephalitis in a renal transplant recipient. J Neurol 239:205–208, 1992.

12. Békássy, NA, Cronqvist, S, Garwicz, S, and Wiebe, T: Arterial occlusion due to Listeria meningoencephalitis in an immunocompromised boy. Scand J Infect Dis 19:485–489, 1987.

13. Bird, GLA, Meadows, J, Goka, J, et al: Cyclosporin-associated akinetic mutism and extrapyramidal syndrome after liver transplantation. J Neurol Neurosurg Psychiatry 53:1068–1071, 1990.

14. Bohlin, A-B, Berg, U, Englund, M, et al: Central nervous system complications in children treated with ciclosporine after renal transplantation. Child Nephrol Urol 10:225–230, 1990.

15. Bolger, GB, Sullivan, KM, Spence, AM, et al: Myasthenia gravis after allogeneic bone marrow transplantation: Relationship to chronic graft-versus-host disease. Neurology 36:1087–1091, 1986.

16. Boon, AP, Adams, DH, Buckels, J, and McMaster, P: Cerebral aspergillosis in liver transplantation. J Clin Pathol 43:114–118, 1990.

17. Byrne, WR and Wajszczuk, CP: Cryptococcal meningitis in the acquired immunodeficiency syndrome (AIDS): Successful treatment with fluconazole after failure of amphotericin B. Ann Intern Med 108:384–385, 1988.

18. Capone, PM and Cohen, ME: Seizures and cerebritis associated with administration of OKT3. Pediatr Neurol 7:299–301, 1991.

19. Champlin, RE and Gale, RP: The early complications of bone marrow transplantation. Semin Hematol 21:101–108, 1984.

20. Chan, GL, Weinstein, SS, Wright, CE, et al: Encephalopathy associated with OKT3 administration: Possible interaction with indomethacin. Transplantation 52:148–150, 1991.

21. Coleman, AE and Norman, DJ: OKT3 encephalopathy. Ann Neurol 28:837–838, 1990.

22. Cox, J, Murtagh, FR, Wilfong, A, and Brenner, J: Cerebral aspergillosis: MR imaging and histopathologic correlation. AJNR Am J Neuroradiol 13:1489–1492, 1992.

23. Crous Tsanaclis, AM and de Morais, CF: Cerebral toxoplasmosis after renal transplantation: Case report. Pathol Res Pract 181:339–341, 1986.

24. Davenport, C, Dillon, WP, and Sze, G: Neuroradiology of the immunosuppressed state. Radiol Clin North Am 30:611–637, May 1992.

25. Davis, D, Henslee, PJ, and Markesbery, WR: Fatal adenovirus meningoencephalitis in a bone marrow transplant patient. Ann Neurol 23:385–389, 1988.

26. Dee, RR and Lorber, B: Brain abscess due to Listeria monocytogenes: Case report and literature review. Rev Infect Dis 8:968–977, 1986.

27. de Groen, PC: Cyclosporine, low-density lipoprotein, and cholesterol. Mayo Clin Proc 63:1012–1021, 1988.

28. de Groen, PC: Cyclosporine: A review and its specific use in liver transplantation. Mayo Clin Proc 64:680–689, 1989.

29. de Groen, PC, Aksamit, AJ, Rakela, J,

et al: Central nervous system toxicity after liver transplantation: The role of cyclosporine and cholesterol. N Engl J Med 317:861–866, 1987.

30. De Klippel, N, Sennesael, J, Lamote, J, et al: Cyclosporin leucoencephalopathy induced by intravenous lipid solution (letter). Lancet 339:1114, 1992.

31. Delattre, J-Y and Posner, JB: Neurological complications of chemotherapy and radiation therapy. In Aminoff, MJ (ed): Neurology and General Medicine. Churchill Livingstone, New York, 1989, pp 365–387.

32. Denning, DW, Tucker, RM, Hanson, LH, et al: Itraconazole therapy for cryptococcal meningitis and cryptococcosis. Arch Intern Med 149:2301–2308, 1989.

33. de Prada, JAV, Martín-Duran, R, Garcia-Monco, C, et al: Cyclosporine neurotoxicity in heart transplantation. J Heart Transplant 9:581–583, 1990.

34. Derouin, F, Devergie, A, Auber, P, et al: Toxoplasmosis in bone marrow-transplant recipients: Report of seven cases and review. Clin Infect Dis 15:267–270, 1992.

35. DeVault, GA Jr, King, JW, Rohr, MS, et al: Opportunistic infections with *Strongyloides stercoralis* in renal transplantation. Rev Infect Dis 12:653–671, 1990.

36. Drutz, DJ and Catanzaro, A: Coccidioidomycosis. Part II. Am Rev Respir Dis 117:727–771, 1978.

37. Eidelman, BH, Abu-Elmagd, K, Wilson, J, et al: Neurologic complications of FK 506. Transplant Proc 23:3175–3178, 1991.

38. Emmons, C, Smith, J, and Flanigan, M: Cerebrospinal fluid inflammation during OKT3 therapy (letter). Lancet ii:510–511, 1986.

39. Estol, CJ, Pessin, MS, and Martinez, AJ: Cerebrovascular complications after orthotopic liver transplantation: A clinicopathologic study. Neurology 41:815–819, 1991.

40. Fisher, MA, Levy, J, Helfrich, M, et al: Detection of *Toxoplasma gondii* in the spinal fluid of a bone marrow transplant recipient. Pediatr Infect Dis J 6:81–83, 1987.

41. Flomenbaum, MA, Jarcho, JA, and Schoen, FJ: Progressive multifocal leukoencephalopathy fifty-seven months after heart transplantation. J Heart Lung Transplant 10:888–893, 1991.

42. Freise, CE, Rowley, H, Lake, J, et al: Similar clinical presentation of neurotoxicity following FK 506 and cyclosporine in a liver transplant recipient. Transplant Proc 23:3173–3174, 1991.

43. Ghalie, R, Fitzsimmons, WE, Bennett, D, and Kaizer, H: Cortical blindness: A rare complication of cyclosporine therapy. Bone Marrow Transplant 6:147–149, 1990.

44. Ghany, AM, Tutschka, PJ, McGhee, RB Jr, et al: Cyclosporine-associated seizures in bone marrow transplant recipients given busulfan and cyclophosphamide preparative therapy. Transplantation 52:310–315, 1991.

45. Grant, JW and von Deimling, A: Primary T-cell lymphoma of the central nervous sytem. Arch Pathol Lab Med 114:24–27, 1990.

46. Grau, JM, Casademont, J, Monforte, R, et al: Myasthenia gravis after allogeneic bone marrow transplantation: Report of a new case and pathogenetic considerations. Bone Marrow Transplant 5:435–437, 1990.

47. Grigg, MM, Costanzo-Nordin, MR, Celesia, GG, et al: The etiology of seizures after cardiac transplantation. Transplant Proc 20 Suppl 3:937–944, 1988.

48. Gryn, J, Goldberg, J, and Viner, E: Propranolol for the treatment of cyclosporine-induced headaches. Bone Marrow Transplant 9:211–212, 1992.

49. Hacker, SM, Knight, BP, Lunde, NM, et al: A primary central nervous system T cell lymphoma in a renal transplant patient. Transplantation 53:691–692, 1992.

50. Hall, WA, Martinez, AJ, and Dummer, JS: Progressive multifocal leukoencephalopathy after cardiac transplantation. Neurology 38:995–996, 1988.

51. Hochberg, FH and Miller, DC: Primary central nervous system lymphoma. J Neurosurg 68:835–853, 1988.

52. Hochberg, FH, Miller, G, Schooley, RT, et al: Central-nervous-system lymphoma related to Epstein-Barr virus. N Engl J Med 309:745–748, 1983.

53. Jack, CR Jr, O'Neill, BP, Banks, PM, and Reese, DF: Central nervous system lymphoma: Histologic types and CT appearance. Radiology 167:211–215, 1988.

54. Jerman, MR, and Fick, RB Jr: Nonbacterial thrombotic endocarditis associated with bone marrow transplantation. Chest 90:919–922, 1986.

55. Kaplan, RS and Wiernick, PH: Neurotoxicity of antineoplastic drugs. Semin Oncol 9:103–130, 1982.

56. Kauffman, CA, Israel, KS, Smith, JW, et al: Histoplasmosis in immunosuppressed patients. Am J Med 64:923–932, 1978.

57. Kong, NCT, Shaariah, W, Morad, Z, et al: Cryptococcosis in a renal unit. Aust N Z J Med 20:645–649, 1990.

58. Kunzendorf, U, Brockmöller, J, Jochimsen, F, et al: Cyclosporin metabolites and central-nervous-system toxicity (letter). Lancet i:1223, 1988.

59. Larner, AJ, Conway, MA, Mitchell, RG, and Forfar, JC: Recurrent Listeria monocytogenes meningitis in a heart transplant recipient. J Infect 19:263–266, 1989.

60. Lefvert, AK and Björkholm, M: Antibodies against the acetylcholine receptor in hematologic disorders: Implications for the development of myasthenia gravis after bone marrow grafting (letter). N Engl J Med 317:170, 1987.

61. Lind, MJ, McWilliam, L, Jip, J, et al: Cyclosporin associated demyelination following allogeneic bone marrow transplantation. Hematol Oncol 7:49–52, 1989.

62. Lopez, OL, Martinez, AJ, and Torre-Cisneros, J: Neuropathologic findings in liver transplantation: A comparative study of cyclosporine and FK 506. Transplant Proc 23:3181–3182, 1991.

63. Löwenberg, B, van Gijn, J, Prins, E, and Polderman, AM: Fatal cerebral toxoplasmosis in a bone marrow transplant recipient with leukemia. Transplantation 35:30–33, 1983.

64. Marks, WH, Perkal, M, Bia, M, and Lorber, MI: Aseptic encephalitis and blindness complicating OKT3 therapy. Clin Transpl 5:435–438, 1991.

65. Martin, MA, Massanari, M, Nghiem, DD, et al: Nosocomial aseptic meningitis associated with administration of OKT3. JAMA 259:2002–2005, 1988.

66. Martinez, AJ and Puglia, J: The neuropathology of liver, heart, and heart-lung transplantation. Transplant Proc 20:806–809, 1988.

67. McManus, RP, O'Hair, DP, Schweiger, J, et al: Cyclosporine-associated central neurotoxicity after heart transplantation. Ann Thorac Surg 53:326–327, 1992.

68. Melms, A, Faul, C, Sommer, N, et al: Myasthenia gravis after BMT: Identification of patients at risk? Bone Marrow Transplant 9:78–79, 1992.

69. Miksits, K, Stoltenburg, G, Neumayer, H-H, et al: Disseminated infection of the central nervous system caused by Nocardia farcinica. Nephrol Dial Transplant 6:209–214, 1991.

70. Mohrmann, RL, Mah, V, and Vinters, HV: Neuropathologic findings after bone marrow transplantation: An autopsy study. Hum Pathol 21:630–639, 1990

71. Myers, SE, and Williams, SF: Guillain-Barré syndrome after autologous bone marrow transplantation for breast cancer: Report of two cases. Bone Marrow Transplant 13:341–344, 1994.

72. Nau, R, Brück, W, Bollensen, E, and Prange, HW: Meningoencephalitis with septic intracerebral infarction: A new feature of CNS listeriosis. Scand J Infect Dis 22:101–103, 1990.

73. Nelson, KR and McQuillen, MP: Neurologic complications of graft-versus-host disease. Neurol Clin 6:389–403, 1988.

74. Palmer, BF and Toto, RD: Severe neurologic toxicity induced by cyclosporine A in three renal transplant patients. Am J Kidney Dis 18:116–121, 1991.

75. Parker, SL, Laszewski, MJ, Trigg, ME, and Smith, WL: Spinal cord aspergillosis in immunosuppressed patients. Pediatr Radiol 20:351–352, 1990.

76. Patchell, RA, White, CL III, Clark, AW, et al: Neurologic complications of bone marrow transplantation. Neurology 35:300–306, 1985.

77. Penn, I: Cancers complicating organ transplantation (editorial). N Engl J Med 323:1767–1769, 1990.

78. Penn, I: The changing pattern of post-transplant malignancies. Transplant Proc 23:1101–1103, 1991.

79. Polo, JM, Fábrega, E, Casafont, F, et al: Treatment of cerebral aspergillosis after liver transplantation. Neurology 42:1817–1819, 1992.

80. Popovich, MJ, Arthur, RH, and Helmer, E: CT of intracranial cryptococcosis. AJNR Am J Neuroradiol 11:139–142, 1990.

81. Raby, N, Forbes, G, and Williams, R: *Nocardia* infection in patients with liver transplants or chronic liver disease: Radiologic findings. Radiology 174:713–716, 1990.

82. Randhawa, PS, Markin, RS, Starzl, TE, and Demetris, AJ: Epstein-Barr virus-associated syndromes in immunosuppressed liver transplant recipients: Clinical profile and recognition on routine allograft biopsy. Am J Surg Pathol 14:538–547, 1990.

83. Reece, DE, Frei-Lahr, DA, Shepherd, JD, et al: Neurologic complications in allogeneic bone marrow transplant patients receiving cyclosporin. Bone Marrow Transplant 8:393–401, 1991.

84. Reyes, J, Gayowski, T, Fung, J, et al: Expressive dysphasia possibly related to FK506 in two liver transplant recipients. Transplantation 50:1043–1045, 1990.

85. Reyes, MG, Noronha, P, Thomas, W Jr, and Heredia, R: Myositis of chronic graft versus host disease. Neurology 33:1222–1224, 1983.

86. Riether, AM, Smith, SL, Lewison, BJ, et al: Quality-of-life changes and psychiatric and neurocognitive outcome after heart and liver transplantation. Transplantation 54:444–450, 1992.

87. Roden, J, Klintmalm, GBG, Husberg, BS, et al: Cerebrospinal fluid inflammation during OKT3 therapy (letter). Lancet ii:272, 1987.

88. Rubin, AM: Transient cortical blindness and occipital seizures with cyclosporine toxicity. Transplantation 47:572–573, 1989.

89. Rubin, AM and Kang, H: Cerebral blindness and encephalopathy with cyclosporin A toxicity. Neurology 37:1072–1076, 1987.

90. Sanders, J, Sale, GE, Ramberg, R, et al: Glioblastoma multiforme in a patient with acute lymphoblastic leukemia who received a marrow transplant. Transplant Proc 14:770–774, 1982.

91. Scheinman, SJ, Reinitz, ER, Petro, G, et al: Cyclosporine central neurotoxicity following renal transplantation: Report of a case using magnetic resonance images. Transplantation 49:215–216, 1990.

92. Schmidley, JW and Galloway, P: Polymyositis following autologous bone marrow transplantation in Hodgkin's disease. Neurology 40:1003–1004, 1990.

93. Seely, E, Drachman, D, Smith, BR, et al: Post bone marrow transplantation (BMT) myasthenia gravis: Evidence for acetylcholine receptor (ACh R) abnormality (abstr). Blood 64 Suppl 1:221a, 1984.

94. Sila, CA: Spectrum of neurologic events following cardiac transplantation. Stroke 20:1586–1589, 1989.

95. Skogberg, K, Syrjänen, J, Jahkola, M, et al: Clinical presentation and outcome of listeriosis in patients with and without immunosuppressive therapy. Clin Infect Dis 14:815–821, 1992.

96. Slatkin, NE, Sheibani, K, Forman, SJ, et al: Myositis as the major manifestation of chronic graft versus host disease (abstr). Neurology 37 Suppl 1:205, 1987.

97. Smith, CIE, Aarli, JA, Biberfeld, P, et al: Myasthenia gravis after bone-marrow transplantation: Evidence for a

donor origin. N Engl J Med 309:1565–1568, 1983.

98. Smith, CIE, Hammarström, L, and Lefvert, A-K: Bone-marrow grafting induces acetylcholine receptor antibody formation (letter). Lancet i:978, 1985.

99. Spitzer, ED, Spitzer, SG, Freundlich, LF, and Casadevall, A: Persistence of initial infection in recurrent *Cryptococcus neoformans* meningitis. Lancet 341:595–596, 1993.

100. Spitzer, PG, Tarsy, D, and Eliopoulos, GM: Acute transverse myelitis during disseminated cytomegalovirus infection in a renal transplant recipient. Transplantation 44:151–153, 1987.

101. Starzl, TE, Demetris, AJ, and Van Thiel, D: Liver transplantation (first of two parts). N Engl J Med 321:1014–1021, 1989.

102. Starzl, TE, Demetris, AJ, and Van Thiel, D: Liver transplantation (second of two parts). N Engl J Med 321:1092–1099, 1989.

103. Steg, RE and Garcia, EG: Complex visual hallucinations and cyclosporine neurotoxicity. Neurology 41:1156, 1991.

104. Stein, DP, Lederman, RJ, Vogt, DP, et al: Neurological complications following liver transplantation. Ann Neurol 31:644–649, 1992.

105. Sullivan, KM, Shulman, HM, Storb, R, et al: Chronic graft-versus-host disease in 52 patients: Adverse natural course and successful treatment with combination immunosuppression. Blood 57:267–276, 1981.

106. Swinnen, LJ, Costanzo-Nordin, MR, Fisher, SG, et al: Increased incidence of lymphoproliferative disorder after immunosuppression with the monoclonal antibody OKT3 in cardiac-transplant recipients. N Engl J Med 323:1723–1728, 1990.

107. Thistlethwaite, JR Jr, Stuart, JK, Mayes, JT, et al: Complications and monitoring of OKT3 therapy. Am J Kidney Dis 11:112–119, 1988.

108. Thomas, DM, Nicholls, AJ, Feest, TG, and Riad, H: OKT3 and cerebral oedema (letter). Br Med J 295:1486, 1987.

109. Tien, RD, Chu, PK, Hesselink, JR, et al: Intracranial cryptococcosis in immunocompromised patients: CT and MR findings in 29 cases. AJNR Am J Neuroradiol 12:283–289, 1991.

110. Todo, S, Fung, JJ, Starzl, TE, et al: Liver, kidney, and thoracic organ transplantation under FK 506. Ann Surg 212:295–307, 1990.

111. Torre-Cisneros, J, Lopez, OL, Kusne, S, et al: CNS aspergillosis in organ transplantation: A clinicopathological study. J Neurol Neurosurg Psychiatry 56:188–193, 1993.

112. Treseler, CB and Sugar, AM: Fungal meningitis. Infect Dis Clin North Am 4:789–808, 1990.

113. Truwit, CL, Denaro, CP, Lake, JR, and DeMarco, T: MR imaging of reversible cyclosporin A-induced neurotoxicity. AJNR Am J Neuroradiol 12:651–659, 1991.

114. Urbano-Márques, A, Estruch, R, Grau, JM, et al: Inflammatory myopathy associated with chronic graft-versus-host disease. Neurology 36:1091–1093, 1986.

115. Viscoli, C, Garaventa, A, Ferrea, G, et al: *Listeria monocytogenes* brain abscesses in a girl with acute lymphoblastic leukaemia after late central nervous system relapse. Eur J Cancer 27:435–437, 1991.

116. Vogt, DP, Lederman, RJ, Carey, WD, and Broughan, TA: Neurologic complications of liver transplantation. Transplantation 45:1057–1061, 1988.

117. White, M, Cirrincione, C, Blevins, A, and Armstrong, D: Cryptococcal meningitis: Outcome in patients with AIDS and patients with neoplastic disease. J Infect Dis 165:960–963, 1992.

118. Wijdicks, EFM, Borleffs, JCC, Hoepelman, AIM, and Jansen, GH: Fatal disseminated hemorrhagic toxoplasmic encephalitis as the initial manifestation of AIDS. Ann Neurol 29:683–686, 1991.

119. Wijdicks, EFM, de Groen, P, Wiesner, RH, and Krom, RAF: Intracranial hemorrhage following liver transplantation (abstr). Neurology 44 Suppl 2:A227, 1994.

120. Wijdicks, EFM, Jambroes, G, and

Riccardi, VM: De novo astrocytoma following immunosuppression in neurofibromatosis. Neurology 40:1467–1468, 1990.

121. Wijdicks, EFM, Wiesner, RH, Dahlke, LJ, and Krom, RAF: FK 506-induced neurotoxicity in liver transplantation. Ann Neurol 35:498–501, 1994.

122. Wilson, SE, de Groen, PC, Aksamit, AJ, et al: Cyclosporin A-induced reversible cortical blindness. J Clin Neuroophthalmol 8:215–220, 1988.

123. Wiznitzer, M, Packer, RJ, August, CS, and Burkey, ED: Neurologic complications of bone marrow transplantation in childhood. Ann Neurol 16:569–576, 1984.

124. Wszolek, ZK, Aksamit, AJ, Ellingson, RJ, et al: Epileptiform electroencephalographic abnormalities in liver transplant recipients. Ann Neurol 30:37–41, 1991.

Part IV

OUTCOME IN CENTRAL NERVOUS SYSTEM CATASTROPHES

Chapter 17

CLINICAL COURSE AND OUTCOME OF ACUTE INJURY TO THE CENTRAL NERVOUS SYSTEM

The considerable cost of intensive care medicine to society has triggered concern about the benefit of aggressive management. This concern particularly pertains to patients who have illnesses in which the probability of survival is low.

When additional neurologic injury develops in patients in intensive care units (ICUs), outcome is often reassessed. Obviously, the clinical situation in which injury occurs makes a difference. In some patients with severe underlying illness, an acute neurologic event is a final event, but in patients with resolving critical illness, it is an unexpected (and sometimes temporary) setback.

Families of these unfortunate patients should not be left in the dark by overcautious physicians. In such instances, the decision to stop treatment in a hopeless situation may be postponed because family members have only a vague idea of the expected disability. Any considerable central nervous system (CNS) injury in a patient with a critical illness should prompt physicians to identify factors that predict a poor outcome. In many conditions, outcome can be quantified with reasonable probability and subsequently should be discussed in detail with family members. They may carry the burden of care of a severely disabled person and should know what to expect when aggressive treatment is continued. No one can know with certainty what the outcome will be, but in many CNS catastrophes, prognostic factors have been explicitly identified. Ultimately, a decision should be made, and the result almost certainly will be a "do not resuscitate" status, withdrawal of medication, or withdrawal of life-sustaining support. A "do not resuscitate" order includes not only no resuscitation in the event of a cardiac or respiratory arrest but also, as discussed with patient or family members, no blood or plasma products, intravenous drugs for acute cardiac arrhythmias, invasive monitoring devices, hemodialysis, cardiac pacemakers, endotracheal tubes, cardioversion, chest tubes, or bronchoscopy. For patients in whom the outcome is expected to be dismal, withdrawal of support should be strongly considered. A retrospective analysis with historical controls at the Cleveland Clinic showed that the median reduction of length of stay was 22 days after "do not resuscitate" orders were given for patients with end-stage illnesses.[32] Nonetheless, for some families, having a very disabled person nearby is preferable to complete loss.

The ethical aspects of withdrawal of support are not discussed. These vexing problems, which include withdrawal of nutrition and hydration, are described in detail in overview papers.[2,13,48,49] In general, after withdrawal of nutrition and hydration, death can be expected within 2 weeks without any signs of discomfort to the patient. This chapter focuses on outcomes of major neurologic catastrophes and may serve as a reference and guide for management decisions. Only major categories are discussed; specific situations can be found in other chapters.

DESCRIPTION OF OUTCOME CATEGORIES

At its simplest, outcome can be defined as death, persistent vegetative state, moderate or severe disability, and good recovery. These components are frequently used in widely accepted rating systems, including the Glasgow outcome scale. Persistent vegetative state is defined as no awareness of person or surroundings; lack of sustained, reproducible, purposeful, or voluntary behavioral responses to any stimuli; mutism but with occasional sounds or expressions, such as yawning, lip smacking, and grimacing; and withdrawal from painful stimuli. Automatic and stereotypical behavior may occur. Primitive auditory or visual orienting reflex with head turning may perplex family members and can incorrectly suggest awareness. Visual tracking or response to visual threat is absent. Patients with midline brain lesions may have an akinetic mutism, which probably should be considered a variant of the vegetative state. These patients remain mute and motionless; no communication is possible.

Locked-in syndrome, often seen in acute ventral pons destruction, causes almost total deafferentation and is rec-ognized by inability to move or communicate other than by blinking or vertical eye movements and, most importantly, by intact or near-intact level of consciousness.

The differences between the most commonly seen syndromes are shown in Table 17–1, which is adapted from a position paper from a multisociety task force on persistent vegetative state.[40]

"Severe disability" usually is applied to patients with residual cognitive or motor deficits that prevent them from functioning independently. Active rehabilitation training programs may produce significant gains in physical independence, but if no spontaneous improvement has emerged within 1 year, return to gainful employment should be considered an unrealistic expectation. However, continued improvement has been reported in patients with severe disability after head injury, but data in other acute CNS disorders are not available. In the category "moderate disability," the patient may have significant deficits, but these patients are able to return to their previous employers, although adjustments to much lower job levels often are necessary. "Good recovery" refers to complete return to baseline function, but minor fixed, nondisabling deficits may be present. In the following discussion, these broad categories are used. Intermediate categories are less well studied.

OUTCOME IN METABOLIC ENCEPHALOPATHIES

Clinical observation alone most likely remains the mainstay of prognostication in metabolic encephalopathies. Careful neurologic examination with daily follow-up should include cognitive testing, assessment of brain stem reflexes, and motor response to noxious stimuli. In many patients, lack of improvement of the motor component of the Glasgow coma scale alone over a certain observation period is indicative of poor outcome. In a large series of patients with nontraumatic coma caused

Table 17-1 NEUROLOGIC CONDITIONS THAT PRODUCE UNRESPONSIVENESS*

Condition	Self-awareness	Sleep-Wake Cycles	Motor Function	Experiences Suffering	Respiratory Function	EEG	Prognosis for Neurologic Recovery
Persistent vegetative state†	Absent	Intact	No purposeful movement; no visual tracking	No	Normal	Polymorphic delta and theta; sometimes slow alpha	Traumatic PVS (1-yr outcome): PVS, 15% of patients; dead, 33%; GR, 7%; MD, 17%; SD, 28% Nontraumatic PVS (1-yr outcome): PVS, 32% of patients; dead, 53%; GR, 1%; MD, 3%; SD, 11%
Brain death	Absent	Absent	None or only reflex spinal movements	No	Absent	Electrocerebral silence	None
Locked-in syndrome	Present	Intact	Quadriplegia; pseudobulbar palsy; preserved vertical eye movements	Yes	Normal	Normal or mildly abnormal	Recovery unlikely; patients remain quadriplegic; prolonged survival possible
Akinetic mutism	Present	Intact	Paucity of movement	Yes	Normal	Nonspecific slowing	Recovery very unlikely and depends on cause

Modified from Medical Aspects of the Persistent Vegetative State.[40]

*This table was constructed to provide a general overview of PVS and related neurologic conditions. Because of the overlap of clinical and laboratory findings, these generalizations will not apply to every patient. Neuroimaging studies (MRI or CT) may be useful in the clinical evaluation of patients but may not always be helpful in differentiating the above conditions.

†Adults only.

GR = good recovery; MD = moderately disabled; PVS = persistent vegetative state; SD = severely disabled.

by metabolic derangements or hypoxia, longitudinal evaluation for 1 week proved to be successful in the prediction of outcome.[37] In critical illness, however, the underlying disorder determines mortality. Advanced support and treatment may potentially increase the number of survivors with permanent severe disability—patients who otherwise would have died from complications.

Hypoxic Ischemic Encephalopathy

In many patients, a confident decision on withdrawal of support cannot be made within 72 hours after cardiopulmonary resuscitation. In any patient, at least 6 hours must have passed before clinical signs can be used for prognostication. At the time of resuscitation, nonreactive pupils and absent motor responses associated with a dramatic global decrease in cerebral blood flow during cardiac compression do not necessarily indicate permanent neuronal damage in the cortical layers.

Immediate awakening after cardiac resuscitation (incidence of 15% to 20% in large series) predicts good outcome,

and permanent cognitive deficits are unusual.[6,16,42,44] Unfortunately, many patients have underlying cardiac disease that limits their performance, and a significant proportion may still die suddenly in the first year. Patients who remain comatose after resuscitation have a very high chance of dying in the hospital (Fig. 17–1) from withdrawal of support or because of recurrent arrhythmias.

Patients who do not withdraw the upper extremities to pain and who remain comatose after 24 hours have a very small but significant chance (approximately 6%) of recovery to independent function if they survive their hospital stay. After 3 days from the time of cardiopulmonary resuscitation, the number of surviving patients is small, and independent function is achieved only by those who improve to withdrawal to pain. Therefore, the decision to withdraw support usually cannot be made on clinical data alone within the first 3 days after resuscitation, and additional laboratory data are needed to assist in an accurate prediction.

Prognosticators of poor outcome have been identified; if they are present, severe disability, persistent vegetative state, or death is very likely (Table

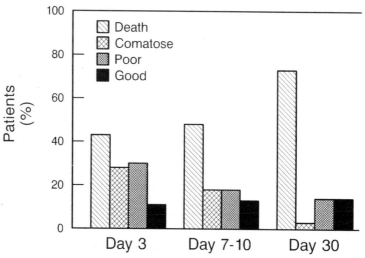

Figure 17–1. Neurologic outcome in postanoxic coma (data were collected from several large series of patients studied after cardiac arrest).

Table 17-2 PROGNOSTICATORS OF POOR OUTCOME IN POSTANOXIC COMA AFTER CARDIAC ARREST*

Clinical	Laboratory
Fixed pupils Myclonus status Sustained upward gaze	Absence of bilateral cortical response on somatosensory evoked potentials Burst-suppression pattern on electro-encephalogram

*When present more than 6 hours after cardio-pulmonary resuscitation.

17-2). (Rules of prognostication may not apply in patients who were resuscitated as a result of submersion and hypothermia; see Chapter 14.) When poor outcome prognosticators are present, and certainly when somatosensory evoked potential cortical responses are bilaterally absent, withdrawal of support should become a strong option. The percentage of patients with these abnormalities in the first day is relatively small (30%), and definitive prognostication often must be postponed until the third day after return of circulation. When myoclonus is absent and cortical somatosensory evoked potentials are present, the guidelines from a prospective study by Levy and associates[37] are useful (Fig. 17-2).

Recovery should be fairly rapid for patients to have a chance of good recovery from anoxic encephalopathy. Good recovery can be expected if, after 72 hours from the time of cardiac arrest, the patient withdraws the arms to pain, localizes pain, or follows simple one-step commands. The chance of awakening decreases remarkably in the first week (50% in the first day, 25% in the third day, and 10% at the end of the first week). Awakening after more than 3 days of coma from anoxia is very frequently associated with severe disability. The neuropsychologic sequelae have only recently been studied in detail. Of 54 survivors of cardiac arrest, 26 (48%) had severe deficits and 22 (41%) had evidence of depression.[51]

Patients with severe disability after postanoxic coma are often in a tragic state. Dramatic recovery from a severely disabled state after 1 month is not often seen, and 6-month outcome is not much different from that in the first month. Occasionally, cognitive function may be relatively spared, but then action myoclonus may determine disability. These patients who have been comatose for some time but awaken are unable to stand or walk without support. Action myoclonus never appears while the patient is comatose and emerges only after awakening. In addition, an electroencephalogram (EEG) shows slowing of background rhythm and not the characteristic burst-suppression abnormality in myoclonus status.

Action myoclonus was discussed in the landmark paper by Lance and Adams in 1963.[35] This entity, perhaps more often seen in asphyxia, must be differentiated from myoclonus status. Myoclonus status is frequently seen in patients who survive cardiac resuscitation, and mortality is very high. Myoclonus status should strongly influence resuscitation orders and decisions to withdraw support, because it reflects very severe anoxic damage. Neuromuscular blockade to control twitching is necessary in many patients, also because vigorous facial twitching may suggest patient discomfort to visiting family members.

Action myoclonus, however, often occurs with severe ataxia caused by anoxic damage to cerebellar hemispheres. Sudden shocklike involuntary movements in all limbs, caused by active muscular contractions, are precipitated by movement or action. Imaging studies are rare, but in most patients, computed tomography (CT) and magnetic resonance imaging (MRI) scans are normal. Treatment with polytherapy may be helpful, but failures have been reported.[11,17,32,46] Administration of clonazepam or 5-hydroxytryptophan with carbidopa is the first line of treatment. Additional treatment with valproate sodium, primidone, or fluoxetine may be

Initial Examination

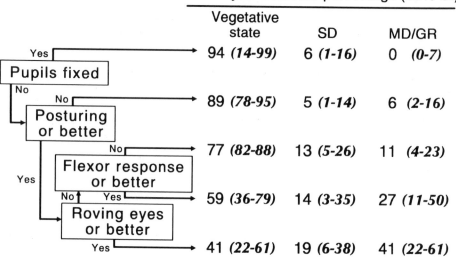

3 Days After CPR

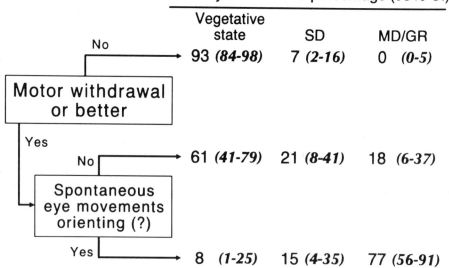

Figure 17–2. Algorithms for prognostication after cardiopulmonary resuscitation (CPR). Data are based on 210 prospectively studied patients. The percentage of patients is given in each subcategory. (Note the wide confidence intervals [CI] caused by the small number of studied patients in each outcome category.) SD = severely disabled; MD = moderately disabled; GR = good recovery. (Data from Levy, et al.[37])

tried, but sedation often becomes a limiting factor. A 1993 placebo-controlled, randomized study that included many causes of cortical myoclonus found that piracetam (median dose, 16.8 g/day) significantly improved disability from motor impairment, in some patients with dramatic results, when used in combination with other drugs.[11]

Isolated cognitive deficits, including an amnesic syndrome, may occur in the first weeks after resuscitation but are very uncommon. Amnesic syndromes that have been described are usually transient but at times permanent.[21] Patients with normal intellectual function but impaired free recall, intact short-term memory, and intact recognition have been recognized.[60] Confabulations are absent and orientation is spared, so that the resemblance to Korsakoff's syndrome is only superficial. Very frequently in amnesic syndrome, a combination of apraxia and motor aphasia is found, and this condition does not notably improve over the years. Although extrapyramidal syndromes have been largely reported with cyanide or carbon monoxide poisoning associated with hypoxia,[28,53,59] it is also noted after cardiac arrest.[7,9] An akinetic rigid syndrome develops as early as 1 week after the ictus and may evolve into surprisingly progressive generalized dystonia with severe bulbar involvement (oromandibular dystonia and blepharospasms) or disablement necessitating a wheelchair or confinement in bed.[9]

Uremic Encephalopathy

When uremic encephalopathy occurs with acute renal failure, associated systemic conditions determine outcome. Mortality from acute renal failure is low (approximately 8%) when serious complications such as sepsis, massive gastrointestinal bleeding, acute myocardial infarction, and acute respiratory failure are absent. Outcome in uremic encephalopathy can be excellent. The clinical signs of uremic encephalopathy may completely disappear after dialysis. In a few patients, the dramatic improvement in the grade of uremic encephalopathy is offset by generalized muscle weakness and muscle cramps. Transient muscle cramps that often occur immediately after dialysis are not related to electrolyte abnormalities. Profound weakness may be caused by hypophosphatemia related to antacid administration and hemodialysis.

Systematic clinical neurologic studies of recovery in patients with acute renal failure have not been published, but anecdotal experience suggests that most patients, if not all, recover without sequelae. Patients may vividly remember a psychotic state at the time of maximal renal failure. Resolution of the clinical signs and symptoms of uremic encephalopathy, often in reverse order of appearance, has also been noted during the diuretic phase of acute renal failure but only when the concentrating ability of the kidney decreases urea and creatinine levels. In the early polyuric phase of recovery, the excretion of urea and creatinine is not yet established and an increase in serum levels is more common.

Failure to improve should point to additional hypoxic-ischemic damage from conditions that are secondary to acute renal failure. During dialysis, hypotension may occur in 30% of the patients and may be, despite immediate intervention, an additional challenge to cerebral perfusion pressure. Failure to recover from uremic encephalopathy also occurs when acute renal failure is associated with systemic disease, which also affects the central or peripheral nervous system. Potential causes are the systemic vasculitides (see Chapter 11), thrombotic thrombocytopenic purpura (see Chapter 10), hemolytic uremic syndrome, and severe intoxication with heavy metals. In all these conditions and in patients with renal failure who do not awaken within 1 week after resolution of uremia by dialysis, outcome is poor. Bilateral subdural hematoma is a very unusual cause but may halt recovery and must be considered when severe coagulopathy is present or when heparin is used during hemodialysis. Thrombocytopenia is common during dialysis and is induced either by heparin treatment or from contact with the dialysis membrane.

Long-term outcome in patients with chronic renal failure is determined by the potential development of dialysis encephalopathy.

Dialysis dementia is rare, occurring only after 2 years of dialysis treatment. It is characterized by severe dysarthria, apraxia of speech, and rapid decline in cognitive function until death 6 months after diagnosis. Although serum levels of aluminum correlate poorly with occurrence, aluminum probably causes this devastating complication. In general, intellectual deterioration is uncommon in patients undergoing long-term dialysis, and many patients do not have significant changes in neuropsychologic performance when tested over the years. A comprehensive review of dialysis dementia, which is rarely seen in the ICU, is found in Bolton and Young's monograph on renal disease.[8]

Hepatic Encephalopathy

Outcome in patients with hepatic encephalopathy depends on the underlying liver disease.[34] Many patients with hepatic encephalopathy admitted to ICUs have either fulminant hepatic failure, in which case the fatality rate is considerable, or long-standing cirrhosis with an acute episode of gastrointestinal bleeding that evolves into acute portosystemic encephalopathy.[12]

Fulminant hepatic failure is frequently fatal without emergency liver transplantation, and the quality of supportive care is of crucial importance. Outcome may be more favorable in patients with drug-induced hepatitis (e.g., acetaminophen overdose) and non-A, non-B associated hepatic necrosis, but outcome in patients with rapid progression to stage III or IV encephalopathy is poor. Recent evidence suggests that the associated brain edema in higher stages of encephalopathy in fulminant hepatic failure is important in its clinical course (see Chapter 9). Despite aggressive treatment of intracranial pressure and additional resolution of clinical and radiologic signs, short-term outcome may still be devastating from complications of liver transplantation and immunosuppression. Even though mortality is high in fulminant hepatic necrosis, patients who survive do well and are expected to have normal intellectual performance. Patients in whom encephalopathy reaches stage IV tend to have a greater chance of severe cognitive deficits, but data on long-term outcome in patients within this category are only anecdotal.

More frequently, hepatic encephalopathy in patients admitted to medical ICUs has been precipitated by gastrointestinal bleeding, spontaneous bacterial peritonitis, or use of diuretic agents. Therefore, correction of associated metabolic abnormalities and administration of lactulose and neomycin may result in a striking improvement in level of consciousness. As mentioned previously, a weak linear relationship exists between stages of encephalopathy and arterial level of ammonia,[56] but increased arterial ammonia level may precede coma by several days, and a decrease in ammonia concentration may precede improvement in the stage of hepatic encephalopathy (see Chapter 9).

Of patients who become comatose or stuporous from hepatic encephalopathy, only one third regain independent function; the remaining 60% of patients die without regaining consciousness.[5,37] In a 1989 study, outcome in patients comatose from hepatic encephalopathy was worse when it was caused by gastrointestinal bleeding than when it was associated with other triggers.[12] Prognosticators of poor outcome in hepatic coma in patients with cirrhosis are ascites, low prothrombin index, and development of hepatorenal syndrome. Even though several episodes of hepatic encephalopathy can be sustained without major cognitive deficits, most patients are now offered liver transplantation despite the cause.

Many patients who recover from hepatic encephalopathy remain impaired in alertness and performance. Much of the day may be spent sleeping, and response to questions is sluggish.

Septic Encephalopathy

When acute respiratory distress syndrome, disseminated intravascular coagulation, or multiorgan failure becomes a consequence of sepsis, mortality is high. In addition, increased arterial lactate levels and low oxygen uptake (VO_2) are associated with increased mortality. It is not clear whether septic encephalopathy is an independent predictor of mortality. Brain function most likely fails with multiple organ failure, and recently it became more evident that severe hypotension is an important, if not crucial, contributor to septic encephalopathy in contrast to the assumption that the brain is a separate organ system that fails in sepsis.

In a series of 14 patients with severe septic encephalopathy, only 3 recovered but all had drowsiness or generalized seizures as presenting symptoms.[63] All patients who lacked motor responses died. (In the assessment of outcome in these patients, however, one should be aware of the long-standing effects of the neuromuscular blocking agents frequently used in this situation.) In these patients, EEG recordings, although nonspecific, may be helpful to assess brain damage. Mortality in septic encephalopathy has been shown to correlate with EEG abnormalities. Young and colleagues[64] reported no deaths in patients with normal EEG findings, 19% mortality with theta activity, 36% with delta activity, 50% with triphasic waves, and 67% with burst-suppression activity. Periodic lateralized epileptiform discharges did not have a predictive value. Results of CT scanning are normal in most patients with septic encephalopathy and very occasionally may demonstrate either multiple watershed infarcts consistent with marked hypotension for hours or multiple subcortical hematomas from disseminated intravascular coagulation. Systematic studies of outcome in septic encephalopathy are needed, but in all likelihood, the rules in hypoxic ischemic encephalopathy probably apply to septic encephalopathy as well.

Failure to awaken after sepsis syndrome is associated with a poor outcome, and EEG or somatosensory evoked potentials may be used for further confirmation.

Diabetic Comas

Mortality in patients with hyperosmolar nonketotic derangement varies from 20% to 60%, and death occurs in half the patients in the first 3 days.[23,55,61,62] Patients in hyperosmolar coma are severely hypovolemic, and cardiogenic shock may complicate the clinical picture. Prognosticators of poor outcome have not been consistently identified, but severity of hyperglycemia, hyperosmolarity, or uremia at presentation does not have predictive value.[61]

In contrast to nonketotic diabetes, diabetic ketoacidosis seldom produces coma.[18] Many patients, often young, completely recover after treatment. On the other hand, hypoglycemic coma can be devastating and may result in a persistent vegetative state or severe disability.[1,39,41] Selective hippocampal damage may occur in hypoglycemia, but in many patients hypoxia plays an additional role and is associated with a poor outcome[31,54] (see Chapter 7). Nevertheless, many patients recover, even after long episodes of hypoglycemia. In addition, a 1991 cohort study found that cognitive decline did not occur in patients with frequent hypoglycemic episodes.[50]

OUTCOME IN STROKE

In patients with a sudden major stroke who are critically ill, ventilator-dependent, and hemodynamically difficult to manage, further immobilization hampers weaning from the ventilator, and if weaning is successful, difficulty with swallowing may lead to aspiration. Patients may also have inadequate understanding of the goals of rehabilitation as a result of aphasia or apraxia, which adds importantly to the misery.

Prognostic factors have been identified in various types of stroke but remain largely unexplored in patients in whom critical illness was complicated by a stroke.

Intracerebral Hematoma

Factors that influence outcome in intracerebral hemorrhage are summarized in Table 17–3.[14,20,29,65] Mortality is high in patients with hematoma of large volume, intraventricular extension, and midline shift. Coma caused by intracerebral hemorrhage with volumes of more than 50 mL is likely to result in death. It is not known how many patients deteriorate from continued bleeding, but increase in volume up to 400% has been noted.[4,22] The total volume of intraventricular clot, however, is equally important.[65] Hyperglycemia in intracerebral hematoma may cause ad-

Table 17–3 PROGNOSTICATORS OF POOR OUTCOME IN INTRACEREBRAL HEMORRHAGE

- Intracranial hemorrhage volume >60 mL*
- Age older than 70 years
- Decreased level of consciousness after ictus (each grade)
- Limb paresis (each grade)
- Intraventricular blood volume of ≥ 20 mL
- Midline shift on computed tomography scan
- Hyperglycemia after ictus

Data from Fieschi, et al.,[20] Helweg-Larsen, et al.,[29] and Daverat, et al.[14]

*The volume of intracerebral hemorrhage may be determined by the ellipsoid method. In brief, ellipsoid volume is ⅘ τ 0.5 A × 0.5 B × 0.5 C. A is the largest diameter of the hemorrhage. B is the diameter at 90° to this measurement. C is the vertical diameter estimated by the number of slices in which the hemorrhage is seen times slice thickness. The slice in which the hemorrhage is barely seen counts as ½.[10]

ditional management difficulties in patients with insulin drips. Normoglycemia should be maintained, but whether outcome is significantly influenced by these measures is not known.

Drowsiness, limb weakness, and advanced age are all factors that determine low probability of good recovery. Patients who are comatose when transferred out of the ICU have virtually no chance of recovery unless other systemic factors are depressing the level of consciousness. Factors that do not predict poor outcome are seizures at onset, location of the hemorrhage, and history of hypertension. The mechanism of hemorrhage probably does not influence survival, although hemorrhages associated with tissue plasminogen activator and anticoagulation are very often associated with brain death or severe disability. Bleeding into multiple intracranial compartments and continued bleeding may account for this association. Of the surviving patients with supratentorial intracerebral hematomas, half will have major cognitive deficits and 25% will recover without major sequelae. Patients with pontine and cerebellar hemorrhages do poorly. Aggressive neurosurgical treatment in a patient with cerebellar hematoma of more than 3 cm is warranted, because the chance of rapid secondary deterioration is great. Pontine hemorrhages are managed conservatively.

Ischemic Stroke

Outcome in patients with infarcts in the anterior circulation is not worse than that in patients with infarcts in the posterior circulation. Many infarcts in the posterior circulation are from small artery disease, and the area of the infarcted tissue is smaller. In anterior circulation infarcts, mortality is high, with stem occlusions of the middle cerebral artery. Prognosticators of poor outcome have been identified, and these factors may also predict brain swelling, in which mortality is high despite aggressive treatment of increased intracranial

Table 17–4 PROGNOSTICATORS OF POOR OUTCOME IN CAROTID TERRITORY ISCHEMIC STROKE

- Decreased level of consciousness after ictus
- Gaze palsy, pupillary asymmetry
- Aphonia
- Hyperdense middle cerebral artery sign[38]
- Brain swelling or early midline shift on computed tomography scan

Table 17–5 PROGNOSTICATORS OF POOR OUTCOME IN VERTEBROBASILAR TERRITORY ISCHEMIC STROKE

- Basilar thrombosis causing locked-in syndrome or coma
- Cerebellar infarction with brain stem compression and hydrocephalus
- Thalamic stroke

Data from Nadeau, et al.[43]

pressure (Table 17–4). Hemorrhagic transformation on CT scan does not necessarily imply clinical worsening or higher risk of permanent disability. Patients with aphonia have recently been found to have a high risk of aspiration, which greatly influences outcome in critical illness or underlying pulmonary disease. Middle cerebral artery territory stroke may remit within the first 3 months, but major functional improvement is not expected after the first 3 to 6 months. Intensive rehabilitation programs, however, may produce improvement of functional ability beyond this time limit.[19] In nondominant hemispheric strokes, neglect disappears within 1 year. Recovery of motor function may begin 2 weeks after onset. Hand and arm movement within 1 to 2 weeks in a previously plegic extremity predicts a high likelihood of recovery to a functional state. Aphasia may be supplanted by increasing fluency, but deficits are likely to persist in patients who presented with global aphasia.[58]

Early seizure in acute stroke is associated with a significant chance of recurrence,[25,33] and anticonvulsants are therefore recommended. In a 1992 study, however, most of the patients who had recurrent seizures had phenytoin coverage, a finding that questions the efficacy of treatment after a single seizure.[33] In patients with vertebrobasilar strokes, outcome is determined by localization[43] (Table 17–5).

Thrombosis of the basilar or vertebral artery that causes coma or locked-in syndrome (ventral pontine infarction causing total deafferentation with preservation of vertical eye movements and blinking) is associated with high mortality and no recovery to independent function. Outcome in locked-in syndrome from any cause is very poor, and significant improvement has been reported only very occasionally. A review of 117 patients from the literature noted a mortality of 67%.[26] Functional recovery is extremely rare. Home placement, permanent gastrostomy, tracheostomy, indwelling urine catheters, and bowel programs, all requiring 24-hour skilled nursing care, are possible, with survival up to 12 years.[27] Communication is achieved only through very sophisticated electronic devices that signal vertical eye movements.

Central pontine myelinolysis, in contrast, may have an identical presentation but a reasonable potential for recovery. MRI shows the characteristic abnormalities that differentiate pontine infarcts from demyelination (see Chapter 7). Syndromes that involve small perforating arteries are associated with a good chance of survival and recovery to independent function.[45]

OUTCOME IN HEAD INJURY

Although numerous clinical variables determine the outcome in head injuries, trauma data banks have consistently identified factors with high predictive power. The Glasgow coma scale, since its introduction in the early 1970s, remains a strong clinical predictor, and many of the laboratory tests do not add any value.[30] In addition, attempts to modify the Glasgow coma scale have not

Table 17-6 PROGNOSTICATORS OF POOR OUTCOME IN CLOSED HEAD INJURY

- Postresuscitation Glasgow coma score of 3
- Age older than 65 years
- Abnormal pupil or pupils for at least one observation
- Shock on admission (blood pressure < 80 mm Hg) and during hospital stay
- Persistent increased intracranial pressure (> 20 mm Hg)
- Hypoxia on admission (PO_2 < 60 mm Hg)
- Computed tomography scan abnormalities (absent cisterns, intraventricular hemorrhage, midline shift, shearing in corpus callosum, bilateral epidural hematomas)

Data from Alberico, et al.,[3] Pal, et al.,[47] Ross, et al.,[52] Trieschman,[57] and Choi, SC, Muizelaar, JP, Barnes, TY, et al: Prediction tree for severely head-injured patients. J Neurosurg 75:251–255, 1991.

increased the predictive value.[47] Poor outcome can be expected in patients who have the clinical features and CT scan abnormalities outlined in Table 17-6.

Patients with postresuscitation minimal Glasgow coma scores after stabilization of airway and hemodynamic resuscitation in the emergency room have a poor outcome irrespective of mass lesions or shift on CT scan. In many data banks, prediction of good or poor outcome (death, vegetative state) was more powerful than prediction of moderate to severe disability. Moreover, continued improvement over the first 6 months can be expected. Three recovery subtypes in patients with initial Glasgow coma scale rates of 8 or less have been identified. One third of these patients have significant improvement in 6 months that is followed by some deterioration in performance that may be linked to depressive symptoms. Half the patients improved in the first 6 months and had only minimal gains in 6 to 12 months. No improvement was seen in approximately 20% of the patients, who had additional documented hypoxia, again suggesting that the initial traumatic impact may be worsened by other factors such as hypoxia and hypothermia.

Advanced age has been consistently identified as an independent predictor of poor outcome in patients with severe injury. Elderly patients do very poorly. In a recent retrospective analysis of a series of 195 patients older than 65 years of age, comatose patients had only a 10% chance of survival and a 4% chance of independent functional outcome.[52] Elderly patients more often have extradural hematomas, associated vascular disease, or multitrauma that jeopardizes recovery.

CT scan abnormalities have also been described as potential indicators of poor outcome, and the finding of compressed cisterns with some midline shift and without an identifiable mass is an independent predictor of poor outcome.[3] Intraventricular hemorrhage also predicts poor outcome but is not an independent prognostic factor.[36]

Outcome in large data banks has shown that the overall percentage of patients in the vegetative state is low (3% to 5%), an observation previously made by Jennett and associates.[30] They found that an initial diagnosis of persistent vegetative state is unlikely to change after 3 months and that mortality is high. Patients can remain in a vegetative state for 15 to 20 years, a situation extremely disruptive for families. In most patients, however, the mortality rate for persistent vegetative state is 82% at 3 years and 95% at 5 years. Patients who become severely disabled after severe head injury may be able to return to work in sheltered workplaces, usually with responsibilities far inferior to those before the injury; only a relative minority are cared for in nursing homes.[24]

Many prediction trees in diffuse brain injury have been developed to determine outcome. A recent example is shown in Figure 17-3.

OUTCOME IN TRAUMATIC SPINE INJURY

Prognostication in spine injury is extraordinarily difficult. Reliable predic-

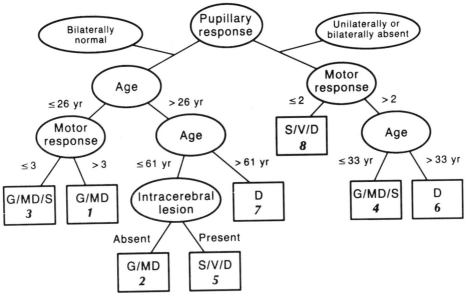

Figure 17–3. Outcome in severe head injury. Prediction tree is based on 555 patients with head injury. The predicted 12-month outcome is defined by the Glasgow coma scale. G, good recovery; MD, moderately disabled; S, severely disabled; V, persistent vegetative state; D, death. The number in each terminal prognostic subgroup (square) represents the prognostic rank of that subgroup according to the proportion of good (G or MD) outcomes. Subgroup 1 is the group with the best prognostic pattern, and subgroup 8 is the group with the worst prognostic pattern. (From Choi, SC, Muizelaar, JP, Barnes, TY, et al: Prediction tree for severely head-injured patients. J Neurosurg 75:251–255, 1991, with permission of the American Association of Neurological Surgeons.)

tive factors are not available, and only general estimates apply. High C-1 to C-3 level lesions abolish respiration, and mechanical ventilation is permanently needed. It has been observed that in a patient with complete cord lesion, some motor or sensory function must return within 2 days or there is no chance of clinically significant recovery.[15] Complete thoracic spine lesions also have less potential for recovery than complete cervical or lumbar lesions. It may take 3 months to decide whether a complete lesion remains complete. In incomplete lesions, recovery can still be expected up to 18 months.

Bladder function is permanently lost. Suprapubic catheters must be placed, because intermittent catheterization requires appropriate hand function and becomes an issue in patients with thoracic lesions. Lumbar lesions result in hyperreflexic bladders, and voiding can be accomplished with manual external pressure. Anticholinergic agents may improve bladder capacity if reflex bladder is too easily triggered. Bowel function can be accomplished by use of suppositories and digital stimulation. Sexual function is lost, but many modifications can result in acceptable alternatives. A comprehensive discussion can be found in Trieschman's text.[57]

CONCLUSIONS

Undoubtedly, the next decade will strongly focus on outcome in and utilization of ICUs. Physicians and family members caring for critically ill patients have begun to recognize that withdrawal of life support can be justifiable and well considered and may put an end to years of ambivalence.

Neurologic complications in critically ill patients make the implementation of a decision to withdraw support (often withdrawal of the ventilator and extubation) more difficult. Neurologists should know exactly what kind of outcome can be expected from critical illness alone, although in some situations, outcome studies are either conflicting or simply not yet available. A practical approach is early identification of signs of very poor or very favorable prognosis. In any outcome study, many patients remain with indeterminate outcome. High probability of poor outcome (persistent vegetative state, severe disability) should influence decisions on death and further management and must reduce prolongation of futile treatments. Ethicists should offer further insight and moral support.

REFERENCES

1. Agardh, C-D, Rosén I, and Ryding, E: Persistent vegetative state with high cerebral blood flow following profound hypoglycemia. Ann Neurol 14:482–486, 1983.

2. Ahronheim, JC and Gasner, MR: The sloganism of starvation. Lancet 335: 278–279, 1990.

3. Alberico, AM, Ward, JD, Choi, SC, et al: Outcome after severe head injury: Relationship to mass lesions, diffuse injury, and ICP course in pediatric and adult patients. J Neurosurg 67:648–656, 1987.

4. Bae, HG, Lee, KS, Yun, IG, et al: Rapid expansion of hypertensive intracerebral hemorrhage. Neurosurgery 31:35–41, 1992.

5. Bates, D, Caronna, JJ, Cartlidge, NEF, et al: A prospective study of nontraumatic coma: Methods and results in 310 patients. Ann Neurol 2:211–220, 1977.

6. Bertini, G, Margheri, M, Giglioli, C, et al: Prognostic significance of early clinical manifestations in postanoxic coma: A retrospective study of 58 patients resuscitated after prehospital cardiac arrest. Crit Care Med 17:627–633, 1989.

7. Bhatt, MH, Obeso, JA, and Marsden, CD: Time course of postanoxic akinetic-rigid and dystonic syndromes. Neurology 43:314–317, 1993.

8. Bolton, CF and Young, GB: Neurological Complications of Renal Disease. Butterworths, Boston, 1990.

9. Boylan, KB, Chin, JH, and DeArmond, SJ: Progressive dystonia following resuscitation from cardiac arrest. Neurology 40:1458–1461, 1990.

10. Broderick, JP, Brott, TG, Duldner, JE, et al: Volume of intracerebral hemorrhage: A powerful and easy-to-use predictor of 30-day mortality. Stroke 24:987–993, 1993.

11. Brown, P, Steiger, MJ, Thompson, PD, et al: Effectiveness of piracetam in cortical myoclonus. Mov Disord 8:63–68, 1993.

12. Christensen, E, Krintel, JJ, Hansen, SM, et al: Prognosis after the first episode of gastrointestinal bleeding or coma in cirrhosis: Survival and prognostic factors. Scand J Gastroenterol 24:999–1006, 1989.

13. Curran, WJ: Defining appropriate medical care: Providing nutrients and hydration for the dying. N Engl J Med 313:940–942, 1985.

14. Daverat, P, Castel, JP, Dartigues, JF, and Orgogozo, JM: Death and functional outcome after spontaneous intracerebral hemorrhage: A prospective study of 166 cases using multivariate analysis. Stroke 22:1–6, 1991.

15. Donovan, WH: Spinal cord injury. In Evans, RW, Baskin, DS, and Yatsu, FM (eds): Prognosis of Neurological Disorders. Oxford University Press, New York, 1992, pp 109–118.

16. Edgren, E, Hedstrand, ULF, Nordin, M, et al: Prediction of outcome after cardiac arrest. Crit Care Med 15:820–825, 1987.

17. Fahn, S: New drugs for posthypoxic action myoclonus: Observations from a well-studied case. Adv Neurol 43:197–199, 1986.

18. Faich, GA, Fishbein, HA, and Ellis, SE: The epidemiology of diabetic acidosis: A population-based study. Am J Epidemiol 117:551–558, 1983.

19. Ferrucci, L, Bandinelli, S, Guralnik, JM, et al: Recovery of functional status after stroke: A postrehabilitation follow-up study. Stroke 24:200–205, 1993.

20. Fieschi, C, Carolei, A, Fiorelli, M, et al: Changing prognosis of primary intracerebral hemorrhage: Results of a clinical

and computed tomographic follow-up study of 104 patients. Stroke 19:192–195, 1988.

21. Finklestein, S and Caronna, JJ: Amnestic syndrome following cardiac arrest (abstr). Neurology 28:389, 1978.

22. Fulgham, J and Wijdicks, EFM: Acute deterioration in supratentorial hypertensive hemorrhage. Mayo Clin Proc (in press).

23. Greene, DA: Acute and chronic complications of diabetes mellitus in older patients. Am J Med 80:39–53, 1986.

24. Groswasser, Z and Sazbon, L: Outcome in 134 patients with prolonged post-traumatic unawareness. Part 2: Functional outcome of 72 patients recovering consciousness. J Neurosurg 72:81–84, 1990.

25. Gupta, SR, Haneedy, MH, Elias, D, and Rubino, FA: Postinfarction seizures: A clinical study. Stroke 19:1477–1481, 1988.

26. Haig, AJ, Katz, RT, and Sahgal, V: Locked-in syndrome: Review. Curr Concepts Rehabil Med 2:12–16, 1986.

27. Haig, AJ, Katz, RT, and Sahgal, V: Mortality and complications of the locked-in syndrome. Arch Phys Med Rehabil 68:24–27, 1987.

28. Hawker, K and Lang, AE: Hypoxic-ischemic damage of the basal ganglia: Case reports and a review of the literature. Mov Disord 5:219–224, 1990.

29. Helweg-Larsen, S, Sommer, W, Strange, P, et al: Prognosis for patients treated conservatively for spontaneous intracerebral hematomas. Stroke 15:1045–1048, 1984.

30. Jennett, B, Teasdale, G, Braakman, R, et al: Prognosis of patients with severe head injury. Neurosurgery 4:283–288, 1979.

31. Kalimo, H and Olsson, Y: Effects of severe hypoglycemia on the human brain: Neuropathological case reports. Acta Neurol Scand 62:345–356, 1980.

32. Kanoti, GA, Gombeski, WR Jr, Gulledge, AD, et al: The effect of do-not-resuscitate orders on length of stay. Cleve Clin J Med 59:591–594, 1992.

33. Kilpatrick, CJ, Davis, SM, and Hopper, JL: Early seizures after acute stroke: Risk of late seizures. Arch Neurol 49:509–511, 1992.

34. Komori, H, Hirasa, M, Takakuwa, H, et al: Concept of the clinical stages of acute hepatic failure. Am J Gastroenterol 81:544–549, 1986.

35. Lance, JW and Adams, RD: The syndrome of intention or action myoclonus as a sequel to hypoxic encephalopathy. Brain 86:111–136, 1963.

36. Lee, J-P, Lui, T-N, and Chang, C-N: Acute post-traumatic intraventricular hemorrhage analysis of 25 patients with emphasis on final outcome. Acta Neurol Scand 84:85–90, 1991.

37. Levy, DE, Bates, D, Caronna, JJ, et al: Prognosis in nontraumatic coma. Ann Intern Med 94:293–301, 1981.

38. Leys, D, Pruvo, JP, Godefroy, O, et al: Prevalence and significance of hyperdense middle cerebral artery in acute stroke. Stroke 23:317–324, 1992.

39. Malouf, R and Brust, JCM: Hypoglycemia: Causes, neurological manifestations, and outcome. Ann Neurol 17:421–430, 1985.

40. Medical Aspects of the Persistent Vegetative State: The Multisociety Task Force on PVS statement of a multi-society task force. N Engl J Med 330:1499–1508, 1994.

41. Miller, SI, Wallace, RJ Jr, Musher, DM, et al: Hypoglycemia as a manifestation of sepsis. Am J Med 68:649–654, 1980.

42. Mullie, A, Verstringe, P, Buylaert, W, et al: Predictive value of Glasgow coma score for awakening after out-of-hospital cardiac arrest: Cerebral Resuscitation Study Group of the Belgian Society for Intensive Care. Lancet i:137–140, 1988.

43. Nadeau, S, Jordan, J, and Mishra, S: Clinical presentation as a guide to early prognosis in vertebrobasilar stroke. Stroke 23:165–170, 1992.

44. Niskanen, M, Kari, A, Nikki, P, et al: Acute physiology and chronic health evaluation (APACHE II) and Glasgow coma scores as predictors of outcome from intensive care after cardiac arrest. Crit Care Med 19:1465–1473, 1991.

45. Norrving, B and Cronqvist, S: Lateral medullary infarction: Prognosis in an unselected series. Neurology 41:244–248, 1991.

46. Obeso, JA, Artieda, J, Rothwell, JC, et

al: The treatment of severe action myoclonus. Brain 112:765–777, 1989.

47. Pal, J, Brown, R, and Fleiszer, D: The value of the Glasgow Coma Scale and injury severity score: Predicting outcome in multiple trauma patients with head injury. J Trauma 29:746–748, 1989.

48. Paris, JJ and Reardon, FE: Court responses to withholding or withdrawing artificial nutrition and fluids. JAMA 253:2243–2245, 1985.

49. Printz, LA: Is withholding hydration a valid comfort measure in the terminally ill? Geriatrics 43:84–88, Nov 1988.

50. Reichard, P, Berglund, A, Britz, A, et al: Hypoglycaemic episodes during intensified insulin treatment: Increased frequency but no effect on cognitive function. J Intern Med 229:9–16, 1991.

51. Roine, RO, Kajaste, S, and Kaste, M: Neuropsychological sequelae of cardiac arrest. JAMA 269:237–242, 1993.

52. Ross, AM, Pitts, LH, and Kobayashi, S: Prognosticators of outcome after major head injury in the elderly. J Neurosci Nurs 24:88–93, 1992.

53. Schwartz, A, Hennerici, M, and Wegener, OH: Delayed choreoathetosis following acute carbon monoxide poisoning. Neurology 35:98–99, 1985.

54. Simon, RP, Meldrum, BS, Schmidley, JW, et al: Mechanisms of selective vulnerability: Hypoglycemia. Cerebrovasc Dis 15:13–24, 1987.

55. Small, M, Alzaid, A, and MacCuish, AC: Diabetic hyperosmolar non-ketotic decompensation. Q J Med 66:251–257, 1988.

56. Stahl, J: Studies of the blood ammonia in liver disease: Its diagnostic, prognostic, and therapeutic significance. Ann Intern Med 58:1–24, 1963.

57. Trieschman, RB: Spinal Cord Injuries: Psychological, Social, and Vocational Rehabilitation, ed 2. Demos Publications, New York, 1988, pp 158–185.

58. Turney, TM, Garraway, WM, and Whisnant, JP: The natural history of hemispheric and brain stem infarction in Rochester, Minnesota. Stroke 15:790–794, 1984.

59. Uitti, RJ, Rajput, AH, Ashenhurst, EM, and Rozdilsky, B: Cyanide-induced parkinsonism: A clinicopathologic report. Neurology 35:921–925, 1985.

60. Volpe, BT and Hirst, W: The characterization of an amnesic syndrome following hypoxic ischemic injury. Arch Neurol 40:436–440, 1983.

61. Wachtel, TJ, Silliman, RA, and Lamberton, P: Prognostic factors in the diabetic hyperosmolar state. J Am Geriatr Soc 35:737–741, 1987.

62. Wachtel, TJ, Tetu-Mouradjian, LM, Goldman, DL, et al: Hyperosmolarity and acidosis in diabetes mellitus: A three-year experience in Rhode Island. J Gen Intern Med 6:495–502, 1991.

63. Wijdicks, EFM and Stevens, M: The role of hypotension in septic encephalopathy following surgical procedures. Arch Neurol 49:653–656, 1992.

64. Young, GB, Bolton, CF, Austin, TW, and Archibald, Y: The electroencephalogram (EEG) in sepsis (abstr). Can J Neurol Sci 13:164, 1986.

65. Young, WB, Lee, KP, Pessin, MS, et al: Prognostic significance of ventricular blood in supratentorial hemorrhage: A volumetric study. Neurology 40:616–619, 1990.

Chapter 18

DIAGNOSIS AND MANAGEMENT OF BRAIN DEATH IN THE INTENSIVE CARE UNIT

CLINICAL DIAGNOSIS OF BRAIN
  DEATH
BASIS OF THE APNEA TEST
  PROCEDURE
CLINICAL OBSERVATIONS
  COMPATIBLE WITH THE
  DIAGNOSIS OF BRAIN DEATH
CONFIRMATORY LABORATORY
  TESTS
RECOMMENDATIONS AFTER THE
  DIAGNOSIS OF BRAIN DEATH

Brain death is commonly a consequence of severe head injury, aneurysmal subarachnoid hemorrhage, or large cerebral artery territory infarction with edema.[47] Brain death is less frequently diagnosed in medical or surgical intensive care units (ICUs) but may occur from a severe anoxic injury associated with prolonged cardiac resuscitation, smoke inhalation, or asphyxia, or from edema associated with fulminant hepatic necrosis, stroke, or rapidly progressing bacterial meningitis. In hospitals with a trauma center, multisystem trauma may be a more common cause of brain death. Progression to brain death in medical ICUs is often expected in patients with a major central nervous system (CNS) catastrophe and may be signaled by a sudden marked drop in blood pressure or core temperature.

The clinical diagnosis of brain death requires expertise from a consulting neurologist. It has been suggested that misinterpretation of clinical signs may be a common error in the diagnosis of brain death.[70,72] Therefore, neurologists should also have a major part in the clinical diagnosis of brain death to eliminate potential confusion with locked-in syndrome, persistent vegetative state,[48] and akinetic mutism[66] (see Chapter 17). If a patient meets the clinical criteria and confounding factors have been excluded, it is reasonable to allow organ donation, although the severity of medical illness may preclude the harvesting of several organs.

CLINICAL DIAGNOSIS OF BRAIN DEATH

Brain death is equivalent to irreversible loss of all brain stem function.[2,12,13,19,54,67,70,73,100] This definition implies (1) documentation of loss of consciousness, (2) no motor response to pain stimuli, (3) no brain stem reflex, and (4) apnea. A structural central nervous system abnormality compatible with brain death should be demonstrated by computed tomography (CT) scan. The diagnosis of brain death must be in doubt if results of CT scan or cerebrospinal fluid studies are normal unless an obvious other pathophysiologic mechanism for brain death is present (e.g., hypoxic ischemic encephalopathy after asphyxia or cardiac arrest). In medical ICUs, the proportion of patients with normal CT findings may be higher when cardiac arrest or asphyxia is an important instigator of brain death.

Pitfalls of diagnosing brain death should be recognized. Hypothermia may blunt brain stem responses only when core temperatures are below 32°C and may mimic brain death below 27°C[28] (see Chapter 14). Any drug intoxication should be excluded. In a newly admitted patient, drug screening may not identify drug overdose or poisoning, and screening is helpful only when the request is for a specific drug or poison. The number of poisons or drugs that cause CNS depression associated with absence of some brain stem reflexes is obviously very large. Drugs that cause complete but reversible absence of brain stem reflexes or isoelectric electroencephalograms have occasionally been reported[41,76,96,102,103] (Table 18-1). If a history of drug intoxication is in doubt, the diagnosis of brain death cannot be made with certainty. At the other extreme, therapeutic levels of barbiturates (e.g., in patients with epilepsy) should not delay the clinical diagnosis of brain death. Any metabolic or endocrine crisis may make the diagnosis of brain death questionable, particularly in patients without a demonstrated structural lesion in the CNS. The diag-

nosis of brain death cannot be made with certainty in patients with coma of undetermined origin, and these patients probably should not be considered candidates for organ donation.

The clinical diagnosis of brain death may be very difficult immediately after surgery. Volatile anesthetic agents usually wash out in several minutes, but when clearance is in doubt, they can be measured in end-tidal volume. The activity of neuromuscular junction blocking agents can be determined with a peripheral nerve stimulator. Large doses of narcotics are typically used in complicated operations (e.g., cardiovascular repairs). Naloxone reverses the manifestations of opioids. The effects of benzodiazepines can be reversed with flumazenil.

To overcome the possible pitfalls of making the diagnosis of brain death, the directions outlined in Figure 18-1 are proposed. Testing for brain death can proceed only after these precautions have been taken. Clinical examination of the brain stem includes testing of brain stem reflexes, evaluation of motor response to pain, and evaluation of the patient's ability to breathe spontaneously.

Pupils. The pupillary response to bright light should be absent in both eyes. Round, oval, or irregularly shaped pupils are all compatible with brain death. Most pupils are in mid position (4 to 6 mm), but dilated pupils (6 to 8 mm) are compatible with brain death. Sympathetic cervical pathways[90] connected with the radially arranged fibers of the dilator muscle remain intact. The mid position of the pupils at postmortem examination therefore can be explained by loss of the remainder of sympathetic tone. Maximally dilated pupils (9 mm) or miosis (<4 mm) is most likely incompatible with the clinical diagnosis of brain death, but reported data on these extremes of pupil size are not available.[89,90] (In a small number of patients in whom we measured change in pupil size after cardiac standstill, pupil size decreased.)

**Table 18-1 DRUGS THAT MAY
MIMIC BRAIN DEATH OR
PRODUCE ISOELECTRIC
ELECTROENCEPHALOGRAMS**

Barbiturates
Tricyclic antidepressants
Neuromuscular blocking agents
Methaqualone
Opiates
Benzodiazepines
Mecloqualone
Meprobamate
Bretylium

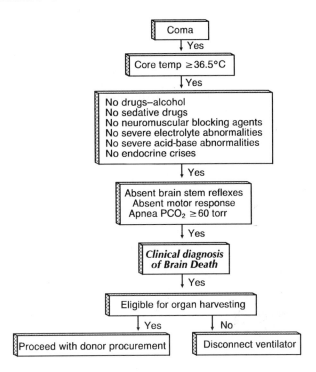

Figure 18–1. Proposed guidelines for the clinical diagnosis of brain death.

Many drugs can influence the size of the pupil, although the response to light often remains intact.[38] Intravenously administered atropine traditionally has been reported to dilate pupils, but a 1991 study in children[34] found that dilation was minimal and pupillary response was retained with conventional doses. The relatively frequent observation of mydriasis after cardiac resuscitation may, therefore, be due to the combined effect of epinephrine and atropine and, perhaps, sympathetic stress response. One report described fixed, dilated pupils after high doses of dopamine,[69] but this observation has not been confirmed. Most patients in shock on high-dose dopamine regimens indeed have dilated pupils, but the pupils never become fixed to light. Because many patients with brain death require dopamine to increase blood pressure, dopamine treatment should not confound the clinical diagnosis of brain death.

Topical instillation of drugs and trauma to the cornea or bulbus oculi may cause reactive mydriasis, but more often reactive miosis is present in the acute stage of direct trauma. (Obviously, preexisting anatomic abnormalities of the iris should be excluded.) Neuromuscular blocking drugs do not noticeably influence pupil size, because nicotine receptors are absent.

Ocular Movements. Ocular movements should be absent after head turning and caloric testing with ice water. Head turning (oculocephalic reflex, doll's head phenomenon), accomplished by fast and vigorous turning of the head from middle position to 90° on both sides, results in eye deviation to the opposite side. Vertical eye movements can be tested with brisk neck flexion, which should not produce eyelid retraction or vertical eye movement. Brisk neck flexion, however, can produce spinal reflexes and hemodynamic changes.[58]

Caloric testing should be done with the head elevated to 30°. The tympanum is irrigated with 50 mL of ice water on each side. The procedure is best accomplished by connecting a

50-mL syringe filled with ice water to a small suction catheter that is then inserted into the external auditory canal. To facilitate assessment of subtle eye movement, a pen mark should be placed on the lower eyelid at the level of the center of the pupil before cold water irrigation. No tonic deviation of the eyes toward the cold caloric stimulus should be demonstrated after 1 minute of observation, and at least 5 minutes should be allowed between sides.

Many drugs may diminish or completely abolish the caloric response (aminoglycosides, tricyclic antidepressants; anticholinergics; antiepileptic drugs; and chemotherapeutic agents).[65,92] In one report, ophthalmoplegia persisted for 3 weeks after intravenous administration of high doses of methylprednisolone and pancuronium was discontinued.[91] In closed head injury, eyelid edema and chemosis of the conjunctiva may restrict movement of the globes. Clotted blood or cerumen may diminish the caloric response. Basal fracture of the petrous bone only unilaterally abolishes the caloric response and may be identified by an ecchymotic mastoid process.

Facial Sensation and Facial Motor Response. Corneal reflexes, which should be absent, are tested with a throat swab. Grimacing to pain can be tested by application of deep pressure with a blunt object on the nail bed, pressure on the supraorbital ridge, and deep pressure on both condyles at the level of the temporomandibular joint. Because the reaction to these three pain stimuli may vary, all should be tested in examination of the motor response to pain.

Pharyngeal and Tracheal Reflexes. Cranial nerves IX and X can be tested by stimulation of the posterior pharynx with a tongue blade, but the response in orally intubated patients can be difficult to interpret. Lack of tracheal response to bronchial suctioning should be demonstrated. Chest movement or cough response must be absent.

Motor Responses. Motor responses of the limbs to pain stimuli should be absent after forceful supraorbital or temporomandibular pressure. Motor response other than decorticate or decerebrate response can be present (Lazarus sign) in arms and legs, may occur spontaneously during hypoxic or hypotensive episodes, and is of spinal origin.[49,50,63,83]

BASIS OF THE APNEA TEST PROCEDURE

Breathing is terminated when respiratory neurons, located near the origin of the glossopharyngeal and vagal nerves in the medulla oblongata, stop firing. The respiratory neurons are controlled by separate central chemoreceptors that sense changes in PCO_2 and pH of the cerebrospinal fluid that accurately reflect changes in plasma PCO_2. The upper and lower limits of PCO_2 for respiratory stimulation are not exactly known and may be different in patients with severe structural CNS damage. There are many other mechanical and chemical stimuli and inhibitory influences to the respiratory neurons of the brain stem.

Hypocapnia should be corrected before formal apnea testing. Many patients with acute catastrophic structural CNS damage are hypocapnic. Hypocapnia is often a result of mechanical ventilation itself, but other causes are hyperventilation induced to decrease intracranial pressure and hypothermia resulting from loss of temperature regulation. Both hypocapnia and hypothermia may unnecessarily prolong apnea testing.[97] Hypothermia may also partly be caused by large-volume infusion at room temperature in an attempt to balance urinary output in patients who have diabetes insipidus.

Hypocapnia can be corrected by a reduction in minute volume (tidal volume or respiratory rate). Because administration of 5% CO_2 in oxygen increases PCO_2 by 17.3 mm Hg in 1 to 2 minutes and may rapidly lead to severe hypercapnia and respiratory acidosis, it is not recommended as a measure to increase PCO_2.

It is not known which PCO_2 level is needed to maximally stimulate the chemoreceptors of the respiratory center in hyperoxygenated patients with severe brain stem destruction.[15] Guideline target arterial PCO_2 levels are derived from a very small number of patients that indeed have respiratory efforts after disconnection of the ventilator but otherwise fulfill all criteria for the diagnosis of brain death. PCO_2 levels in these patients vary from 30 to 56 mm Hg.[88] The medical consultants to the President's Commission for the Study of Ethical Problems in Medicine and Biomedical and Behavioral Research issued advisory guidelines for the determination of death that are based on these observations and recommended that $PaCO_2$ be equal to or greater than 60 mm Hg. Less restrictive guidelines (PCO_2 of 44 mm Hg), which would facilitate the apnea procedure, were suggested by Ropper and associates.[85]

In 4 of 36 patients who otherwise fulfilled brain death criteria, normal breaths occurred at relatively low PCO_2 values (range, 30 to 37 mm Hg; mean, 34 mm Hg). Respiratory-like movements, however, were observed at PCO_2 levels between 41 and 51 mm Hg. These respiratory-like movements could not be reproduced and were ineffective for ventilation. They consisted of shoulder elevation and adduction, back arching, and intercostal expansion and produced virtually no tidal volume or significant inspiratory force.

Respiratory-like movements can be seen at the end of the apnea test, particularly when O_2 saturation reaches critical values. Retained breathing in a patient who otherwise has the clinical criteria for brain death is very rare. When it occurs, it is observed almost immediately after disconnection, with initial PCO_2 in the 40s.

Other, less reliable targets for PCO_2 can be obtained from anesthetized patients (approximately 30 mm Hg)[29,46] or in publications on breath-holding (approximately 40 to 45 mm Hg).[25,77] In the past decade, only one patient was seen at Saint Marys Hospital, Rochester, Minn, with absent brain stem reflexes,

an immediate normal respiratory pattern when the ventilator was disconnected, and an initial PCO_2 in the 40s. In this patient, blood pressure was normal or at times increased to a mean arterial pressure of 125 mm Hg. This finding corroborates the previous observation that in patients who had breathing efforts after disconnection, blood pressures were pharmacologically unsupported, which suggested that respiratory and vasomotor centers were intact.[85]

Target PCO_2 levels are presumably higher in patients with chronic hypercapnia, typically patients with chronic obstructive pulmonary disease, bronchiectasis, or sleep apnea and morbid obesity.[33] Chronic hypercapnia may be suspected in patients with increased initial serum bicarbonate concentrations, assuming that no metabolic acidosis is present. In these patients, there is evidence of abnormal ventilatory drive and tidal volumes may be muted, but there is no evidence that respiratory efforts are completely absent at normal PCO_2 levels. Confirmatory tests are indicated.

The practice of apnea testing is not consistent among neurologists and needs further refinement and strict criteria.[23] The procedure is facilitated when the test is begun with a baseline PCO_2 of 40 mm Hg or more. With a median increase of 3 mm Hg/h, the target level of PCO_2 of 60 mm Hg is usually reached 8 minutes after disconnection.[7,10,11,64,81] Side effects of hypercapnia are related to the degree of hypoxia. Oxygenation with 100% O_2 through a catheter at the level of the carina secures adequate oxygenation during the test and in my experience is much better than a T-piece alone. The apnea test procedure is based on the mechanism of apneic mass movement oxygenation, and PO_2 in the alveoli decreases as fast as PCO_2 increases. Oxygenation, therefore, prevents hypoxia in the test period, but because preexisting severe pulmonary disease, bilateral pneumonia, acute respiratory distress syndrome, or neurogenic edema creates a large dead space, oxygenation may be inadequate in patients with these conditions.

Severe respiratory acidosis without hypoxia is usually tolerated but may cause arrhythmias in patients with coronary artery disease or a history of cardiac arrhythmias. The most common manifestations are ventricular premature contractions, ventricular tachycardia, and mild hypotension and invariably occur in patients who become hypoxemic. However, in a 1989 series in which 50% of the patients had underlying cardiac disease, only nonsignificant cardiac arrhythmias were seen.[10] The apnea test precautions and procedure are summarized in Figure 18–2.

CLINICAL OBSERVATIONS COMPATIBLE WITH THE DIAGNOSIS OF BRAIN DEATH

Some clinical observations can cause delayed assessment of donors, mainly because their insignificance is not appreciated by nonneurologists. Deep tendon reflexes and plantar reflexes (including clonus and Babinski's reflex) are compatible with the diagnosis of brain death. Spontaneous movements of the limbs, more frequent in young adults, include rapid flexion in arms, raising of all limbs off the bed, grasping movements, spontaneous jerking of one leg, walking-like movements, and movements of the arms that may reach the level of the endotracheal tube.[49,50,63,83] Respiratory-like movements also may occur, consisting of shoulder elevation and adduction, back arching, and intercostal expansion characteristic of an agonal breathing pattern.

Other responses are profuse sweating, blushing, tachycardia, and a sudden increase in blood pressure.[18,24,101] These responses can sometimes be elicited by neck flexion and can be eliminated by ganglion blocking agents (e.g., trimethaphan). Diabetes insipidus may not develop in every patient with brain death,[71] and some patients have normal blood pressure.

CONFIRMATORY LABORATORY TESTS

The standard for diagnosis of brain death is repeat clinical diagnosis after an (arbitrary) interval of at least 6 hours. A confirmatory test is not mandatory except in patients who are not amenable to reliable evaluation of specific components of clinical testing. In countries other than the United States, confirmatory tests may be required by law (e.g., in Germany).

In many reports on confirmatory tests, blind assessment, interobserver variation, and, most important, control studies are not consistently addressed. Many tests require costly equipment and well-trained technicians. Clinical experience with confirmatory tests other than cerebral angiography, nuclear scan, electroencephalography, and transcranial Doppler ultrasonography is limited.

Confirmatory tests that are generally accepted are conventional angiography and electroencephalography. Brain death has recently been accepted as a clinical indication for transcranial Doppler ultrasonography by the Therapeutics and Technology Assessment Subcommittee of the American Academy of Neurology.[3] Each of the confirmatory tests is reviewed.

Conventional Angiography

A selective four-vessel angiogram is done in the radiology suite. Iodinated contrast medium is injected under high pressure in both the anterior and the posterior circulations.[14] The procedure, which takes a few hours, should result in no intracerebral filling at the level of the carotid bifurcation or the circle of Willis. The external carotid circulation is patent, and delayed filling of the superior longitudinal sinus may occur.[39,44,59] However, the procedure has been shown to yield conflicting results, largely because no guidelines for interpretation exist and the high injection pressure may overcome increased intracranial pressure.

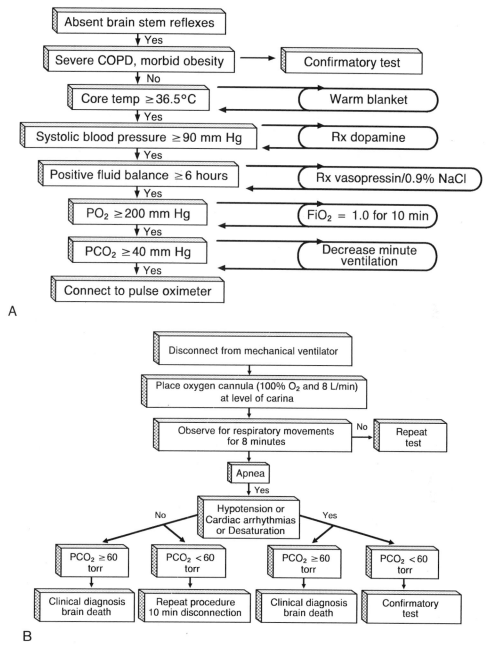

Figure 18–2. Apnea testing in brain death. *A*, Precautions. *B*, Procedure. COPD = chronic obstructive pulmonary disease.

Isotope Angiography

The technique consists of rapid intravenous injection of serum albumin labeled with technetium 99m and bedside imaging with a portable gamma camera.[55,56,59] Intracranial radioisotope activity is absent in brain death. In delayed images, filling of sagittal and transverse sinuses may occur through connections between the extracranial circulation and the venous system. The sensitivity and specificity of absence of intracranial radioisotope are not exactly known, but no false-positive scan results have yet been reported. One of the disadvantages of the technique is that the posterior circulation is not visualized.

Electroencephalography

The technique of electroencephalographic recording in brain death has been well described.[9,16,40,51,57,86] Most institutions use an 18-channel instrument and apply standards suggested by the American Electroencephalographic Society for recording brain death. In brain-dead patients, no activity above 2 μV for 30 minutes of recording is found at a sensitivity of 2 μV/mm with a filter setting of 0.1 or 0.3 second and 70 Hz. Persistent electroencephalographic activity may occur.[22,45] In a consecutive series of 56 patients fulfilling the criteria for brain death, 20% had electroencephalographic activity that lasted up to 168 hours.[40] These patterns were low-voltage background beta activity, spindle-like potentials, and alpha-like potentials.

The ^{99m}Tc-HMPAO Brain Scan

The technetium 99m hexamethylpropyleneamineoxime (^{99m}Tc-HMPAO) brain scan is a relatively new procedure that can be performed at the bedside in many institutions. It takes from 15 to 20 minutes, but the technique is not widely available.[1,32,36,37,80,82,104] The isotope should be injected within 30 minutes of

reconstitution. A portable gamma camera produces planar views within 5 to 10 minutes. Correct intravenous injection should be verified by chest and abdominal films. Imaging of brain uptake of the tracer can be done at any convenient time. No uptake should be demonstrated in the brain parenchyma (hollow skull) (Fig. 18–3). Experience with this technique is limited. Sensitivity has been reported to be as low as 94%, but specificity is 100%.[60] Reproducibility has been tested in only a few patients. Correlation between cerebral angiography and ^{99m}Tc-HMPAO scintigraphy is excellent. The disadvantages of this technique are that the isotope must be injected immediately after preparation, the cost is high, and expertise is needed to rule out artifacts.

Transcranial Doppler Ultrasonography

A portable 2-MHz pulsed Doppler instrument can be used at the bedside for transcranial Doppler (TCD) ultrasonography.[43,53,74,75,84,87,98] At least two intracranial arteries should be insonated (the middle cerebral artery through the temporal bone above the zygomatic arch *and* the vertebral and basilar arteries through the suboccipital transcranial window *or* the ophthalmic artery and intracavernous internal carotid artery through the transorbital window).

Several patterns compatible with no forward flow and no cerebral perfusion have been reported (Fig. 18–4). Ab-

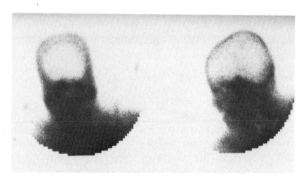

Figure 18–3. Nuclear scan demonstrating hollow skull from lack of ^{99m}Tc-HMPAO uptake in brain death.

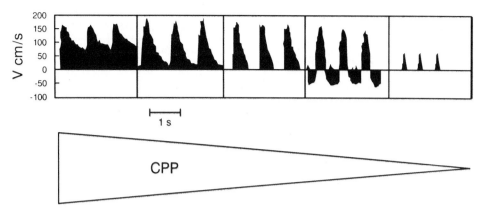

Figure 18–4. Transcranial Doppler patterns associated with increased intracranial pressure evolving into brain death. CPP = cerebral perfusion pressure. (From Hassler, et al.,[43] with permission of American Association of Neurological Surgeons.)

sence of TCD signals should not be interpreted as compatible with brain death, because in up to 10% of the patients, a temporal window is not present for intonation. Nonetheless, disappearance of TCD signals in patients with progressive deterioration to brain death should be considered valid confirmation. TCD study results should be considered inadequate if no signal can be obtained on both temporal windows despite demonstration of characteristic signals through other windows.

Transcranial Doppler signals consistently found in brain death are (1) absent or reversed diastolic flow, indicating either retrograde diastolic flow or flow only through systole (retrograde diastolic flow is caused by the contractive forces of the arteries) and (2) small systolic peaks in early systole with absent or reversed diastolic flow, indicating very high vascular resistance associated with greatly increased intracranial pressure.

Experience with TCD sonography in the confirmation of brain death is substantial. The sensitivity and specificity are, respectively, 91.3% and 100% in patients with demonstrated TCD signals in at least two insonated arteries. TCD ultrasonography occasionally demonstrates "brain death patterns" in patients who are clinically brain dead and who have electroencephalographic

activity. Small systolic peaks and increased diastolic flow have been demonstrated as transient phenomena during aneurysmal rebleeding[43] and in a patient with occlusion of a middle cerebral artery ipsilateral to the main occlusion.[74] TCD signals can be normal in patients with primary infratentorial lesions leading to brain stem death and in patients with anoxic-ischemic damage after cardiac arrest or asphyxia. TCD patterns of brain death reflect increased intracranial pressure[52,53] and, therefore, are useless in conditions not associated with increased pressure, such as asphyxia and cardiac resuscitation. TCD velocities can be affected by PCO_2, hematocrit, and cardiac output, but these concerns are insignificant in the diagnosis of brain death.

Miscellaneous Tests

Many tests are variants or modifications of the tests mentioned previously. In general, the number of tested patients is very small; more disturbing, these tests may produce similar results in neurologic disorders of the CNS that lead to coma without the clinical diagnosis of brain death (e.g., lack of cortical response of somatosensory evoked potentials in postanoxic encephalopathy). Contrast CT scanning with meglumine diatrizoate (Angiografin) as a bolus of 1 mL/kg of body weight followed by drip infusion of 0.02 mL/kg per minute in brain-dead patients does not visualize intracranial vessels.[79] Correlation with cerebral angiography is good,[5] but exposure of the donor's kidneys to contrast medium and the potential for anaphylaxis make this technique unsuitable.

Brain stem and somatosensory evoked potentials have been tested in brain-dead patients, most of whom have no response. However, any major acute CNS catastrophe that does not produce brain death may result in absent cortical responses, so that this test seems invalid in the diagnosis of brain death.[4,6,8,17,26,27,30,42,62,93,94,99]

Nevertheless, Goldie and associates[35] claimed that absent brain stem auditory evoked potentials combined with lack of somatosensory evoked potentials beyond Erb's point were unique in brain-dead patients, a pattern not found in comatose patients who had sparing of parts of the brain stem. These results have not yet been confirmed, and somatosensory evoked potentials have not gained universal acceptance as a reliable confirmatory test.

RECOMMENDATIONS AFTER THE DIAGNOSIS OF BRAIN DEATH

Discussion with family members about organ donation should be initiated only after the clinical diagnosis of brain death has been made. The following approach is suggested. The family should be unequivocally told that the patient is dead. Mechanical ventilation, fluids, and blood pressure medication are administered so that organs can be preserved until the decision about donation is made. Refusal by the family to have organs harvested removes the rationale for supportive therapy, and mechanical ventilation is immediately discontinued after the family has been allowed adequate time for consideration.

Table 18–2 GUIDELINES FOR ADEQUATE DONOR MANAGEMENT

Fluid resuscitation	Colloids 5% dextrose
Hypotension (systolic pressure <100 mm Hg)	Dopamine, up to 10 μg/kg per minute (or lower dose in combination with norepinephrine)
Diabetes insipidus	Vasopressin, 0.5 U/h 1-Desamino-8-D-arginine vasopressin, 1 to 4 μg Desmopressin, 0.5 to 2 μg IV (every 8 to 12 h)

Data from Darby, et al.,[20] and Debelak, et al.[21]

Donor procurement requires notification of a local transplantation coordinator. Management of a brain-dead patient is complex.[20,21] Major immediate threats[20,21,31,61] are (1) pulmonary edema, requiring pulmonary artery catheter placement and positive end-expiratory pressure ventilation, (2) hypotension, requiring adequate volume resuscitation and vasopressors (dopamine, 2 to 10 μg/kg),[71] and (3) polyuria from diabetes insipidus, requiring 1-desamino-8-D-arginine vasopressin, 1 to 4 μg intravenously every 8 hours, or desmopressin (0.5 to 2 μg) intravenously (Table 18–2). Prophylactic use of antibiotics and hormone substitution are controversial. A recent study, however, noted that triiodothyronine therapy was not warranted, although others noted improvement in myocardial function and reduction of inotropic requirement.[68,78,95]

CONCLUSIONS

Brain death in surgical and medical ICUs occurs in clinical situations such as anoxic-ischemic coma, fulminant hepatic failure, near-drowning, hypothermia, smoke inhalation, head injury, major hemorrhagic stroke (usually in anticoagulated patients), and bacterial meningitis. The severity of underlying critical illness may preclude organ donation, although several organs (e.g., skin, bone, cornea, heart valves, inner ear) are still very useful. The diagnosis of brain death has never been easy for physicians, including neurologists. Brain death can be defined as documentation of loss of consciousness, lack of motor response to pain stimuli, absence of brain stem reflexes, and demonstrated apnea to a PCO_2 of 60 mm Hg or more. Confounding factors (usually drug intoxication) should be excluded, and CT scanning or spinal fluid examination should in general demonstrate abnormalities that are compatible with the diagnosis of brain death. In patients who fulfill the clinical criteria of brain death but have normal findings on CT scanning of the brain, repeated evaluation hours apart and demonstration that cerebral blood flow is absent (cerebral angiogram or nuclear scan) should allow the decision to withdraw life-sustaining measures or to initiate donor procurement.

REFERENCES

1. Abdel-Dayem, HM, Bahar, RH, Sigurdsson, GH, et al: The hollow skull: A sign of brain death in Tc-99m HM-PAO brain scintigraphy. Clin Nucl Med 14:912–916, 1989.
2. Ad Hoc Committee of the Harvard Medical School to Examine the Definition of Brain Death: A definition of irreversible coma. JAMA 205:337–340, 1968.
3. American Academy of Neurology, Therapeutics and Technology Assessment Subcommittee: Assessment: Transcranial Doppler. Neurology 40:680–681, 1990.
4. Anziska, BJ and Cracco, RQ: Short latency somatosensory evoked potentials in brain dead patients. Arch Neurol 37:222–225, 1980.
5. Arnold, H, Kühne, D, Rohr, W, and Heller, M: Contrast bolus technique with rapid CT scanning: A reliable diagnostic tool for the determination of brain death. Neuroradiology 22:129–132, 1981.
6. Barelli, A, Corte, FD, Calimici, R, et al:

Do brainstem auditory-evoked potentials detect the actual cessation of cerebral functions in brain dead patients? Crit Care Med 18:322–323, 1990.
7. Belsh, JM, Blatt, R, and Schiffman, PL: Apnea testing in brain death. Arch Intern Med 146:2385–2388, 1986.
8. Belsh, JM and Chokroverty, S: Short-latency somatosensory evoked potentials in brain-dead patients. Electroencephalogr Clin Neurophysiol 68:75–78, 1987.
9. Bennett, DR: The EEG in determination of brain death. Ann N Y Acad Sci 315:110–120, 1978.
10. Benzel, EC, Gross, CD, Hadden, TA, et al: The apnea test for the determination of brain death. J Neurosurg 71:191–194, 1989.
11. Benzel, EC, Mashburn, JP, Conrad, S, and Modling, D: Apnea testing for the determination of brain death: A modified protocol. J Neurosurg 76:1029–1031, 1992.
12. Black, P: Comments. Neurosurgery 18:567, 1986.
13. Black, P McL: Brain death (Parts 1 and 2). N Engl J Med 299:338–344, 393–401, 1978.
14. Bradac, GB and Simon, RS: Angiography in brain death. Neuroradiology 7:25–28, 1974.
15. Bruce, EN and Cherniack, NS: Central chemoreceptors. J Appl Physiol 62:389–402, 1987.
16. Cantu, RC: Brain death as determined by cerebral arteriography (letter). Lancet i:1391–1392, 1973.
17. Chancellor, AM, Frith, RW, and Shaw, NA: Somatosensory evoked potentials following severe head injury: Loss of the thalamic potential with brain death. J Neurol Sci 87:255–263, 1988.
18. Conci, F, Proccacio, F, Arosio, M, and Boselli, L: Viscero-somatic and viscero-visceral reflexes in brain death. J Neurol Neurosurg Psychiatry 49:695–698, 1986.
19. Conference of Medical Royal Colleges and Their Faculties in the United Kingdom: Diagnosis of brain death. Br Med J 2:1187–1188, 1976.

20. Darby, JM, Stein, K, Grenvik, A, and Stuart, SA: Approach to management of the heartbeating 'brain dead' organ donor. JAMA 261:2222–2228, 1989.

21. Debelak, L, Pollak, R, and Reckard, C: Arginine vasopressin versus desmopressin for the treatment of diabetes insipidus in the brain dead organ donor. Transplant Proc 22:351–352, 1990.

22. Deliyannakis, E, Ioannou, F, and Davaroukas, A: Brain stem death with persistence of bioelectric activity of the cerebral hemispheres. Clin Electroencephalogr 6:75–79, 1975.

23. Earnest, MP, Beresford, HR, and McIntyre, HB: Testing for apnea in suspected brain death: Methods used by 129 clinicians. Neurology 36:542–544, 1986.

24. Ebata, T, Watanabe, Y, Amaha, K, et al: Haemodynamic changes during the apnea test for diagnosis of brain death. Can J Anaesth 38:436–440, 1991.

25. Engel, GL, Ferris, EB, Webb, JP, and Stevens, CD: Voluntary breathholding. II. The relation of the maximum time of breathholding to the oxygen tension of the inspired air. J Clin Invest 25:729–733, 1946.

26. Facco, E, Liviero, MC, Munari, M, et al: Short latency evoked potentials: New criteria for brain death? J Neurol Neurosurg Psychiatry 53:351–353, 1990.

27. Firsching, R: The brain-stem and 40 Hz middle latency auditory evoked potentials in brain death. Acta Neurochir (Wien) 101:52–55, 1989.

28. Fischbeck, KH and Simon, RP: Neurological manifestations of accidental hypothermia. Ann Neurol 10:384–387, 1981.

29. Frumin, MJ, Epstein, RM, and Cohen, G: Apnoeic oxygenation in man. Anesthesiology 20:789–798, 1959.

30. Garcia-Larrea, L, Bertrand, O, Artru, F, et al: Brain-stem monitoring. II. Preterminal BAEP changes observed until brain death in deeply comatose patients. Electroencephalogr Clin Neurophysiol 68:446–457, 1987.

31. Gelb, AW and Robertson, KM: Anaesthetic management of brain dead for organ donation. Can J Anaesth 37:806–812, 1990.

32. George, MS: Establishing brain death: The potential role of nuclear medicine in the search for a reliable confirmatory test. Eur J Nucl Med 18:75–77, 1991.

33. Glauser, FL, Fairman, RP, and Bechard, D: The causes and evaluation of chronic hypercapnea. Chest 91:755–759, 1987.

34. Goetting, MG and Contreras, E: Systemic atropine administration during cardiac arrest does not cause fixed and dilated pupils. Ann Emerg Med 20:55–57, 1991.

35. Goldie, WD, Chippa, KH, Young, RR, and Brooks, EB: Brainstem auditory and short-latency somatosensory evoked responses in brain death. Neurology 31:248–256, 1981.

36. Goodman, JM and Heck, LL: Confirmation of brain death at bedside by isotope angiography. JAMA 238:966–968, 1977.

37. Goodman, JM, Heck, LL, and Moore, BD: Confirmation of brain death with portable isotope angiography: A review of 204 consecutive cases. Neurosurgery 16:492–497, 1985.

38. Greenan, J and Prasad, J: Comparison of the ocular effects of atropine or glycopyrrolate with two I.V. induction agents. Br J Anaesth 57:180–183, 1985.

39. Greitz, T, Gordon, E, Kolmodin, G, and Widén, L: Aortocranial and carotid angiography in determination of brain death. Neuroradiology 5:13–19, 1973.

40. Grigg, MA, Kelly, MA, Celesia, GG, et al: Electroencephalographic activity after brain death. Arch Neurol 44:948–954, 1987.

41. Haider, I, Matthew, H, and Oswald, I: Electroencephalographic changes in acute drug poisoning. Electroencephalogr Clin Neurophysiol 30:23–31, 1971.

42. Hall, JW III, Mackey-Hargadine, JR, and Kim, EE: Auditory brain-stem response in determination of brain death. Arch Otolaryngol 111:613–620, 1985.

43. Hassler, W, Steinmetz, H, and Gawlowski, J: Transcranial Doppler ultrasonography in raised intracranial pressure and in intracranial circula-

tory arrest. J Neurosurg 68:745–751, 1988.

44. Hazratji, SM, Singh, BM, and Strobos, RJ: Angiography in brain death. N Y State J Med 81:82–83, 1981.

45. Hughes, JR: Limitations of the EEG in coma and brain death. Ann N Y Acad Sci 315:121–136, 1978.

46. Ivanov, SD and Nunn, JF: Methods of elevation of PCO_2 for restoration of spontaneous breathing after artificial ventilation of anaesthetized patients. Br J Anaesth 41:28–37, 1969.

47. Jennett, B, Gleave, J, and Wilson, P: Brain death in three neurosurgical units. Br Med J 282:533–539, 1981.

48. Jennett, B and Plum, F: Persistent vegetative state after brain damage; a syndrome in search of a name. Lancet i:734–737, 1972.

49. Jordan, JE, Dyess, E, and Cliett, J: Unusual spontaneous movements in brain-dead patients (letter). Neurology 35:1082, 1985.

50. Jørgensen, EO: Spinal man after brain death: The unilateral extension-pronation reflex of the upper limb as an indication of brain death. Acta Neurochir (Wien) 28:259–273, 1973.

51. Jørgensen, EO: Requirements for recording the EEG at high sensitivity in suspected brain death. Electroencephalogr Clin Neurophysiol 36:65–69, 1974.

52. Klingelhöfer, J, Conrad, B, Benecke, R, and Sander, D: Intracranial flow patterns at increasing intracranial pressure. Klin Wochenschr 65:542–545, 1987.

53. Klingelhöfer, J, Conrad, B, Benecke, R, et al: Evaluation of intracranial pressure from transcranial Doppler studies in cerebral disease. J Neurol 235:159–162, 1988.

54. Korein, J: Diagnosis of brain death (letter). Br Med J 281:1424, 1980.

55. Korein, J, Braunstein, P, George, A, et al: Brain death. I. Angiographic correlation with a radioisotope bolus technique for evaluation of critical deficit of cerebral blood flow. Ann Neurol 2:195–205, 1977.

56. Korein, J, Braunstein, P, Kricheff, I, et al: Radioisotopic bolus technique as a test to detect circulatory deficit associated with cerebral death: 142 studies on 80 patients demonstrating the bedside use of an innocuous IV procedure as an adjunct in the diagnosis of cerebral death. Circulation 51:924–939, 1975.

57. Korein, J and Maccario, M: A prospective study on the diagnosis of cerebral death (abstr). Electroencephalogr Clin Neurophysiol 31:103–104, 1971.

58. Kuwagata, Y, Sugimoto, H, Yoshioka, T, and Sugimoto, T: Hemodynamic response with passive neck flexion in brain death. Neurosurgery 29:239–241, 1991.

59. Langfitt, TW and Kassell, NF: Non-filling of cerebral vessels during angiography: Correlation with intracranial pressure. Acta Neurochir (Wien) 14:96–104, 1966.

60. Laurin, NR, Driedger, AA, Hurwitz, GA, et al: Cerebral perfusion imaging with technetium-99m HM-PAO in brain death and severe central nervous system injury. J Nucl Med 30:1627–1635, 1989.

61. Lindop, MJ: Basic principles of donor management for multiorgan removal. Transplant Proc 23:2463–2464, 1991.

62. Machado, C, Valdés, P, García-Tigera, J, et al: Brain-stem auditory evoked potentials and brain death. Electroencephalogr Clin Neurophysiol 80:392–398, 1991.

63. Mandel, S, Arenas, A, and Scasta, D: Spinal automatism in cerebral death (letter). N Engl J Med 307:501, 1982.

64. Marks, SJ and Zisfein, J: Apneic oxygenation in apnea tests for brain death: A controlled trial. Arch Neurol 47:1066–1068, 1990.

65. Matz, GJ: Aminoglycoside ototoxicity. Am J Otolaryngol 7:117–119, 1986.

66. Molinari, GF: Brain death, irreversible coma, and words doctors use. Neurology 32:400–402, 1982.

67. National Institutes of Neurological Diseases and Stroke (a collaborative study): An appraisal of the criteria of cerebral death: A summary statement. JAMA 237:982–986, 1977.

68. Novitzky, D, Cooper, DKC, and Reichert, B: Hemodynamic and metabolic responses to hormonal therapy in

brain-dead potential organ donors. Transplantation 43:852–854, 1987.

69. Ong, GL and Bruning, HA: Dilated fixed pupils due to administration of high doses of dopamine hydrochloride. Crit Care Med 9:658–659, 1981.

70. Pallis, C: ABC of brain stem death. Br Med J 285:1409–1412, 1487–1490, 1558–1560, 1641–1644, 1720–1722, 1982; 286:39, 123–124, 209–210, 284–287, 1983.

71. Pallis, C: Diabetes insipidus with brain death (letter). Neurology 35:1086–1087, 1985.

72. Pallis, C: Brainstem death. In Vinken, PJ, Bruyn, GW, and Klawans, HL (eds): Handbook of Clinical Neurology. Vol 57: Head Injury. Elsevier Science Publishers, Amsterdam, 1990, pp 441–496.

73. Pallis, CA and Prior, PF: Guidelines for the determination of death (letter). Neurology 33:251–252, 1983.

74. Petty, GW, Mohr, JP, Pedley, TA, et al: The role of transcranial Doppler in confirming brain death: Sensitivity, specificity, and suggestions for performance and interpretation. Neurology 40:300–303, 1990.

75. Powers, AD, Graeber, MC, and Smith, RR: Transcranial Doppler ultrasonography in the determination of brain death. Neurosurgery 24:884–889, 1989.

76. Powner, DJ: Drug-associated isoelectric EEGs: A hazard in brain-death certification. JAMA 236:1123, 1976.

77. Prechter, GC, Nelson, SB, and Hubmayr, RD: The ventilatory recruitment threshold for carbon dioxide. Am Rev Respir Dis 141:758–764, 1990.

78. Randall, TT and Höckerstedt, KAV: Triiodothyronine treatment in brain-dead multiorgan donors: A controlled study. Transplantation 54:736–738, 1992.

79. Rappaport, ZH, Brinker, RA, and Rovit, RL: Evaluation of brain death by contrast-enhanced computerized cranial tomography. Neurosurgery 2:230–232, 1978.

80. Reid, RH, Gulenchyn, KY, and Ballinger, JR: Clinical use of technetium-99m HM-PAO for determination of

brain death. J Nucl Med 30:1621–1626, 1989.

81. Rohling, R, Wagner, W, Mühlberg, J, et al: Apnea test: Pitfalls and correct handling. Transplant Proc 18:388–390, 1986.

82. Roine, RO, Launes, J, Lindroth, L, and Nikkinen, P: ^{99m}Tc hexamethyl-propyleneamine oxime scans to confirm brain death (letter). Lancet ii:1223–1224, 1986.

83. Ropper, AH: Unusual spontaneous movements in brain-dead patients. Neurology 34:1089–1092, 1984.

84. Ropper, AH, Kehne, SM, and Wechsler, L: Transcranial Doppler in brain death. Neurology 37:1733–1735, 1987.

85. Ropper, AH, Kennedy, SK, and Russell, L: Apnoea testing in the diagnosis of brain death: Clinical and physiological observations. J Neurosurg 55:942–946, 1981.

86. Rosoff, SD and Schwab, RS: The EEG in establishing brain death: A 10-year report with criteria and legal safeguards in the 50 states (abstr). Electroencephalogr Clin Neurophysiol 24:283–284, 1968.

87. Saunders, FW and Cledgett, P: Intracranial blood velocity in head injury: A transcranial ultrasound Doppler study. Surg Neurol 29:401–409, 1988.

88. Schafer, JA and Caronna, JJ: Duration of apnea needed to confirm brain death. Neurology 28:661–666, 1978.

89. Schwartz, BA and Vendrely, E: One of the problems posed by the diagnosis of irreversible coma: The flat EEG and pupil diameter (abstr). Electroencephalogr Clin Neurophysiol 28:648, 1970.

90. Sims, JK and Bickford, RG: Non-mydriatic pupils occurring in human brain death. Bull Los Angeles Neurol Soc 38:24–32, 1973.

91. Sitwell, LD, Weinshenker, BG, Monpetit, V, and Reid, D: Complete ophthalmoplegia as a complication of acute corticosteroid- and pancuronium-associated myopathy. Neurology 41:921–922, 1991.

92. Snavely, SR and Hodges, GR: The neu-

rotoxicity of antibacterial agents. Ann Intern Med 101:92–104, 1984.

93. Starr, A: Auditory brain-stem responses in brain death. Brain 99:543–554, 1976.

94. Stöhr, M, Riffel, B, Trost, E, and Ullrich, A: Short-latency somatosensory evoked potentials in brain death. J Neurol 234:211–214, 1987.

95. Taniguchi, S, Kitamura, S, Kawachi, K, et al: Effects of hormonal supplements on the maintenance of cardiac function in potential donor patients after cerebral death. Eur J Cardiothorac Surg 6:96–102, 1992.

96. Thompson, AE and Sussmane, JB: Bretylium intoxication resembling clinical brain death. Crit Care Med 17:194–195, 1989.

97. Van Donselaar, CA, Meerwaldt, JD, and Van Gijn, J: Apnoea testing to confirm brain death in clinical practice. J Neurol Neurosurg Psychiatry 49:1071–1073, 1986.

98. Van Velthoven, V and Calliauw, L: Diagnosis of brain death. Transcranial Doppler sonography as an additional method. Acta Neurochir (Wien) 95:57–60, 1988.

99. Wagner, W: SEP testing in deeply comatose and brain dead patients: The role of nasopharyngeal, scalp and earlobe derivations in recording the P14 potential. Electroencephalogr Clin Neurophysiol 80:352–363, 1991.

100. Walker, AE: Cerebral Death, ed 2. Urban & Schwarzenberg, Baltimore, 1981.

101. Wetzel, RC, Setzer, N, Stiff, JL, and Rogers, MC: Hemodynamic responses in brain dead organ donor patients. Anesth Analg 64:125–128, 1985.

102. White, A: Overdose of tricyclic antidepressants associated with absent brain-stem reflexes. Can Med Assoc J 139:133–134, 1988.

103. Yang, KD and Dantzker, DR: Reversible brain death: A manifestation of amitriptyline overdose. Chest 99:1037–1038, 1991.

104. Yatim, A, Mercatello, A, Coronel, B, et al: ^{99m}Tc-HMPAO cerebral scintigraphy in the diagnosis of brain death. Transplant Proc 23:2491, 1991.

INDEX

Numbers followed by an "F" indicate figures; numbers followed by a "T" indicate tabular material.